MUSCULOSKELETAL ASSESSMENT

Joint Range of Motion and Manual Muscle Strength

■ *Second Edition*

MUSCULOSKELETAL ASSESSMENT

Joint Range of Motion and Manual Muscle Strength

■ *Second Edition*

HAZEL M. CLARKSON M.A., B.P.T.

Formerly Assistant Professor, Department of Physical Therapy, Faculty of
Rehabilitation Medicine, University of Alberta, Edmonton, Alberta, Canada

Photography by Jacques Hurabielle, P.P.O.C., Ph.D
Illustrations by Heather K. Doy, B.A., B.F.A. and Joy D. Marlowe, M.A., C.M.I.

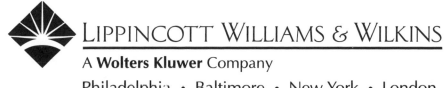

LIPPINCOTT WILLIAMS & WILKINS
A **Wolters Kluwer** Company

Philadelphia • Baltimore • New York • London
Buenos Aires • Hong Kong • Sydney • Tokyo

Editor: Margaret Biblis
Managing Editor: Linda S. Napora
Marketing Manager: Debby Hartman
Senior Production Manager: Helen Ewan
Senior Production Coordinator: Michael Carcel
Senior Project Editor: Sandra Cherrey Scheinin
Art Director: Carolyn O'Brien
Interior Design: Joan Wendt
Cover Design: Kuronen & Michaels
Indexer: Maria Coughlin

Copyright © 2000 Lippincott Williams & Wilkins

351 West Camden Street
Baltimore, Maryland 21201-2436 USA

227 East Washington Square
Philadelphia, Pennsylvania 19106-3780 USA

Printed in the United States of America

First Edition, 1989

Library of Congress Cataloging–in–Publication Data

Clarkson, Hazel M.
  Musculoskeletal assessment : joint range of motion and manual
muscle strength / Hazel M. Clarkson ; photography by Jacques
Hurabielle ; illustrations by Heather K. Doy and Joy D. Marlowe.—
2nd ed.
    p. cm.
  Includes bibliographical references and index.
  ISBN 0-683-30384-8 (alk. paper)
  1. Musculoskeletal system—Diseases—Diagnosis. 2. Joints—Range
of motion—Measurement. 3. Muscle strength—Testing. I. Title.
  [DNLM: 1. Musculoskeletal Diseases—diagnosis. 2. Musculoskeletal
Physiology. 3. Musculoskeletal System—anatomy & histology.
4. Physical Examination—methods.   WE 141 C613m 2000]
RC925.7.C53   2000
616.7′2075—dc21
DNLM/DLC
for Library of Congress   99-33414
                                                                               CIP

The publishers have made every effort to trace the copyright holders for borrowed material. If they have inadvertently overlooked any, they will be pleased to make the necessary arrangements at the first opportunity.

  To purchase additional copies of this book, call our customer service department at **(800) 638-0672** or fax orders to **(800) 447-8438.** For other book services, including large quantity sales, ask for the Special Sales department.

  Canadian customers should call **(800) 665-1148,** or fax **(800) 655-0103.** For all other calls originating outside of the United States, please call **(410) 528-4223** or fax us at **(410) 528-8550.**

  Visit Lippincott Williams & Wilkins on the Internet: http://www.lww.com or contact our customer service department at **custserv@lww.com.** Lippincott Williams & Wilkins customer service representatives are available from 8:30 am to 6:00 pm, EST, Monday through Friday, for telephone access.

*Dedicated to the late Gail Gilewich,
a dear friend and colleague.*

PREFACE

The first edition of this text proved useful as an educational tool that promoted independent student learning and as a reference book for clinicians. The preface to the first edition provided an outline of the format. The format for this edition is essentially the same. Changes made in this second edition are based on feedback from students and colleagues and from my teaching.

The text has been updated. In Chapter One, the reliability and validity of the assessment of joint range of motion, using the universal goniometer, and of manual muscle testing have been added. Appendix A, at the back of the text, includes a description of the OB "Myrin" goniometer and how to use it. Illustrations of the muscles of the eye and the neck flexors have been added to the sections dealing with muscle strength assessment for the face and neck.

Numerous changes have been made to the sections on range of motion, including the addition of photographs and illustrations. Procedures used to scan the active range of motion of the extremities and hand are illustrated and described. The description of the assessment and measurement of the range of motion for each joint motion begins with a reminder to assess active range of motion and identifies the substitution/trick movements to be avoided, when applicable. This is followed by description and illustration of the methods used to assess, then measure the passive range of motion using the universal goniometer or tape measure. Assessment of the length of selected muscles is included following the assessment and measurement of passive range of motion. The muscle(s) placed on stretch are illustrated to show muscle attachments.

A final chapter has been added to demonstrate that the methods used for assessment are basically the same methods used for treatment. Through the use of description and illustration, the principles and methodology of joint range of motion, muscle length, and manual muscle strength evaluation are shown to be the same as those used for selected treatment techniques. Thus, this textbook can be used to learn assessment and treatment methods. Presentation of the chapter content in table form, simplifies the content and facilitates learning. It might be useful for the reader to review this information before learning specific methods of assessment and treatment, to get an overview of assessment and treatment methodology.

Hazel M. Clarkson, M.A., B.P.T.

PREFACE

TO THE FIRST EDITION

This book has evolved in response to a perceived need for a textbook that contains the principles and methodology of joint range of motion and manual muscle strength evaluation in one volume. The work is primarily intended for undergraduate students in occupational and physical therapy programs. The content was written on the assumption that the students possess prerequisite knowledge of the anatomy of the musculoskeletal system.

Measurement of joint range of motion and assessment of muscle strength are important clinical skills in the practice of occupational and physical therapy. These evaluations form two component parts of the physical assessment of a patient with a musculoskeletal disorder. The methods used to assess range and strength are based on the principles of assessment, articular function, and movement.

The first chapter of this volume focuses on the principles and methodology of evaluation. The overview of the principles and methods provided here contains knowledge prerequisite for the remaining chapters. Chapters 2 through 8 focus on the specific methodology of range of motion and muscle strength evaluation of the head, neck, trunk, and extremities. These chapters are each devoted to a specific joint complex, and all are organized in an identical format.

• **Surface Anatomy.** Each chapter begins with a review of the surface anatomy of the region. Through illustration and description, the pertinent landmarks for assessment purposes are identified. Muscles are excluded from this description, as precise points of palpation are presented later in the chapter. Surface anatomy and other anatomical references provided in the chapter are presented in sufficient depth to promote a review for the student, as the knowledge of anatomy forms the basis of understanding joint articulation, movement, and function.

• **Range of Motion Assessment.** Following the surface anatomy, the assessment of range of motion of the particular joint is presented. The joint articulations and axes are illustrated. The "visualization" of the articulations and axes is particularly relevant in the measurement process as the student needs to visualize the shape of the articulating surface that permits movement and the axis about which movement takes place. A summary of joint structure and movements is presented in table form. This table provides reference information pertinent to assessment, measurement, and interpretation of findings.

Following the relevant anatomy, the methodology for measuring each movement at the joint is presented. A consistent method of measuring joint range of motion is essential for accurate assessment of a patient's present status, progress, and effectiveness of the treatment program. Learning is promoted through consistency in documentation and illustration of methods.

• **Muscle Strength Assessment.** The next section of the chapter focuses on manual muscle strength assessment. The section begins with a review of the relevant anatomy of the region, including muscle actions, attachments, and nerve supply.

In each chapter the muscle strength tests are described under the main headings of joint movements. The prime mover(s) and accessory muscle(s) are identified. Through illustration and description, the against-gravity tests are presented, followed by the gravity-eliminated tests. The sequence is consistent for each movement.

For each muscle strength test, the first against-gravity photograph illustrates the start position and stabilization. The next photograph illustrates the patient's position at the end of the range of motion and the best point for muscle palpation. The resistance test follows with a photograph of the therapist applying manual resistance.

An illustration of the muscle being tested and the location of the therapist's hand relative to deep anatomical structures when applying resistance accompanies the resistance photograph. The illustration also provides a visual review of muscle attachments and direction of muscle fibers to assist the student in visualizing the deep structures.

The first gravity-eliminated test photograph illustrates the start position and stabilization. A second photograph illustrates the end position for the gravity-eliminated test and the best point for palpation of the muscle(s) being assessed.

All muscle tests illustrated first show the optimal start position that could be used to test the muscle(s), based on the position that offers the best stabilization. In some instances, there may be more than one position that could be used to test the muscle. These positions are termed alternate positions and are documented if they are common in clinical practice or if the preferred start position is impractical or contraindicated for some patients.

• **Functional Application.** The final section of each chapter is devoted to the functional application of assessment. The specific function of the joint complex is described. The functional range of motion at the joint is documented. Emphasis is placed on those ranges required for performance of daily activities. The function of the muscles is described according to biomechanical principles and daily activities. Assessments of joint range of motion and muscle strength are not performed in isolation of function. Through knowledge of the range of motion and muscle function required in daily activities, the therapist can elicit meaningful information from the assessments. The therapist correlates the assessment findings with the patient's ability to perform daily activities and, in conjunction with other physical assessment measures, plans an appropriate treatment plan to restore or maintain function.

Throughout the book, extensive use is made of visual material. The purpose of this format is to provide the student with a visual orientation of techniques. Although learning a clinical skill needs the classroom and laboratory environment, it is our hope that the presentation style will serve as a valuable adjunct to classroom teaching.

Hazel M. Clarkson
Gail B. Gilewich

ACKNOWLEDGMENTS

Let me first of all thank again those who contributed to the first edition of this book.

It is a pleasure to thank both Jacques Hurabielle and Troy Lorenson for teaming up with me again to produce the photographs and Joy Marlowe for the additional artwork for this edition.

Because of their invaluable constructive criticism and encouragement, I am grateful to and thank all of the following who assisted with this second edition:

- All colleagues who provided reviews and suggestions for change

- The physical therapy and occupational therapy students I taught at the University of Alberta who provided valuable feedback on the first edition of this text, and who later did the same as clinicians.

- My former colleagues at the University of Alberta who supported this work

- The reference librarians at the John W. Scott Health Sciences Library, University of Alberta—a special thanks for their ever-accommodating assistance

- Liza Chan and the students who assisted her in collecting reference materials

Thanks to the entire Lippincott Williams & Wilkins team who worked to make this second edition a reality.

My father, Dr. Graham Clarkson, I thank for reviewing the manuscripts and offering helpful suggestions. My mother, June Clarkson, I thank for her diligent proofreading and helpful suggestions from her perpsective as an occupational therapist. Finally, I wish to thank my husband Hans Longerich and the rest of my family for their continued support and encouragement.

CONTENTS

CHAPTER 1

PRINCIPLES AND METHODS

A fundamental requisite to the study of evaluation of joint range of motion (ROM) and muscle strength is the knowledge of evaluation principles and methodology. This chapter discusses the factors pertinent to evaluation of ROM and strength. A firm foundation in the principles, methods, and associated terminology presented in this chapter is necessary knowledge for the specific techniques presented in subsequent chapters.

VISUAL OBSERVATION

Visual observation is an integral part of assessment of joint ROM and muscle strength. Throughout the initial assessment of the patient, the therapist gathers visual information that contributes to determining the patient's problem(s) and formulating an appropriate assessment plan. Information that is gained visually includes such factors as symmetrical or compensatory motion in functional activities, body posture, muscle contours, body proportions, and color, condition, and creases of the skin. The body part being assessed should be adequately exposed for visual inspection.

PALPATION

Palpation is the examination of the body surface by touch. Palpation is performed to assess bony and soft tissue contours, soft tissue consistency, and skin temperature and texture. The therapist uses visual observation and palpation to "visualize" the deep anatomy.[1]

To assess and treat patients, palpation is an essential skill. The therapist must be able to locate bony landmarks to align a goniometer correctly when assessing joint ROM. Bony landmarks are used as reference points to assess limb or trunk circumference. A therapist must be proficient in palpation to determine the presence or absence of muscle contraction when assessing strength or conducting reeducation exercises. Palpation is also used to locate structures that need to be sta-

bilized to isolate joint movement when mobilizing a joint. Palpation is used to identify bony or soft tissue irregularities and to localize structures that require direct treatment.

Proficiency at palpation is gained through practice and experience. There is such individual variation in human anatomy that it is necessary to practice palpation on as many subjects as possible.

Palpation Technique

The patient is made comfortable, kept warm, and the body or body part is well supported to relax the muscles. This allows palpation of deep or inert (noncontractile) structures such as ligaments and bursae.

The therapist visually observes the area to be palpated and notes any deformity or abnormality.

The therapist palpates with the pads of the index and middle fingers and occasionally uses the thumb pad. Fingernails should be kept short.

The therapist's fingers are in direct contact with the skin, and palpation is not attempted through clothing.

To instill a feeling of security the therapist uses a sensitive but firm touch. Prodding is uncomfortable and may elicit tension in the muscles.

To palpate muscles and tendons, the patient isometrically contracts the muscle against resistance followed by relaxation of the muscle. The muscle is palpated during contraction and relaxation.

To palpate tendons, the tips of the index and middle fingers are placed across the long axis of the tendon and gently rolled forward and backward across the tendon.

THERAPIST POSTURE

When performing assessment techniques the therapist needs to apply correct biomechanical principles of posture and lifting. The therapist's posture and support of the patient's limb are described.

Posture. Balance and effective weight shifting from one leg to the other is attained by maintaining a broad base of support. The therapist stands with the head and trunk upright, feet shoulder width apart, knees slightly flexed, and one foot slightly ahead of the other. The stance is in the line of the direction of movement.

When performing movements that are parallel to the side of the plinth, the therapist stands beside the plinth with the leg furthest from the plinth ahead of the other leg (Fig. 1-1). When performing movements that are perpendicular to the side of the plinth, the therapist faces the plinth with one foot slightly in front of the other (Fig. 1-2). When performing diagonal movements, the therapist's stance is in line with the diagonal movement and one foot is slightly ahead of the other.

Protection for the therapist's lumbar spine is acquired through assuming a posterior pelvic tilt. The lumbar spine is flattened through tightening of the abdominal and gluteal muscles. Additional protection is gained by keeping as close to the patient as possible, avoiding spinal rotation by moving the feet to turn and using the leg musculature to perform the work by flexing and extending the joints of the lower extremity.

Supporting the Patient's Limb. To move a limb or limb segment easily the therapist supports the part at the level of its center of gravity, approximately located at the junction of the upper and middle third of the segment.[2] Ensure all joints are adequately supported when lifting or moving a limb or limb segment.

A relaxed hand grasp, where the hand conforms to the contour of the part is used to support or lift a body part (Fig. 1-3).[2] The therapist gives additional support by cradling the part with the forearm.

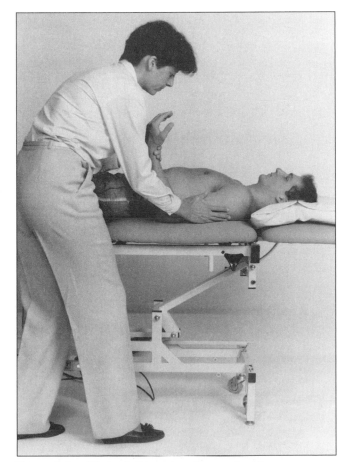

Figure 1-1. Therapist's stance when performing movements parallel to the side of the plinth.

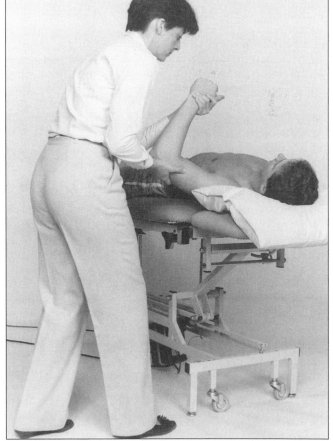

Figure 1-2. Therapist's stance when performing movements perpendicular to the side of the plinth.

MOVEMENT DESCRIPTION

The amount of movement that occurs at a joint is the ROM of the joint. To perform active ROM (AROM), the patient voluntarily moves the body part through the ROM without assistance. To perform a passive ROM (PROM), the therapist or another external force moves the body part through the ROM.

To assess the ROM at a joint, the therapist must have a sound knowledge of anatomy. This includes a knowledge of joint articulations, motions, and normal limiting factors. These factors are isolated for discussion.

JOINT ARTICULATIONS AND CLASSIFICATION

An anatomical joint or articulation is formed when two bony articular surfaces, lined by hyaline cartilage meet[3] and movement is allowed to occur at the junction. The movements that occur at a joint are partly determined by the shape of the articular surfaces. Anatomical articulations are classified as described and illustrated in Table 1-1.

In addition to classifying a joint according to the anatomical relationship of the articular surfaces, a joint may also be classified as a syndesmosis or a physiological or functional joint. A *syndesmosis* is a joint in which the bones are held together by fibrous connective tissue that forms an interosseous ligament or membrane (Fig. 1-11).[5] Movement is possible around one axis. A *physiological*[3] or *functional*[6] joint consists of two surfaces, muscle and bone (scapulothoracic joint) or bursa and bone (subdeltoid joint), moving one with respect to the other (Fig. 1-12).

JOINT MOVEMENTS: PLANES AND AXES

Joint movements are more easily described and understood using a coordinate system that has its central point located just anterior to the second sacral vertebra, with the subject standing in the anatomical position. The anatomical position is illustrated in Figures 1-13, 1-14, and 1-15. The start positions for assessing ranges of movement described in this text are understood to be the anatomical position of the joint, unless otherwise indicated.

The coordinate system consists of three imaginary cardinal planes and axes. This same coordinate system can be transposed so that its central point is located at the center of any joint in the body (Fig. 1-16). Movement in, or parallel to, the cardinal planes occurs around the axis that lies perpendicular to the plane of movement. Many functional movements occur in diagonal planes located between the cardinal planes. Table 1-2 describes the planes and axes of the body.

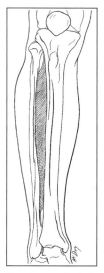

Figure 1-11.   Syndesmosis (Tibiofibular joint).

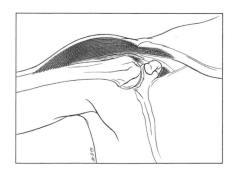

Figure 1-12.   Physiological or functional joint (subdeltoid joint).

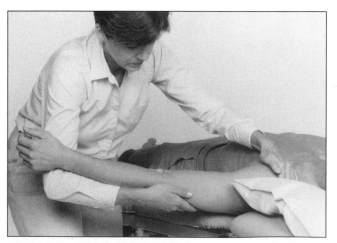

Figure 1-3.   The limb supported at the center of gravity using a relaxed hand grasp.

TABLE 1-1 ▼ CLASSIFICATION OF ANATOMICAL ARTICULATIONS[4]

Ball and socket (spheroidal)

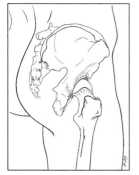

Figure 1-4. Ball and socket articulation (hip joint). A ball-shaped surface articulates with a cup-shaped surface; movement is possible around innumerable axes.

Hinge (ginglymus)

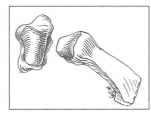

Figure 1-5. Hinge articulation (humeroulnar joint). Two articular surfaces that restrict movement largely to one axis; usually have strong collateral ligaments.

Plane

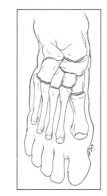

Figure 1-6. Plane articulation (intertarsall joints). This articulation is formed by the apposition of two relatively flat surfaces; gliding movements occur at these joints.

Ellipsoidal

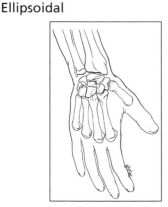

Figure 1-7. (Top) Ellipsoidal articulation (radiocarpal joint). This articulation is formed by an oval convex surface in apposition with an elliptical concave surface; movement is possible around two axes.

Saddle (sellar)

Figure 1-8. (Bottom) Saddle articulation (first carpometacarpal joint). Each joint surface has a convexity at right angles to a concave surface; movement is possible around two axes.

Bicondylar

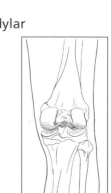

Figure 1-9. Bicondylar articulations (femorotibial joint). Most movement occurs around one axis; some degree of rotation is also possible around an axis set at 90° to the first; formed by one surface having two convex condyles, the corresponding surface having two concave reciprocal surfaces.

Pivot (trochoid)

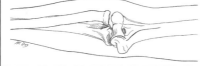

Figure 1-10. Pivot articulation (superior radioulnar joint). Formed by a central bony pivot surrounded by an osteoligamentous ring; movement is restricted to rotation.

MOVEMENT TERMINOLOGY

Visual depiction of the following movement terminology is provided in subsequent chapters.

Angular Movements. Angular motions refer to movements that produce an increase or a decrease in the angle between the adjacent bones and include flexion, extension, abduction, and adduction.[4]

Flexion—bending of a part so the anterior surfaces come closer together. Special considerations:

Flexion of the thumb—the thumb moves across the palm of the hand.
Knee and toe flexion—the posterior or plantar surfaces of the body parts, respectively, come closer together.
Ankle flexion—when the dorsal surface of the foot is brought closer to the anterior aspect of the leg, the movement is termed dorsiflexion.

Lateral flexion of the neck and trunk—bending movements that occur in a lateral direction either to the right or left side.

Extension—the straightening of a part and movement is in the opposite direction to flexion movements. Special consideration:

Ankle extension—when the plantar aspect of the foot is extended toward the posterior aspect of the leg, the movement is termed plantarflexion.

Hyperextension—movement that goes beyond the normal anatomical joint position of extension.

Abduction—movement away from the midline of the body or body part. The midline of the hand passes through the third digit and the midline of the foot passes through the second digit. Special considerations:

Abduction of the scapula is referred to as protraction and is movement of the vertebral border of the scapula away from the vertebral column.

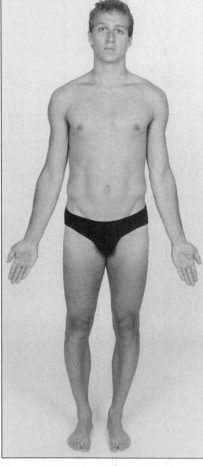

Figure 1-13.   Anatomical position—anterior view. The individual is standing erect with the arms by the sides, toes, palms of the hand and eyes facing forward and fingers extended.

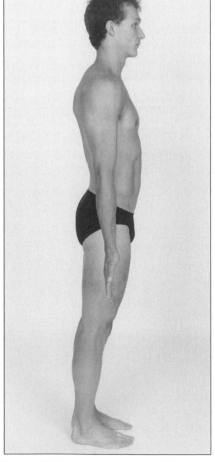

Figure 1-14.   Anatomical position—lateral view.

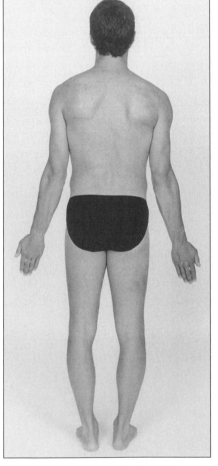

Figure 1-15.   Anatomical position—posterior view.

Abduction of the thumb—the thumb moves in an anterior direction in a plane perpendicular to the palm of the hand.

Abduction of the wrist is referred to as wrist radial deviation.

Eversion of the foot—the sole of the foot is turned outward; it is not a pure abduction movement because it includes abduction and pronation of the forefoot.

Adduction—movement toward the midline of the body or body part. Special considerations:

Adduction of the scapula is referred to as retraction and is movement of the vertebral border of the scapula toward the vertebral column.

Adduction of the thumb—the thumb moves back to anatomical position from a position of abduction.

Adduction of the wrist is referred to as wrist ulnar deviation.

Inversion of the foot—the sole of the foot is turned inward; it is not a pure adduction movement because it includes adduction and supination of the forefoot.

Shoulder elevation—movement of the arm above shoulder level (90°) to a vertical position alongside the head (180°). The vertical position is arrived at by moving either through shoulder flexion or through shoulder abduction and the movement is referred to as shoulder elevation through flexion or shoulder elevation through abduction, respectively. In the clinical setting these movements may be referred to as shoulder flexion and shoulder abduction.

Rotation Movements. These movements generally occur around a longitudinal or vertical axis.

Internal (medial, inward) rotation—turning of the anterior surface of a part toward the midline of the body. Special considerations:

Internal rotation of the forearm is referred to as pronation.

External (lateral, outward) rotation—turning of the anterior surface of a part away from the midline of the body. Special considerations:

External rotation of the forearm is referred to as supination.

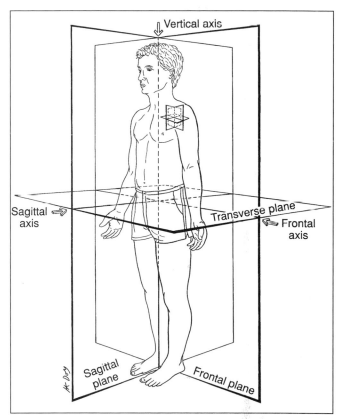

Figure 1-16. Planes and axes illustrated in anatomical position.

TABLE 1-2 ▼ PLANES AND AXES OF THE BODY

Plane	Description of Plane	Axis of Rotation	Description of Axis	Most Common Movement
Frontal (coronal)	Divides body into anterior and posterior sections	Sagittal	Runs anterior/posterior	Abduction, adduction
Sagittal	Divides body into right and left sections	Frontal (transverse)	Runs medial/lateral	Flexion, extension
Transverse (horizontal)	Divides body into upper and lower sections	Longitudinal (vertical)	Runs superior/inferior	Internal rotation, external rotation

Neck or trunk rotation—turning around a vertical axis to either the right or left side.

Scapular rotation—described in terms of the direction of movement of either the inferior angle of the scapula or the glenoid cavity of the scapula (Fig. 1-17).

    Medial (downward) rotation of the scapula—movement of the inferior angle of the scapula toward the midline and movement of the glenoid cavity in a caudal or downward direction.

    Lateral (upward) rotation of the scapula—movement of the inferior angle of the scapula away from the midline and movement of the glenoid cavity in a cranial or upward direction.

Circumduction—a combination of the movements of flexion, extension, abduction, and adduction.

Opposition of the thumb and little finger—the tips of the thumb and little finger come together.

Reposition of the thumb and little finger—the thumb and little finger return to anatomical position from a position of opposition.

Horizontal abduction (extension)—occurs at the shoulder and hip joints. With the shoulder joint in 90° of either abduction or flexion or the hip joint in 90° flexion, the arm or the thigh, respectively, is moved in a direction either away from the midline of the body or in a posterior direction.

Horizontal adduction (flexion)—occurs at the shoulder and hip joints. With the shoulder joint in 90° of either abduction or flexion, or the hip joint in 90° flexion, the arm or the thigh, respectively, is moved in a direction either toward the midline of the body or in an anterior direction.

Tilt—describes movement of either the scapula or the pelvis.

    Anterior tilt of the scapula—"the coracoid process moves in an anterior and caudal direction while the inferior angle moves in a posterior and cranial direction."[7(p16)]

    Posterior tilt of the scapula—the coracoid process moves in a posterior and cranial direction while the inferior angle of the scapula moves in an anterior and caudal direction.

    Anterior tilt of the pelvis—the anterior superior iliac spines of the pelvis move in an anterior and caudal direction.

    Posterior pelvic tilt—the anterior superior iliac spines of the pelvis move in a posterior and cranial direction.

    Lateral pelvic tilt—movement of the ipsilateral iliac crest in the frontal plane in either a cranial direction (elevation or hiking of the pelvis) or a caudal direction (pelvic drop).

Shoulder girdle elevation—movement of the scapula and lateral end of the clavicle in a cranial direction.

Shoulder girdle depression—movement of the scapula and lateral end of the clavicle in a caudal direction.

Hypermobility—an excessive amount of movement; joint ROM that is greater than the normal ROM expected at the joint.

Hypomobility—a reduced amount of movement; joint ROM that is less than the normal ROM expected at the joint.

Passive insufficiency—of a muscle occurs when the length of a muscle prevents full ROM at the joint or joints that the muscle crosses over (Fig. 1-18).[8]

ASSESSMENT CONTRAINDICATIONS AND PRECAUTIONS— RANGE OF MOTION

Active ROM or PROM must not be assessed if any contraindications to this form of assessment exist. In special instances the assessment techniques must be performed with a modified approach.

    Both AROM and PROM assessment techniques are contraindicated:

1. In the region of a dislocation or unhealed fracture
2. Immediately after surgery if motion to the part will interrupt the healing process
3. If myositis ossificans or ectopic ossification is sus-

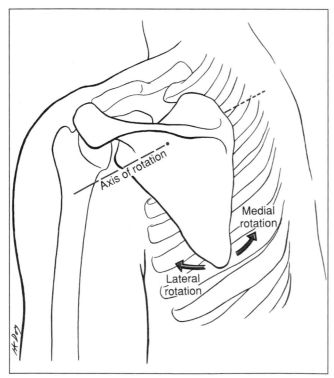

Figure 1-17. Rotation of the scapula.

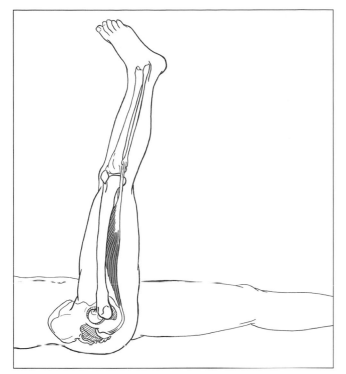

Figure 1-18. Passive insufficiency of the hamstring muscles. Hip flexion ROM is limited by the length of the hamstring muscles when the knee joint is held in extension.

pected or present, AROM and PROM should not be undertaken without first ensuring the patient is assessed by a professional who has expertise in the management of these conditions.[9]

The therapist must take extra care when performing AROM and PROM assessment where motion to the part might aggravate the condition, such as:

1. In the presence of an infectious or inflammatory process in a joint or the region around a joint
2. In patients taking medication for pain or muscle relaxants, because the patient may not be able to respond appropriately and movement may be performed too vigorously
3. In the region of marked osteoporosis or in conditions where bone fragility is a factor. PROM must be performed with extreme care or not at all.
4. In assessing a hypermobile or subluxed joint
5. In painful conditions where the assessment technique might aggravate the condition
6. In patients with hemophilia
7. In the region of a hematoma, most notably at the elbow, hip, or knee
8. In assessing joints if bony ankylosis is suspected
9. Immediately after an injury where there has been a disruption of soft tissue (ie, tendon, muscle, ligament)
10. In the region of a newly united fracture
11. After prolonged immobilization of a part

Note: Contraindications and precautions to be taken when treating the cervical spine and other regions of the spine are not discussed here and are beyond the scope of this text but should be studied before the therapist or student attempts to assess and treat the spine.

ASSESSMENT OF ACTIVE RANGE OF MOTION

An overview of the AROM available at the joints of the upper or lower limb can be attained using tests that include movement at several joints simultaneously. For a detailed assessment of the AROM, the patient performs all of the active movements that normally occur at the affected joint(s) and at the joints immediately proximal and distal to the affected joint(s). The therapist observes as the patient performs each active movement one at a time, and if possible, bilaterally and symmetrically. Assessment of the AROM provides the therapist with information about the patient's willingness to move, coordination, level of consciousness, attention span, joint ROM, movements that cause or increase pain, muscle strength, and ability to follow instructions and perform functional activities. AROM may be decreased due to the patient's restricted joint mobility, muscle weakness, pain, inability to follow instructions, or unwillingness to move.

When assessing AROM ensure that movement occurs only at the joint being assessed. Trick or substitute movements may take the form of additional movements at the joint being assessed or at other joints, thus giving the appearance of having a greater AROM than is actually present. The therapist must try to eliminate trick or substitute movements through adequate explanation and instruction to the patient regarding the movement to be performed and the trick movements to be avoided, proper patient positioning, adequate stabilization of the proximal joint segment as required, and practice in assessing AROM. To assess joint ROM accurately the therapist must know and recognize all of the trick or substitute movements the patient could use. If the patient's use of trick or substitute movements results in inaccurate AROM assessment this may lead to an inappropriate treatment plan. Observation of AROM is followed by an assessment of PROM.

MEASUREMENT OF ACTIVE RANGE OF MOTION

The patient uses active movement to perform functional activities. If AROM is decreased, it may be difficult or impossible to perform these activities. For an objective measure of the patient's ability to perform functional activity, the therapist measures the AROM using a universal goniometer (see Fig. 1-19). The measurement procedure for the universal goniometer is described in the section for measurement of PROM.

ASSESSMENT OF PASSIVE RANGE OF MOTION

Passive ROM is assessed to determine the amount of movement possible at the joint. PROM is usually slightly greater than AROM due to the slight elastic stretch of tissues and in some instances the decreased bulk of relaxed muscles. The therapist takes the body segments through a PROM to estimate each joint's ROM, determine the quality of the movement throughout the ROM and the end feel, note the presence of pain, and determine whether a capsular or noncapsular pattern of movement is present. After this assessment of the PROM, the therapist repeats the PROM to measure and record the PROM using a goniometer or tape measure.

The following concepts and terms are important to understanding joint motion restriction when assessing PROM.

Normal Limiting Factors and End Feels. The unique anatomical structure of a joint determines the direction and magnitude of its PROM. The factors that normally limit movement and determine the magnitude of the PROM at a joint include:

The stretching of soft tissues, that is, muscles, fascia, and skin

The stretching of ligaments or the joint capsule

The apposition of soft tissues

Bone contacting bone

In assessing the PROM of a joint, the therapist observes whether the range is full or restricted and by feel determines which structure(s) limits the movement. The end feel is the sensation transmitted to the therapist's hands at the extreme end of the PROM and indicates the structures that limit the joint movement.[10] The end feel may be normal (physiological) or abnormal (pathological).[11]

A normal end feel exists when there is full PROM at the joint and the normal anatomy of the joint stops movement. An abnormal end feel exists when there is either a decreased or increased passive joint ROM or when there is a normal PROM but structures other than the normal anatomy stop joint movement. Normal and abnormal end feels are presented in Tables 1-3 and 1-4. The author has documented the end feels in joint movement based on a knowledge of the anatomy of the region, clinical experience, and available references.[3,10–16]

Method to Assess End Feel. Movement is isolated to the joint being assessed. The patient is relaxed and the therapist stabilizes the proximal joint segment, applies slight traction to and moves the distal joint segment to the end of the ROM for the test movement. Slight overpressure is applied at the end of the ROM and the end feel is noted.

Capsular and Noncapsular Patterns. When assessing the PROM at a joint, the therapist visually estimates the available PROM for each movement at the joint, determines the end feels, and establishes the presence or absence of pain. If there is a decreased PROM, the therapist assesses the *pattern of joint movement restriction.* The description of capsular and noncapsular patterns is derived from the work of Cyriax.[10]

• **Capsular Pattern.** If a lesion of the joint capsule or a total joint reaction is present, a characteristic pat-

---

TABLE 1-3 ▼ NORMAL (PHYSIOLOGICAL) END FEELS[10–12]

End Feel General Terminology (Specific Terminology)	Description
Hard (Bony)	An abrupt, hard stop to movement when bone contacts bone; for example, passive elbow extension, the olecranon process contacts the olecranon fossa.
Soft (Soft tissue apposition)	When two body surfaces come together a soft compression of tissue is felt; for example, in passive knee flexion, the posterior aspects of the calf and thigh come together.
Firm (Soft tissue stretch)	A firm or springy sensation that has some give when muscle is stretched; for example, passive ankle dorsiflexion performed with the knee in extension is stopped due to tension in the gastrocnemius muscle.
(Capsular stretch)	A hard arrest to movement with some give when the joint capsule or ligaments are stretched. The feel is similar to stretching a piece of leather; for example, passive shoulder external rotation.

End Feel	Description
Hard	An abrupt hard stop to movement, when bone contacts bone, or a bony grating sensation, when rough articular surfaces move past one another, for example, in a joint that contains loose bodies, degenerative joint disease, dislocation, or a fracture.
Soft	A boggy sensation that indicates the presence of synovitis or soft tissue edema.
Firm	A springy sensation or a hard arrest to movement with some give, indicating muscular, capsular, or ligamentous shortening.
Springy block	A rebound is seen or felt and indicates the presence of an internal derangement; for example, the knee with a torn meniscus.
Empty	If considerable pain is present, there is no sensation felt before the extreme of passive ROM as the patient requests the movement be stopped, this indicates pathology such as an extra articular abscess, a neoplasm, acute bursitis, joint inflammation, or a fracture.
Spasm	A hard sudden stop to passive movement that is often accompanied by pain, is indicative of an acute or subacute arthritis, the presence of a severe active lesion, or fracture. If pain is absent a spasm end feel may indicate a lesion of the central nervous system with resultant increased muscular tonus.

PRINCIPLES AND METHODS

tern of restriction in the PROM will occur, called the capsular pattern. Only joints that are controlled by muscles exhibit capsular patterns. When painful stimuli from the region of the joint provoke involuntary muscle spasm, a restriction in motion at the joint in the capsular proportions results. Each joint capsule resists stretching in selective ways; therefore, in time, certain aspects of the capsule become more contracted than others. The capsular pattern exhibits as a proportional limitation of joint motions that are characteristic to each joint, for example, the capsular pattern of the shoulder joint is different from the pattern of restriction at the hip joint. The capsular pattern at each joint is similar between individuals. Joints that rely primarily on ligaments for their stability do not exhibit capsular patterns and the degree of pain elicited when the joint is strained at the extreme of movement indicates the severity of the total joint reaction or arthritis. The capsular pattern for each joint is provided in each chapter, with movements listed in order of restriction (most restricted to least restricted).

• Noncapsular Pattern. A noncapsular pattern exists when there is limitation of movement at a joint but not in the capsular pattern of restriction. A noncapsular pattern indicates the absence of a total joint reaction. Ligamentous adhesions, internal derangement, or extra-articular lesions may result in a noncapsular pattern at the joint.

Ligamentous adhesions affect specific regions of the joint or capsule. Motion is restricted and there is pain when the joint is moved in a direction that stretches the affected ligament. Other movements at the joint are usually full and pain free.

Internal derangement occurs when loose fragments of cartilage or bone are present within a joint. When the loose fragment impinges between the joint surfaces, the movement is suddenly blocked and there may be localized pain. All other joint movements are full and pain free. Internal derangements only occur in certain joints such as the knee, jaw, and elbow.

Extra-articular lesions that affect nonarticular structures, such as muscle adhesions, muscle spasm, muscle strains, hematomas, and cysts, may limit joint ROM in one direction while a full and painless PROM is present in all other directions.

MEASUREMENT OF PASSIVE RANGE OF MOTION

Instrumentation. The instrument chosen to assess joint ROM depends on the degree of accuracy required in the measurement and the time and resources available to the clinician. Radiographs, photographs, photocopies, the use of the electrogoniometer, flexometer, or plumb line may give objective, valid, and reliable measures of ROM but are not always practical in the clinical environment. When doing clinical research, the therapist is encouraged to investigate alternate instruments that will offer a more stringent assessment of joint ROM. The universal goniometer, OB "Myrin" goniometer (see Appendix A), and tape measure are the three instruments that are used to directly measure the ROM as presented in this text.

• Universal Goniometer. In a clinical environment the most common device for measuring joint angles or ROM is called a universal goniometer (Fig. 1-19). The universal goniometer is a 180° or 360° protractor with one axis that joins two arms. One arm is stationary and

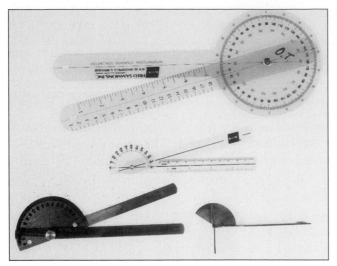

Figure 1-19. Various sizes of 180° and 360° universal goniometers.

the other arm is movable around the axis or fulcrum of the protractor. The size of universal goniometer used is determined by the size of the joint being assessed. Larger goniometers are usually used for measurement of joint range at large joints.

Validity—Universal Goniometer. Validity is "the degree to which an instrument measures what it is supposed to measure."[17(p171)] Validity indicates the accuracy of a measurement. The therapist uses the universal goniometer to provide measurements of the number of degrees of movement or the position of a joint. Measurements must be accurate as the results, taken to be valid representations of actual joint angles, are used to plan treatment, determine treatment effectiveness, patient progress, and degree of disability.

Criterion-related validity is one means of assessing the accuracy of the universal goniometer for assessing joint angles or positions. To establish this validity, the universal goniometer measures are compared to the measures obtained with an instrument, for example an x-ray, that is an accepted standard (criterion), for the measurement of joint angles. If a close relationship is found between the measures obtained with the universal goniometer and the accepted standard, the universal goniometer measures are valid.

Radiographs, "the most accurate means of assessing joint motion,"[18(p116)] and photography are accepted standards used for comparison to determine the accuracy of the universal goniometer. When the supporting evidence from the radiographs or photographs is collected at the same time as the measurement from the universal goniometer, concurrent validity is assessed.

There has been little study of the criterion-related validity of the universal goniometer. Using x-ray bone angle measurements compared to goniometric measurements of knee joint position,[19,20] there is high criterion-related validity, and disparate findings of goniometric accuracy in only a small part of the range,

thought to be due to the increased complexity of movement in approaching terminal extension. Using a photographic reference standard[21] to assess elbow joint positions, the "results indicate that relatively inexperienced raters should be able to use goniometers accurately to measure elbow position when given standardized methods to follow."[21(p1666)]

Content validity is another means of assessing the accuracy of the universal goniometer. Content validity is essentially a judgment of how well an instrument measures what it is purported to measure. "Physical therapists judge the validity of most ROM measurements based on their anatomical knowledge and their applied skills of visual inspection, palpation of bony landmarks, and accurate alignment of the goniometer."[22(p1871)] This provides "sufficient evidence to ensure content validity."[22(p1871)]

Reliability—Universal Goniometer. Reliability is "the extent to which the instrument yields the same measurement on repeated uses either by the same operator (intraobserver reliability) or by different operators (interobserver reliability)."[23(p49)] Reliability indicates the consistency of a measurement.

The therapist measures ROM and compares measurements taken over time to evaluate treatment effectiveness and patient progress. It is important for the therapist to know that joint position and ROM can be measured consistently, that is, without much deviation due to measurement error. If this is possible, then in comparing ROM measures the similarity or difference between the measures can be relied on to indicate whether a true change has occurred that is not due to measurement error or lack of measurement consistency.

Reliability of joint position and ROM using the universal goniometer depends on the joint being assessed but has generally been found to be good to excellent.

Reliability study results indicate that:

1. The universal goniometer is more reliable than visual estimation of joint ROM.[24–27]
2. The reliability of goniometric measurement varies depending on the joint and motion assessed.[25,28–31]
3. Intratester reliability is better than intertester reliability; therefore, the same therapist should perform all measures when possible.[24,25,28,29,32–34] Different therapists should not be used interchangeably to obtain ROM measurements on the same patient unless the intertester reliability is known.[35]
4. The size of the goniometer selected to assess ROM at a joint does not affect measurement reliability.[36,37]
5. The findings are mixed on whether taking the average of repeated measures improves[25,33,38] or makes no difference[30,31,36] to the reliability of goniometric measures.
6. Reliability is low in ROM measurements in the presence of spasticity.[39–41]

Joint ROM can be measured reliably using a universal goniometer when, preferably, the same therapist performs the repeated measures using a "rigid standardized measurement protocol"[32(p57)] in the absence of spasticity. The intratester and intertester reliability should be determined for each clinical facility[11,18] so that the measurement error factor is known, thus allowing therapists to better determine patient progress.

• **Tape Measure.** ROM can also be measured through observation of a change in distance from one segment to another. These observations are measured with a tape measure and recorded in inches or centimeters.

Passive Joint ROM Assessment and Measurement Procedure

• **Expose the Area.** Explain the need to expose the area to be assessed to the patient. Adequately expose the area and drape the patient as required.

• **Explanation and Instruction.** Briefly explain the PROM assessment and measurement procedure to the patient. The therapist explains and demonstrates the movement to be performed and/or passively moves the patient's uninvolved limb through the ROM.

• **Assessment of the Normal ROM.** Initially assess and record the PROM of the uninvolved limb to determine the patient's normal PROM and normal end feels and to demonstrate the movement to the patient before performing the movement on the involved side. If there is bilateral limb involvement, the therapist can use the tables of normal AROM values provided by the American Academy of Orthopedic Surgeons[42] and clinical experience to judge the patient's normal PROM, keeping in mind that the PROM is usually slightly greater than the AROM.

The "normal" ROMs are presented in table form at the beginning of each chapter. "Normal" ranges can be misleading because joint ROM can vary between individuals depending on gender, age, occupation, and health status.[43] Therefore, "normal" ranges should be used only as a guide when treating patients.

• **Assessment and Measurement Procedure.**
a. Patient Position. Ensure the patient is comfortable and well supported, with the joint to be assessed in the anatomical position. The patient is positioned so the proximal joint segment can be stabilized to allow only the desired joint motion, movement can occur through the full ROM unrestricted, and the goniometer can be properly placed to measure the ROM. If the patient's position varies from the standard assessment position outlined in this text, a special note is made on the ROM assessment form.

b. Substitute Movements. When assessing and measuring PROM the therapist must ensure that only the desired movement occurs at the joint being assessed. Substitute movements may take the form of additional movements at the joint being assessed or at other joints, thus giving the appearance of having a greater joint ROM than is actually present. The therapist must try to eliminate substitute movements through proper patient positioning, adequate stabilization of the proximal joint segment, and practice in assessing PROM. To assess joint ROM accurately the therapist must know and recognize the possible substitute movements. If the presence of substitute movements results in inaccurate PROM assessment and measurement the treatment plan may be inappropriate.

c. Stabilization. Stabilize the proximal joint segment to limit movement to the joint being assessed or measured and prevent substitute movement for lack of joint range by making use of (1) the patient's body weight—used to help fix the shoulder or pelvic girdles; (2) the patient's position—for example, when assessing hip abduction ROM with the patient supine, at the end of the hip abduction ROM the pelvis may move toward the side being assessed and give the appearance of a greater range of hip abduction than actually exists. If the contralateral leg is positioned over the opposite side of the plinth with the foot resting on a stool, this leg will act to prevent the unwanted shift of the pelvis; and (3) external forces—external pressure applied directly by the therapist and devices such as belts or sandbags. In stabilizing, ensure that manual contacts or devices avoid tender or painful areas, for example, in some viral diseases (ie, poliomyelitis) muscle bellies may be tender.

d. Assessment of Passive Range and End Feel. Movement is isolated to the joint being assessed. The patient is relaxed and the therapist stabilizes the proximal joint segment, applies slight traction to and moves the distal joint segment to the end of the PROM for the test movement. Slight overpressure is applied at the end of the PROM and the PROM and end feel are noted.

e. Measurement. The method used to assess joint ROM is called the *neutral zero method.*[42] All joint motions are measured from a defined zero position, either the anatomical position or a position specified as zero. Any movement on either side of zero is positive and moves toward 180°.

If the involved joint has a full AROM and PROM the joint ROM does not have to be measured with a goniometer or tape measure. The ROM is recorded as either full, N (normal), or WNL (within normal limits), unless a normal ROM value is required for comparison on the involved side.

• Measurement procedure—universal goniometer
  • *Goniometer placement:* The preferred placement of the goniometer is lateral to the joint, just off the surface of the limb, but it may also be placed over the top of the joint, using only light contact between the goniometer and the skin. If joint

swelling is present this may give erroneous results when assessing joint ROM with the goniometer placed over the top of the joint.

- *Axis:* The axis of the goniometer is placed over the axis of movement of the joint. A specific bony prominence or anatomical landmark can be used to represent the axis of motion even though this may not represent the exact location of the axis of movement throughout the entire ROM.
- *Stationary arm:* The stationary arm of the goniometer usually lies parallel to the longitudinal axis of the fixed proximal joint segment and/or points toward a distant bony prominence.
- *Movable arm:* The movable arm of the goniometer usually lies parallel to the longitudinal axis of the moving distal joint segment and/or points toward a distant bony prominence.

If careful attention is paid to the correct positioning of the two goniometer arms and the positions are maintained as the joint moves through the ROM, the goniometer axis will be aligned approximately with the axis of motion.[43]

The goniometer is first aligned to measure the defined zero position for the PROM at a joint. If it is not possible to attain the defined zero position, the joint is positioned as close as possible to the zero position and the distance the movable arm is positioned away from the 0° start position on the protractor is recorded as the start position. One of the following two techniques is then used to measure the PROM at a joint:

i. The therapist has the patient actively move through the joint ROM and relax at the end of the ROM. The therapist realigns the goniometer at the end of the AROM and passively moves the goniometer and the body part through the final few degrees of the PROM.
ii. The therapist moves the movable arm of the goniometer with the distal limb segment through the entire range of movement to the end of the PROM.

Using either technique, the distance the movable arm moves away from the 0° start position on the protractor is recorded as the joint ROM.

To avoid parallax when reading a goniometer the therapist should look directly onto the scale and view the scale with both eyes open or by closing one eye. The methodology should be consistent on subsequent readings.

Sources of Error in Measuring Joint ROM. The goniometer scale must be read carefully to avoid erroneous ROM measurements. Sources of error to avoid when measuring joint ROM are:[44]

Reading the wrong side of the scale on the goniometer, such as, when the goniometer pointer is positioned midway between 40° and 50°, the value of 55° rather than 45° is read.

A tendency to read values that end in a particular digit, such as zero (ie, "_0°").

Having expectations of what the reading "should be" and allowing this to influence the recorded result. For example, the patient has been attending treatment for 2 weeks and the therapist expects and sees an improvement in the ROM that is not actually present.

A change in the patient's motivation to perform

Taking successive ROM measurements at different times of the day

Measurement procedure error

The therapist should ensure that sources of error do not occur or are minimized, so that ROM measurements will be reliable and the patient's progress can be meaningfully monitored. For reliable measurements, ROM should be assessed at the same time each day, by the same therapist, using the same measuring tool, using the same patient position, and following a standard measurement protocol.[43]

If upper or lower extremity joint ROM is measured by the same therapist, 3° or 4° increase in the ROM indicates improvement.[31] If different therapists measure the ROM, an increase of more than 5° for the upper extremity and 6° for the lower extremity indicates progress.[31]

Recording of Measurement. Pictorial or numerical charts may be used to record ROM. See Appendix B for a sample of a numerical recording form. If the AROM and PROM are full the joint ROM does not have to be measured with a goniometer or tape measure and the ROM may be recorded as either full, N (normal), WNL (within normal limits), or numerically.

If the PROM is either decreased or increased from the normal ROM, the existing ROM is shaded in on a pictorial chart or the number of degrees of motion is recorded on a numerical chart.

On pictorial charts the therapist extends lines from the joint axis on the diagram to the number of degrees on the arc of movement at the beginning and end of each movement. The area between the two lines is shaded in to indicate the ROM. The date is recorded either at the end of each line along the arc or is coded according to the type of shading used on the chart.

Every space on the ROM recording form should include an entry.[6] If the measurement was not performed, NT (not tested) should be entered and a line may be drawn from the first such entry to the end of several adjacent entries so that NT does not have to be recorded in every space.[6]

The ranges of motion are recorded on the numerical chart as follows:

When it is possible to begin the movement at the 0° start position, the ROM is recorded by writing the number of degrees the joint has moved away from 0°, for example, shoulder elevation through flexion 180° or 0° to 180°, knee flexion 75° or 0° to 75°, knee extension 0°.

When it is not possible to begin the movement from the 0° start position, the ROM is recorded by writing the number of degrees the joint is away from the 0° at the beginning of the ROM followed by the number of degrees the joint is away from 0° at the end of the ROM. For example, the patient cannot achieve 0° elbow extension due to a contracture (abnormal shortening) of the elbow flexor muscles, the end feel is firm. The elbow cannot be extended beyond 10° of elbow flexion and can be flexed to 120°. The ROM would be recorded either as elbow flexion 10° to 120° or elbow extension -10°, elbow flexion 120°.

Note: The only time that ROM is recorded as a negative value is when the patient cannot achieve the 0° start position. Any changes from the standard method of assessing joint ROM using the universal goniometer should be noted on the assessment form.

Assessing Joint ROM With a Two-Joint or Multijoint Muscle in the Region. When assessing joint ROM with a two-joint or multijoint muscle in the region, the position of one of the nontest joint(s) the muscle crosses may decrease the ROM possible at the test joint due to passive insufficiency of the muscle. When assessing the amount of movement possible at one joint, place the other joint(s) crossed by the muscle in a position that puts the two-joint or multijoint muscle on slack (ie, by approximating the muscle origin and insertion).

For example, when assessing hip flexion ROM with the knee in extension, passive insufficiency of the hamstring muscles limits hip flexion ROM (see Fig. 1-18). Positioning the knee in flexion places the hamstrings on slack. The hamstring muscles no longer limit hip joint movement.

• Assessment and Measurement of Muscle Length
One-Joint Muscle. To assess and measure the length of a muscle that crosses one joint, the joint crossed by the muscle is positioned so that the muscle is lengthened across the joint.

Two-Joint Muscle. To assess and measure the length of a two-joint muscle one of the joints the muscle crosses is positioned so that the muscle is lengthened across the joint. This joint position is held and the therapist moves the second joint as far as possible through a ROM to maximally lengthen or stretch the muscle.

Multijoint Muscle. To assess and measure the length of a multijoint muscle either the proximal or distal joints the muscle crosses are positioned so that the muscle is lengthened across these joints. These joints are held in this position and the therapist moves the remaining joint crossed by the muscle as far as possible through a PROM to maximally lengthen or stretch the muscle.

When passive insufficiency of the muscle limits the movement at a joint, the end feel will be firm due to the muscle being stretched preventing further joint movement. Placing the muscle on slack and retesting the joint PROM will normally result in an increased PROM. A universal goniometer, OB goniometer, or tape measure is used to measure the PROM possible at the last joint moved to place the muscle on full stretch, or the therapist observes and notes a limitation in joint ROM due to muscle tightness. The PROM measurement represents the length of the shortened muscle. When applicable, the technique of assessing or measuring muscle length is described and illustrated at the end of the ROM section of subsequent chapters.

SUMMARY—JOINT RANGE OF MOTION ASSESSMENT AND MEASUREMENT

The main steps in the assessment and measurement of joint ROM are outlined in Figures 1-20, 1-21, and 1-22 using shoulder extension as an example.

Passive joint ROM must be assessed before assessing muscle strength. The full available PROM at the joint then becomes the range the muscle can be expected to work through and is therefore defined as the full available ROM for the purpose of grading muscle strength.

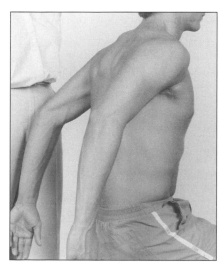

Figure 1-20.   Observation of the AROM.

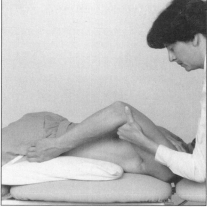

Figure 1-21.   Assessment of the PROM to estimate the joint ROM, determine the end feels, establish the presence or absence of pain, and determine the presence of a capsular or noncapsular pattern of movement.

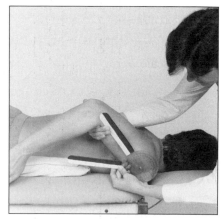

Figure 1-22.   Using an instrument (eg, universal goniometer) to measure the PROM.

DEFINITION—MANUAL MUSCLE TESTING

"Manual muscle testing is a procedure for the evaluation of the function and strength of individual muscles and muscle groups based on effective performance of a movement in relation to the forces of gravity and manual resistance."[45(p466)] Manual muscle testing (MMT) can be used to assess most medical conditions but has limitations in the treatment of neurological disorders where there is an alteration in muscle tone if reflex activity is altered[46] or if there is a loss of cortical control due to lesions of the central nervous system.[47]

To assess muscle strength the therapist must have a sound knowledge of anatomy (including joint motions, muscle origins and insertions, and muscle function) and surface anatomy (to know where a muscle or its tendon is best palpated). The therapist must be a keen observer and be experienced in muscle testing to detect minimal muscle contraction, movement, and muscle wasting and substitutions or trick movements. A consistent method of manually testing muscle strength is essential to assess accurately a patient's present status, progress, and the effectiveness of the treatment program.

MUSCLE TESTING TERMINOLOGY

Muscle Strength. This is the maximal amount of tension or force that a muscle or muscle group can voluntarily exert in one maximal effort,[48] when type of muscle contraction, limb velocity, and joint angle are specified.[49] Use of the term muscle strength in the clinical setting actually represents torque.[50]

Torque. Torque is the tendency of a force (ie, muscle tension) to turn a lever (ie, a limb or limb segment) around an axis of rotation (ie, a joint). Torque is a product of force and the perpendicular distance between the force and the axis of rotation.

Muscle Endurance. Endurance is the ability of a muscle or a muscle group to perform repeated contractions, against a resistance, or maintain an isometric contraction for a period of time.[48]

Muscle Fatigue.[51] Fatigue is a diminished response of the muscle to generate force that may be due to a lack of energy stores or oxygen, a buildup of lactic acid, protective inhibitory influences from the central nervous system, or a decrease in conduction impulses at the myoneural junction.

Overwork/Overtraining.[51] This is a phenomenon that causes a temporary or permanent loss of strength due to excessively vigorous activity or exercise relative to the patient's condition. Patients with certain neuromuscular diseases are more susceptible to this condition because of their lack of the normal sensation of discomfort that accompanies fatigue and puts a natural stop to performance of the activity or exercise before damage occurs.

Ranges of Muscle Work.[52] The full range in which a muscle works refers to the muscle changing from a position of full stretch and contracting to a position of maximal shortening. The full range can be more precisely described if it is divided into parts: outer, inner, and middle ranges (Fig. 1-23). Outer range is from a position where the muscle is on full stretch to a position halfway through the full range. Inner range is from a position halfway through the full range to a position where the muscle is fully shortened. Middle range is the portion of the full range between the midpoint of the outer range and the midpoint of the inner range.

Active Insufficiency. The active insufficiency of a muscle that crosses two or more joints occurs when the muscle produces simultaneous movement at all of the joints it crosses and reaches such a shortened position that it no longer has the ability to develop effective tension (Fig. 1-24).[8] When a muscle is placed in a shortened position of active insufficiency it is described as putting the *muscle on slack.*[7]

Isometric (Static) Contraction. This occurs when tension is developed in the muscle but no movement occurs, the origin and insertion of the muscle do not change position, and the muscle length does not change.[48]

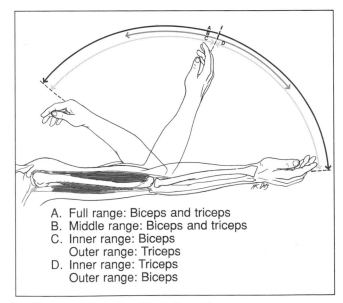

A. Full range: Biceps and triceps
B. Middle range: Biceps and triceps
C. Inner range: Biceps
   Outer range: Triceps
D. Inner range: Triceps
   Outer range: Biceps

Figure 1-23. Ranges of muscle work.

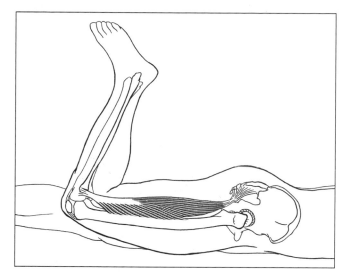

Figure 1-24. Active insufficiency of the hamstring muscles. Knee flexion performed with the hip in extension results in a shortening of the hamstring muscles that in turn decreases the ability of the hamstrings to develop tension.

Isotonic Contraction. The muscle develops constant tension[53] against a load or resistance.

Isokinetic Contraction. The muscle contracts at a constant rate of movement[54] or velocity.

Concentric Contraction. Tension is developed in the muscle and the origin and insertion of the muscle move closer together; the muscle shortens.

Eccentric Contraction. Tension is developed in the muscle and the origin and insertion of the muscle move farther apart; the muscle lengthens.

Functional Classification of Muscle. Muscles work in groups to produce movement. Muscles may be categorized as follows, according to the major role of the muscles in producing the movement.

• Prime Mover or Agonist. This is a muscle or muscle group that makes the major contribution to movement at the joint.

• Antagonist. An antagonist is a muscle or muscle group that has an opposite action to the prime mover(s). The antagonist relaxes as the agonist moves the part through a ROM.

• Synergist. A synergist is a muscle that contracts and works along with the agonist to produce the desired movement. Synergists function in different ways to assist the prime mover to produce the movement. Three types of synergists are described.

Neutralizing or Counteracting Synergists.[8] These are muscles that contract to prevent unwanted movements produced by the prime mover. For example, when the long finger flexors contract to produce finger flexion the wrist extensors contract to prevent wrist flexion from occurring.

Conjoint Synergists.[8] Conjoint synergists are Two or more muscles that work together to produce the desired movement. The muscles contracting alone would be unable to produce the movement. For example, wrist extension is produced by contraction of extensor carpi radialis longus and brevis and extensor carpi ulnaris. If the extensor carpi radialis longus or brevis contract alone, the wrist extends and radially deviates. If the extensor carpi ulnaris contracts alone, the wrist extends and ulnar deviates. When the muscles contract as a group the radial and ulnar deviation actions of the muscles cancel out and the common action of wrist extension results.

Stabilizing or Fixating Synergists.[8] These muscles prevent movement or control the movement at joints proximal to the moving joint to provide a fixed or stable base from which the distal moving segment can effectively work. For example, if the elbow flexors contract to lift an object off a table anterior to the body, the muscles of the scapula and glenohumeral joint must contract to either allow slow controlled movement or no movement to occur at the scapula and glenohumeral joint to provide the elbow flexors with a fixed origin from which to pull. If the scapular muscles do not contract the object cannot be lifted because the elbow flexors would act to pull the shoulder girdle downward toward the table top.

FACTORS AFFECTING STRENGTH

It is commonly recognized that a number of factors affect strength.[8,48,50,55] The therapist must consider these factors when assessing a patient's strength.

Age. Muscle strength increases from birth to a maximum point between 20 and 30 years of age.[54] Following this maximum, a decrease in strength occurs with increasing age due to a deterioration in muscle mass. Muscle fibers decrease in size and number, connective tissue and fat increase, and the respiratory capacity of the muscle decreases.

Gender. Men are generally stronger than women.[56]

Type of Muscle Contraction. The ability to develop tension in a muscle varies depending on the type of muscle contraction. More tension can be developed during an eccentric contraction than during an isometric contraction. The concentric contraction has the smallest tension capability. When assessing strength the same type of contraction should be used on successive tests.

Muscle Size. The larger the cross-sectional area of a muscle, the greater the strength of the muscle. When testing a muscle that is small, the therapist would expect less tension to be developed than if testing a large, thick muscle.

Speed of Muscle Contraction. When a muscle contracts concentrically, the force of contraction decreases as the speed of contraction increases. The patient is instructed to perform each muscle test movement at a moderate pace.

Previous Training Effect. Strength performance depends on the ability of the nervous system to activate the muscle mass. Strength may increase as one becomes familiar with and learns the test situation. The therapist must instruct the patient well and give the patient an opportunity to move through or be passively moved through the test movement at least once before strength is assessed.

Joint Position

• Angle of Muscle Pull. When a muscle contracts it creates a force and causes the body segment in which it inserts to rotate around a particular axis of the joint that the muscle crosses. The turning effect produced by the muscle is called the torque and is the product of the muscle force and the perpendicular distance between the joint axis of rotation and the muscle force. The position of the joint affects the angle of pull of a muscle and therefore changes the perpendicular distance between the joint axis of rotation and the muscle force and the torque. The optimal angle of muscle pull occurs when the muscle is pulling at a 90° angle or perpendicular to the bony segment. At this point, all of the muscle force is acting to rotate the segment and no force is wasted acting as a distracting or stabilizing force on the limb segment.

• Length—Tension Relations. The tension developed within a muscle depends on the initial length of the muscle. Regardless of the type of muscle contraction, a muscle contracts with more force when it is stretched than when it is shortened. The greatest amount of tension is developed when the muscle is stretched to the greatest length possible within the body, that is, if the muscle is in full outer range. Tension decreases as the muscle shortens until the muscle reaches less than 50% of its rest length, at which point it is not able to develop tension. When testing the strength of a two-joint muscle the nontest joint position is important to note. For example, the knee flexors (hamstrings) are able to develop greater tension and demonstrate greater strength if the patient is tested in a position of hip flexion. This position places the muscles in a stretched position, as opposed to a position of hip extension, which places the muscles in a shortened position.

Angle of muscle pull and length—tension relations interact to produce the muscle force curve. Most muscles demonstrate a decrease in force or strength from outer range into inner range, when assessed using isometric contractions at different joint angles.[57] Not all strength curves illustrate a muscle developing maximal tension at the position of full stretch because the angle of pull of the muscle may be small at this point even though the muscle length is optimal for development of tension. Williams and Stutzman,[57] Kulig and coworkers,[58] and Williams and associates[59] give analyses of strength curves for different muscle groups. The therapist must be aware of muscle strength patterns throughout the ROM so that resistance is applied correctly throughout the ROM and graduated when performing a muscle test. When testing isometric strength the position of the joint must be the same on successive tests if comparisons are to be made to assess changes in strength. If the muscle is tested in inner range, it may be graded much weaker than if it had been tested in middle or outer ranges.

Diurnal Variation.[60,61] Muscle strength is variable and this variability follows a regular cycle each day. Therefore, muscle strength should be assessed at the same time of day to accurately compare strength results and determine progress.

Temperature.[62] Strength of a muscle varies depending on the temperature of the muscle at the time of testing. Strength should be assessed when the muscle is at the same temperature on successive tests, preferably at room temperature.

Fatigue. As the patient tires, muscle strength decreases. The therapist determines the strength of the muscle using as few repetitions as possible to avoid fatigue. The functional capability of a muscle is more accurately assessed if endurance is also considered when testing the muscle. After the therapist has determined the muscle strength, the patient remains in the test position and repeats the test movement against the same resistance the muscle was able to move according to the strength grade assigned to the muscle until the patient can no longer move through the ROM, that is, drops to the next lowest whole grade. The number of repetitions until this point may be recorded as a clinical indicator of endurance. Alternatively, the therapist may complete the muscle testing and then repeat only those movements requiring good endurance for activities of daily living (ADL). The number of times the patient would repeat the movement in specific activities is an indicator of functional requirements.

The patient's level of motivation, level of pain, body type, occupation, and dominance are other factors that may affect strength. The therapist must consider the factors that affect strength to select the most appropriate method to use for the strength assessment and ensure consistency of application when performing manual muscle testing.

JOINT POSITIONS

Close-Packed Position. When a joint is in the close-packed position the joint surfaces are fully congruent.[12] In the close-packed position there is maximal tension in the joint capsule and ligaments; the joint surfaces are pressed together firmly and the joint surfaces cannot be pulled apart using traction.[12]

The close-packed position should be avoided when testing muscle strength because the patient can lock the joint and hold the joint in this position against resistance in the presence of a weak prime mover, resulting in an inaccurate assessment of muscle strength. The therapist must be especially careful of this positioning at the elbow, knee, and ankle joints. Close-packed joint positions are listed in Table 1-5.

Loose-Packed Position. The loose-packed position is any position of a joint other than the close-packed position, where the joint surfaces are not congruent and parts of the joint capsule are lax.[63] The position of least stress on the joint,[12] least congruency of joint surfaces and the greatest laxity of the capsule and ligaments is the *resting position* or maximum loose-packed position of the joint.[63] The loose-packed (resting) position may be used to prevent joint pain when testing isometric muscle strength in the region of a painful joint because of the decreased tension on the joint capsule and ligaments and decreased intra-articular pressure provided by this position. Resting joint positions are listed in Table 1-5.

ASSESSMENT CONTRAINDICATIONS AND PRECAUTIONS— MANUAL MUSCLE TESTING

Muscle strength must not be assessed manually if any contraindications to this form of assessment exist. In special instances the assessment techniques must be carried out with a modified approach. The same contraindications and precautions for assessing AROM or PROM apply when manually assessing muscle strength. Additional contraindications and precautions are listed here. The contraindications and precautions presented are based on those described by Kisner and Colby[51] in the application of resistance exercise.

Manual assessment of muscle strength is contraindicated if:

1. Inflammation is present in the region.
2. Pain is present. Pain will inhibit muscle contraction and will not give an accurate indication of muscle strength. Testing muscle strength in the presence of pain may cause further injury.

Extra care must be taken where resisted movements might aggravate the condition, such as:

1. Patients with a history or at risk of cardiovascular problems, such as suspected or known aneurysm, fixed-rate pacemaker, arrhythmias, suspected or known thrombophlebitis, recent embolus, marked obesity, hypertension, angina pectoris, myocardial in-

farctions, and cerebral vascular accident, should be instructed to avoid the *Valsalva maneuver* during the muscle testing procedure. Kisner and Colby[51] describe the sequence of events in the Valsalva procedure. The Valsalva maneuver involves an expiratory effort against a closed glottis that occurs during a strenuous and prolonged effort. A deep breath is taken at the beginning of the effort and held by closing the glottis. The abdominal muscles contract causing an increase in the intra-abdominal and intrathoracic pressures and a decrease in the venous return to the heart. This results in a decreased cardiac output, a temporary decrease in arterial blood pressure, and an increase in heart rate. When the patient relaxes after the effort, an expiration causes an increase in blood pressure and forceful contraction of the heart due to a rapid venous return to the heart. The Valsalva maneuver can be avoided by instructing the patient not to hold the breath during the test. Should this be difficult, the patient may be instructed to breathe out[65] or to talk during the test.[51]

2. Patients who have had abdominal surgery or have herniation of the abdominal wall should be carefully instructed to avoid the Valsalva maneuver to prevent unsafe stress on the abdominal wall.[51]
3. In situations in which fatigue may be detrimental to or exacerbate the patient's condition, such as extreme debility, malnutrition, malignancy, and chronic obstructive pulmonary disease, strenuous testing should not be carried out. Fatigue may exacerbate the patient's condition in cases such as multiple sclerosis, poliomyelitis, postpoliomyelitis syndrome, myasthenia gravis, lower motor neuron disease, and intermittent claudication. Signs of fatigue include complaints of tiredness, pain and muscular spasm, a slow response to contraction, tremor, and a decreased ability to perform AROM.
4. In situations in which overwork may be detrimental to the patient's condition (eg, patients with certain neuromuscular diseases), care should be used.

Instrumentation. The instrument chosen to assess muscle strength depends on the degree of accuracy required in the measurement and the time and resources available to the clinician. Hand-held dynamometers, free weights, the use of the cable tensiometer, the handgrip dynamometer, the pinch meter, or isokinetic dynamometers may give objective, valid, and reliable measures of muscle strength but are not always practical in the clinical environment. When doing clinical research, the therapist is encouraged to investigate alternate instruments that will offer a more stringent assessment of muscle strength. MMT is the method used to assess muscle strength as presented in this text.

• Validity—MMT. The therapist uses MMT to provide information about muscle strength, that is, the maximal amount of tension or force that a muscle or muscle group can voluntarily exert in one maximal effort.[48] Measurements must be accurate because the results, taken to be valid representations of muscle strength, are

TABLE
1-5

▼ CLOSE-PACKED AND LOOSE-PACKED POSITIONS OF SELECTED JOINTS[12,15,63,64]

Joint(s)	Close-Packed Position	Loose-Packed (Resting) Position
Facet (spine)	Extension	Midway between flexion and extension
Temporomandibular	Clenched teeth	Mouth slightly open
Glenohumeral	Abduction and external rotation	55° abduction, 30° horizontal adduction, rotated so that the forearm is in the transverse plane
Acromioclavicular	Arm abducted to 90°	Arm resting by side, shoulder girdle in the physiological position*
Sternoclavicular	Maximum shoulder elevation	Arm resting by side, should girdle in the physiological position*
Ulnohumeral (elbow)	Extension	70° elbow flexion, 10° forearm supination
Radiohumeral	Elbow flexed 90°, forearm supinated 5°	Full extension, full supination
Proximal radioulnar	5° supination	70° elbow flexion, 35° forearm supination
Distal radioulnar	5° supination	10° forearm supination
Radiocarpal (wrist)	Extension with radial deviation	Midway between flexion-extension (so that a straight line passes through the radius and third metacarpal) with slight ulnar deviation
First carpometacarpal	Full opposition	Midway between abduction-adduction and flexion-extension
Metacarpophalangeal (fingers)	Full flexion	Slight flexion
Metacarpophalangeal (thumb)	Full opposition	
Interphalangeal	Full extension	Slight flexion
Hip	Full extension, internal rotation and abduction	30° flexion, 30° abduction, and slight external rotation
Knee	Full extension and external rotation of the tibia	25° flexion
Talocrural (ankle)	Maximum dorsiflexion	10° plantarflexion, midway between maximum inversion and eversion
Subtalar	Full supination	Midway between extremes of inversion and eversion
Midtarsal	Full supination	Midway between extremes of ROM
Tarsometatarsal	Full supination	Midway between extremes of ROM
Metatarsophalangeal	Full extension	Neutral
Interphalangeal	Full extension	Slight flexion

*Physiological position[63] is the term given to the resting position of the shoulder girdle. The scapula is situated over the ribs two through seven and the vertebral border is 5 cm lateral to the spinous processes; the clavicle lies nearly in the horzontal plane. In the physiological position imaginary lines drawn through the long axis of the clavicle, along the plane of the scapula and along the midsagittal plane form the sides of an equilateral triangle having angles of 60°.

used to make a diagnosis, assess patient prognosis, plan treatment, determine treatment effectiveness, and evaluate functional status. There is a lack of evidence to demonstrate the validity of MMT. However, in an effort to establish criterion-related validity, MMT results have been compared to the measures obtained with hand-held dynamometers.[66–68] The close relationship between the measures obtained with MMT and the hand-held dynamometer measures suggest that muscle strength is measured by both techniques.

From the clinicians' judgment, MMT seems to measure the torque-producing capability of the tested muscle(s)[69] and thus MMT appears to have content validity.

• Reliability—MMT. It is important for the therapist to know that muscle strength can be evaluated consistently, so that results taken over time can be compared to evaluate treatment effectiveness and patient progress. If this is possible, then in comparing measures the similarity or difference between the measures can be relied on to indicate a true change in strength due to treatment or over time, and are not simply due to measurement error and lack of measurement consistency.

Most studies assessing the reliability of MMT are based on the use of isometric make or break testing techniques. Using a standardized procedure for testing, reliability of interrater MMT results with complete agreement of muscle grades is low.[70,71] Interrater and intrarater reliability within the range of one whole muscle grade[71–74] and interrater reliability within one half a grade (ie, within a + or − grade)[67,70] is very high. Although this indicates a high level of consistency for MMT, a difference of one whole strength grade may not be adequate for clinical decision-making.[73]

Reliability and validity study results for MMT indicate that:

1. Intratester reliability is better than intertester reliability; therefore, the same therapist should perform all MMTs when possible.[72,74]
2. MMT grading is limited by the strength of the examiner, especially in very strong patients when assessing grades of 5.[75]
3. MMT is not sensitive to strength changes in the higher grades of 4 and 5.[67,68,76]
4. MMT scores tend to overestimate the patient's strength in the higher grades of 4 and 5.[66,67,75–77]
5. MMT scores are most sensitive in lower grades 0 to 3.[78]
6. It is suggested that MMT be supplemented with quantitative means of assessing strength (eg, isokinetic dynamometry, tensiometry) for grades that are greater than 3 and more subjective in nature.[73]
7. MMT grades are not equivalent to linear measurements,[70,79] for example, a grade 3 does not equal 50% muscle strength. Similarly, normal strength does not equal 100% strength and varies depending on the muscle group tested, for example, a grade 5 for the knee extensors equals 53%, the plantarflexors equals 34%, and the hip extensors equals 65% of the actual maximal strength of each muscle group.[76]

To increase the reliability of the assessment of muscle strength, the MMT should be conducted at the same time of day to avoid varying levels of fatigue, by the same therapist, in the same environment, using the same patient position, and following a standard testing protocol, to allow for more accurate comparisons between tests and assessment of the patient's progress.

Manual muscle testing is a convenient, versatile, quick to apply, and inexpensive means of assessing muscle strength. In weaker patients it is not possible to use equipment such as an isokinetic testing device[80,81] or hand-held dynamometer[82] for testing lower grades (ie, < 3). Using MMT, specific stabilization, isolated testing of single muscle actions, and elimination of substitute action and movement are possible.

In the clinical setting, MMT is a common means of assessing strength. Although the validity and reliability of MMT appear to be less than ideal and further research is needed, there is merit in using MMT if the limitations are kept in mind.

MANUAL ASSESSMENT OF MUSCLE STRENGTH

After the visual observation and assessment of AROM and PROM have been completed, the therapist performs a manual assessment of muscle strength.

Individual Versus Group Muscle Test. Muscles with a common action or actions may be tested as a group or a muscle may be tested individually. For example, flexor carpi ulnaris and flexor carpi radialis may be tested together as a group in the action of wrist flexion. Flexor carpi ulnaris may be tested more specifically in the action of wrist flexion with ulnar deviation. Although it is not always possible to isolate a muscle completely, individual muscle tests are illustrated and described in this text.

Muscle Testing Assessment Procedure

• Explanation and Instruction. Briefly explain the manual muscle test assessment procedure to the paient. The therapist explains and demonstrates the movement to be performed and/or passively moves the patient's limb through the test movement.

• Assessment of Normal Muscle Strength. Initially assess and record the strength of the uninvolved limb to determine the patient's normal strength (ie, grade 5) and to demonstrate the movement before assessing the strength of the involved side. If the contralateral limb cannot be used for comparison, the therapist must rely on past experience to judge the patient's normal strength considering the factors that affect strength, such as the patient's age, gender, dominance, and occupation.

• Patient Position. The patient is positioned to isolate the muscle or muscle group to be tested in either a gravity eliminated or against gravity position.[83] Ensure the patient is comfortable and adequately supported. The muscle or muscle group being tested is placed in full outer range, with only slight tension being placed on the muscle. When assessing muscle strength "good control and specificity of body positions chosen during testing is essential to produce valid strength estimates."[84(p509)]

• Stabilization. Stabilize the site of attachment of the origin of the muscle so that the muscle has a fixed point from which to pull. When testing a two-joint or multi-joint muscle, stabilize or fix the segment proximal to the joint where movement occurs to test the muscle action. Prevent substitutions and trick movements by making use of the following methods of stabilization:

1. The patient's body weight—used to help fix the shoulder or pelvic girdles.
2. The patient's normal muscles—(a) having the patient use muscles that are not normally used when performing the test movement, for example, the patient holds the edge of the plinth when hip flexion is tested and/or (b) having the patient use the fixator muscles that would normally act as stabilizers for the movement, for example, the scapular muscles when glenohumeral flexion is performed.
3. The patient's position—for example, when assessing hip abduction muscle strength in the side-lying position, the patient holds the nontest leg in maximal hip and knee flexion to tilt the pelvis posteriorly and fix the pelvis and lumbar spine.
4. External forces—external pressure applied directly by the therapist and devices such as belts and sandbags.

In stabilizing, ensure that manual contacts or devices avoid tender or painful regions, for example, in some viral diseases (ie, poliomyelitis) muscle bellies may be tender. Ensure that manual contacts or devices do not exert too much force directly over the belly of the muscle being tested and inhibit contraction.[85]

Substitution and Trick Movements. When muscles are weak or paralyzed, other muscles may take over or gravity may be used to perform the movements normally carried out by the weak muscles.[86] These vicarious motions are called trick movements[86] or substitution movements.[7] The different types of substitution or trick movements are listed below and are primarily based on the substitution or trick movements described by Kendall and colleagues[7] and Wynn Parry.[86]

1. Direct or indirect substitution by:
   a. Another prime mover that may also result in deviation in the direction of the other actions performed by the substitute prime mover. For example, with weakness or absence of supinator, biceps brachii can contract to perform supination and elbow flexion may occur simultaneously.
   b. The fixator muscles producing movement that appears to have occurred through the site of origin of the weak agonist. For example, the lateral abdominals will contract to stabilize the pelvis during testing of the hip abductor muscles. If the hip abductors are weak, the lateral abdominals may elevate the pelvis and in turn move the lower extremity to give the appearance of hip abduction.
   c. Other favorably placed muscles in the region that may contract to position the joint so that other muscles by virtue of the new joint position can perform the test motion. For example, if the deltoid muscle is paralyzed the external rotators externally rotate the humerus so that the long head of biceps brachii is positioned more laterally with respect to the shoulder joint and is in a position to assist with shoulder abduction.
   d. Other muscles in the total limb pattern that may contract in an attempt to assist the weak muscles. For example, the shoulder flexes when the patient attempts to flex the elbow in the presence of elbow flexor muscle weakness.
2. Accessory insertion—The insertion of a muscle may be such that when the muscle contracts it helps to perform the prime movement of the weak or paralyzed muscle. For example, the flexor pollicis brevis and abductor pollicis brevis muscles insert into the base of the proximal phalanx of the thumb and perform the prime movements of thumb metacarpophalangeal joint flexion and abduction, respectively. These muscles also insert into the extensor expansion of the thumb and when the muscles contract, tension is created on the extensor expansion and extensor pollicis longus tendon, resulting in extension of the thumb in the presence of extensor pollicis longus muscle paralysis.
3. Tendon action—When the antagonist to a weak or paralyzed muscle contracts, it produces movement that places the weaker muscle on stretch. The stretch will produce passive movement at the joints crossed by the weak muscle in the direction of the weak muscle's prime action, giving the appearance of muscle contraction. This passive movement is more pronounced if the weak muscle is shortened and lacks normal extensibility. For example, in the presence of flexor digitorum superficialis and profundus muscle paralysis if the extensors of the wrist contract to produce wrist extension, the finger flexors are placed on stretch. The stretch on the finger flexors results in passive flexion of the fingers giving the appearance of contraction of the long finger flexors.
4. Rebound phenomenon—When an antagonist to a weak or paralyzed muscle contracts and then relaxes quickly, it will produce passive movement in the direction of the prime movement of the weak muscle. This gives the appearance of contraction of the weak muscle. For example, the interphalangeal joint of the thumb is positioned in extension to test the strength of the flexor pollicis longus muscle. In this position the extensor pollicis longus may contract to pull the interphalangeal joint into further extension and then quickly relax. This sudden relaxation results in slight passive flexion of the interphalangeal joint that could be mistaken for movement performed by contraction of the flexor pollicis longus.
5. Gravity—The patient may shift the body part so that gravity may be used to perform the movement of the weak or paralyzed muscle. For example, in sitting with the shoulder abducted 90°, elbow flexed, and the upper limb resting on a table the patient with a weak or paralyzed triceps may not be able to extend the elbow and move the forearm along the table top. The patient may attempt to extend the elbow by performing shoulder girdle depression and shoulder ex-

ternal rotation to position the forearm so that gravity assists the weak triceps.

The therapist must try to eliminate trick movements or substitutions through adequate explanation and instruction to the patient of the movement to be performed and the trick movements that must be avoided, proper patient positioning, adequate stabilization of the muscle origin, palpation of the muscle(s) being tested to ensure contraction, and practice in assessing muscle strength. To grade muscle strength accurately the therapist must be aware of and recognize trick movements or substitutions that may occur.[71] When trick movements are not recognized, the patient's problem will not be identified and treatment planning may be inappropriate.

• **Screen Test.** A screen test is a method used to streamline the muscle strength assessment, avoid unnecessary testing, and avoid fatiguing or discouraging the patient by eliminating as many tests as possible the patient would not be able to successfully complete. A screen test is an arbitrarily assigned starting point.

The therapist may screen the patient through the information gained from:

1. The previous assessment of the patient's AROM
2. Reading the patient's chart or previous muscle test results
3. Observing the patient perform functional activities; for example, shaking the patient's hand may indicate the strength of grasp (ie, the finger flexors).

Based on the available information, the patient is positioned so that the assessment of strength begins at or near the patient's actual level of strength.

Alternatively, the patient may be screened by:

4. Beginning all muscle testing at a particular grade; this is usually a grade of 3. The patient is instructed to actively move the body part through the full ROM against gravity. Based on the results of the initial test the muscle test is either stopped or it proceeds.

METHODS OF ASSESSING AND GRADING MUSCLE STRENGTH

Conventional and alternate methodologies of assessing and grading muscle strength are described. Regardless of the method used when manually assessing muscle strength, a grade is assigned to indicate the strength of a muscle or muscle group. In conventional grading and some alternate grading methods, the grade indicates the strength of a voluntary muscle contraction and the AROM possible within the available PROM, previously assessed.

All methods of assessing muscle strength described are based on the principles of muscle testing that have evolved clinically over time. Lovett (cited in Daniels and Worthingham[87]) developed the concept of using gravity as a factor to assess the strength of a muscle.

Wright[88] was the first to publish a method of classifying muscles according to the ability of the muscle to overcome the resistance of gravity or friction. Further developments have been documented by others including Brunnstrom,[89] Smith and colleagues,[90] Hines,[91] Daniels and Worthingham,[87] and Kendall and Kendall.[92]

Conventional Method

Manual grading of muscle strength is based on three factors[87]:

1. Evidence of contraction—no palpable or observable muscle contraction (grade 0) or a palpable or observable muscle contraction and no joint motion (grade 1)
2. Gravity as a resistance—ability to move the part through the full available ROM: gravity eliminated (grade 2) or against gravity (grade 3)
3. Amount of manual resistance—ability to move the part through the full available ROM against gravity and against: moderate manual resistance (grade 4) or maximal manual resistance (grade 5).

In addition to the whole grades 0 to 5, more detailed grading of muscle strength is achieved by adding a plus or minus to the whole grade to denote variation in the ROM. Movement through less than half of the available ROM is denoted by a plus and movement through greater than half of the available ROM by a minus. The grade gives a general indication of the patient's AROM within the available PROM at the joint. For example, if the patient is stronger than a grade 2 yet weaker than a grade 3 and is able to move the limb through less than half of the available ROM against the resistance of gravity the muscle would be assigned a grade of 2+.

Muscles are graded using a conventional grading system. Numerals or letters are used to indicate grades of muscle strength. The numerical notation is not a precise, graded quantitative determination of muscle strength.[46] Table 1-6 gives a description of each grade.

Beasley[76] found that a grade of 3 (fair) does not necessarily indicate 50% of the normal strength of the muscle or muscle group tested when compared with a standard normal reference. A grade of 3 is well below the 50% mark varying from being approximately 9% for some muscles and slightly greater than 30% for other muscles tested in the study. Therefore, there is a greater range between the grades of 3 and 5 (normal) than between the grades of 3 and 0.

Grading

• **Against Gravity.** In each chapter, the grade of 3 is used as the screen test except for testing of the facial muscles where conventional muscle grading is not applied. The patient is positioned so that gravity resists the muscle's or muscle group's prime movement(s) through as much of the ROM as possible. In most cases it is not possible to move against gravity through the entire ROM as the bone moves from a horizontal to a vertical position or a vertical to a horizontal position. Therefore, the muscle has either little resistance from the pull of gravity at the start or end of motion, or the muscle has

TABLE 1-6 ▼ CONVENTIONAL GRADING

Numerals	Letters	Description
Against gravity tests		The patient is able to actively move through:
5	N (normal)	The full available ROM against gravity and against maximal resistance
4	G (good)	The full available ROM against gravity and against moderate resistance
4−	G−	Greater than one half the available ROM against gravity and against moderate resistance
3+	F+	Less than one half the available ROM against gravity and against moderate resistance
3	F (fair)	The full available ROM against gravity
3−	F−	Greater than one half the available ROM against gravity
2+	P+	Less than one half the available ROM against gravity
Gravity eliminated tests		The patient is able to actively move through:
2	P (poor)	The full available ROM gravity eliminated
2−	P−	Greater than one half the available ROM gravity eliminated
1+	T+	Less than one half the available ROM gravity eliminated
1	T (trace)	None of the available ROM gravity eliminated and there is a palpable or observable flicker of a muscle contraction
0	0 (zero)	None of the available ROM gravity eliminated and there is no palpable or observable muscle contraction

no resistance at the end of motion when gravity assists the movement and the antagonist contracts eccentrically to complete the ROM.[93] The muscle is placed in full outer range. The muscle force exerted during the muscle test can be influenced to a great extent by the therapist's instructions.[53,94] The volume of the therapist's voice can influence voluntary muscle contraction. High-volume commands can elicit a stronger muscle contraction than low-volume commands.[95,96] During each test the therapist gives commands explicitly and consistently to elicit the strongest possible response from the patient. As the patient attempts to move at a moderate pace through the ROM, the therapist palpates the prime mover(s) to ensure contraction and rule out the possibility of substitution or trick movements.

If the patient moves through only part of the ROM against gravity, the muscle is given a grade of 2+ or 3− and this ends the muscle test.

If the patient moves through the full ROM against gravity, the test is repeated against manual resistance to determine the grade. The grade of 3 is given if the patient cannot perform the movement against manual resistance. If the patient can perform the movement against manual resistance, a grade of greater than 3 is assigned depending on the magnitude of the resistance and how far into the ROM the resistance could be applied. The patient is asked to relax at the end of each test movement and the therapist positions the limb for the next test movement.

• **Manual Resistance.** The therapist uses a lumbrical grip, in which the metacarpophalangeal joints are flexed with the interphalangeal joints held in extension and the thumb either adducted or relaxed in slight extension, to apply resistance (Fig. 1-25). Add resistance

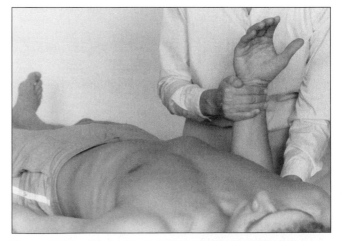

Figure 1-25. Manual resistance applied at a 90° angle to the limb segment using a lumbrical grip.

gradually to allow the patient to "set" the muscles. The resistance force is applied at a 90° angle to the limb segment (see Fig. 1-25).

Apply the resistance force at the distal end of the segment into which the muscle(s) being tested is (are) inserted.[7,97] Allowing a joint to come between the point of application of the resistance and the muscle insertion may increase the chance of substitution. Ensure resistance is not given distal to an unstable or weakly supported joint. Every attempt should be made to keep the length of the resistance arm (ie, the distance between the axis of rotation of the joint and the point of application of the manual resistance) standard for each muscle test. *Note:* The longer the length of the resistance arm, the less the resistance force required by the therapist to counteract the torque produced by the muscle.

Nicholas and coworkers[98] report that if the therapist gives an equal or greater resistance to the limb when testing muscle A but for a shorter period of time than when testing muscle B, it is possible that muscle A could be assessed as being weaker than muscle B. When applying resistance to test a muscle the therapist mentally integrates the time taken to go through the ROM with the magnitude of the resistance force to arrive at a perception of the strength deficit and assign a grade.[98] Because of this and the force—velocity relationships, the therapist should use the same time and the same velocity of movement to go through the ROM when performing comparable muscle tests.

The magnitude of the resistance force is based on the amount of resistance that can be applied and allow the patient to move smoothly through the full ROM. The resistance force applied throughout the movement "should be just a little less than would stop the movement."[88(p568)] The therapist must modify the amount of resistance given throughout the ROM according to the patient's capabilities. If too much resistance is given, the patient will not be able to move through the ROM and this may lead to recruitment of other muscles to perform the movement.

• Gravity Eliminated. If the patient cannot move through any part of the ROM against gravity, the patient is positioned so that gravity is eliminated (ie, the patient performs the movement in the horizontal plane). This position may require that the weight of the limb be supported on a relatively friction-free surface or be supported by the therapist. The muscle origin is stabilized, the muscle(s) is palpated during the test, and the patient attempts to move through the ROM. During the actual test, the therapist gives commands explicitly and consistently from one test to another. Commands should elicit the strongest response possible.

If the patient moves through the full ROM with gravity eliminated, the muscle is assigned a grade of 2.

If the patient is able to move through only a part of the ROM, then a grade of either a 2− or a 1+ is given.

If no movement occurs, the therapist grades the muscle based on the presence or absence of a muscle contraction.

The patient is asked to relax at the end of each test movement and the therapist positions the limb for the next test movement.

Palpation. Palpate a muscle near its tendon attachment or near a bony point using the pads of the index and middle fingers. Always palpate and observe the muscle(s) being tested when assessing grades of 0 through 3, because the muscle may be graded based on the quality of contraction when no movement is possible or the lack of muscle tension with movement may indicate substitution or trick movements. In cases of extreme weakness, a flicker of a contraction may be detected more easily by observing slight movement of the skin than by palpating.

Number of Repetitions Used in Testing. Strength is determined after two to three repetitions of the test movement. Fatigue will become a factor with too many repetitions, resulting in erroneous recording and underestimating the patient's true strength because the grades of manual muscle strength assessment methods do not take endurance into account.

ALTERNATE METHODS AND GRADING OF MUSCLE STRENGTH

Alternate methods and grading of muscle strength may be used in situations in which the patient cannot be positioned as required for conventional grading, it is too tiring or time consuming to change the patient's position, or it would be more appropriate to test a muscle or muscle group taking its normal function into account (eg, a stabilizer with an isometric test, a weight-bearing muscle in a weight-bearing position using body weight as the resistance).

Alternate Gravity Eliminated Methods and Grading

• Assisted Against Gravity Method. This method is used if the patient cannot be positioned so that the movement occurs in a gravity eliminated situation. The patient is positioned so that gravity resists the movement. The patient relaxes and the therapist judges the weight of the limb or limb segments to be moved. The therapist offers assistance equal to the weight of the limb (to approximate the gravity eliminated conventional method), while the patient performs as much of the ROM as possible. Table 1-7 gives a description of assisted against gravity grading.

• Palpation Method. This method is used when testing very weak muscles and muscles that function primarily as stabilizers, for example, the muscles connecting the shoulder girdle to the trunk. The therapist positions the limb segment so that the muscle will contract in inner range against gravity and the patient attempts to hold

TABLE 1-7

▼ ASSISTED AGAINST GRAVITY GRADING

Numeral	Description
	The patient is able to actively move through:
2	The full available ROM assisted against gravity
2−	Greater than one half the available ROM assisted against gravity
1+	Less than one half the available ROM assisted against gravity
1	None of the available ROM assisted against gravity but there is a palpable or observable flicker of a muscle contraction
0	None of the available ROM assisted against gravity and there is no palpable or observable muscle contraction

the position. One of the therapist's hands remains just below the limb to control its fall if the patient is unable to hold the limb in any part of the ROM against gravity. The muscle is palpated and graded according to the feel of the muscle contraction. Table 1-8 gives a description of palpation grading.

Palpation grading may also be used if joint movement causes pain and no absolute contraindications exist. It is extremely difficult if not impossible to perform a static contraction and produce a situation where absolutely no movement occurs at the joint crossed by the muscle. There is always some degree of joint movement, compression, and shearing even with static muscle contraction.[99] Therefore, if joint pain is a factor, it may be preferable to perform palpation grading with the joint placed in a loose-packed (resting) position. The therapist keeps one hand immediately below the patient's limb so that no movement or only slight movement occurs if the patient is unable to hold the limb in any part of the ROM against gravity.

Alternate Against Gravity Methods and Grading

• **Resisted Gravity Eliminated Method.** This method is used when the patient cannot be positioned so that movement occurs against gravity. The patient is positioned so that gravity is eliminated and the therapist gives resistance equal to or greater than the weight of the limb. Table 1-9 gives a description of resisted gravity eliminated grading.

• **Isometric Method.** This method is used when testing muscles that function primarily as stabilizers, that is, the muscles of the trunk and wrist and muscles connecting the shoulder girdle to the trunk. The strength of muscles that perform multiple actions are more easily assessed using the isometric method. This method may be used to assess strength if joint movement causes pain and no contraindications exist. There is always some degree of joint movement, compression, and shearing even with static muscle contraction.[99] Therefore, if joint pain is a

TABLE 1-8

▼ PALPATION GRADING

Numeral	Description
	The patient is unable to actively hold the limb in any part of the ROM against gravity, and the therapist palpates:
2	A prolonged firm muscle contraction
2−	A minimal muscle contraction
1	A slight flicker of a muscle contraction and the muscle can be felt to relax
0	No muscle contraction

TABLE 1-9 ▼ RESISTED GRAVITY ELIMINATED GRADING

Numeral	Description
	The patient is able to actively move through:
5	The full available ROM against resistance equal to the weight of the limb plus maximal resistance
4	The full available ROM against resistance equal to the weight of the limb plus moderate resistance
4−	Greater than one half the available ROM against resistance equal to the weight of the limb plus moderate resistance
3+	Less than one half the available ROM against resistance equal to the weight of the limb plus moderate resistance
3	The full available ROM against resistance equal to the weight of the limb
3−	Greater than one half the available ROM against resistance equal to the weight of the limb
2+	Less than one half the available ROM against resistance equal to the weight of the limb

factor, it may be preferable to place the joint in a loose-packed (resting) position when applying the isometric method.

The isometric method is also used to selectively test the integrity of contractile tissue (ie, muscle and tendon) by applying stress to the tissue by way of muscle contraction. The joint is in resting position and no movement occurs at the joint during the isometric contraction. Thus, no stress is placed on inert or non-contractile tissue (ie, joint capsule, ligaments, and nerves). During the isometric contraction, the therapist notes whether pain is elicited and whether the contraction is weak or strong to determine if there is a muscular lesion. Isometric muscle testing may also be used as a quick method of scanning for muscle weakness before performing more detailed muscle testing, as required.

The therapist positions the limb segment so that the muscle will contract in either middle or inner range against gravity and then gradually takes away any support as the patient attempts to hold the position. Alternatively, the patient actively moves the limb segment into either middle or inner range for the muscle being assessed. If the limb segment is held in the start position against gravity, the therapist gradually applies resistance. The resistance must not "break" the muscle contraction so that the patient cannot hold the position. This isometric testing technique is referred to as a make test.[100] The therapist gradually decreases the resistance as the limb segment is felt to fall toward the muscle's outer range. The therapist has the patient maintain the contraction for about 4 seconds to allow time to establish a maximal isometric contraction.[101] The muscle is graded based on the maximal amount of resistance the muscle can hold against. Table 1-10 gives a description of isometric grading.

When using isometric grading, the therapist considers that the strength needed to hold the test position is the same as the strength needed to move through the test movement[7] although Wilson and Murphy[102] note there is no research to suggest that force measured at any one point in the ROM is representative of muscle force throughout the entire movement. Strength varies throughout the ROM and a more accurate picture of the muscle's capabilities is attained if three isometric muscle tests are performed with the muscle positioned in inner, middle, and outer ranges or better yet the muscle test is performed through the ROM using conventional grading. When using isometric grading, to maintain reliability in testing, the muscle should be tested in the same part(s) of the ROM each time.[87] Isometric testing is an accepted clinical method of assessing muscle strength[103] but predicting dynamic work capabilities from isometric tests is generally not reliable.[53,102] Dynamic tests are superior to isometric tests in their relationship to dynamic activities.[102]

Special Tests

• Hands and Toes. The weight of the fingers and toes is so minimal that the effect of gravity is unimportant and need not be considered when testing the muscles of the fingers and toes.[7] The muscles of the fingers, thumb, and toes may be tested in either a gravity eliminated or an against gravity position for all grades. In the clinic it is common to observe the muscles of the fingers, thumb, and toes being tested isometrically. Table 1-11 gives a description of the grading for the hand and toes.

• Facial Muscles. Conventional grading is not applied to the results of the tests because it is not always practical or possible to palpate the muscle, apply resistance,

Numeral	Description
	The patient:
5	Maintains the test position against gravity and maximal resistance
4	Maintains the test position against gravity and moderate resistance
4−	Maintains the test position against gravity and less than moderate resistance
3+	Maintains the test position against gravity and minimal resistance
3	Maintains the test position against gravity

Note: If the patient is tested in a gravity eliminated position additional resistance equal to the weight of the limb must be added.

or position the patient. The results of the tests can be descriptive or recorded according to a defined set of parameters as follows: *normal* (N, 5) for completion of the test movement with ease and control; *fair* (F, 3) for performance of test movement with difficulty; *trace* (T, 1) for minimal muscle contraction; and *zero* (0) when no contraction can be elicited.[87]

• **Weight-Bearing Muscles.** To be resisted maximally some muscles of the lower extremity require the resistance of body weight. These muscle tests are described for the gastrocnemius and soleus muscles but weight-bearing tests could also be performed for the quadriceps, gluteus medius and minimus, and quadratus lumborum muscles.

Testing With a Two-Joint or Multijoint Muscle in the Region. When applying resistance to a two-joint

muscle either directly or indirectly, take care to avoid positions of excessive shortening of the two-joint muscle because this may lead to painful cramping of the muscle.[7]

1. To test the strength of a one-joint muscle with a two-joint or multijoint muscle in the region that performs the same action at the joint, the contribution of the two-joint or multijoint muscle to the movement must be reduced or eliminated. This is done by passively placing the two-joint or multijoint muscle in a shortened position at the nontest joint(s) to render it more actively insufficient before testing the one-joint muscle.

   Example: When testing the strength of coracobrachialis to flex and adduct the shoulder, the elbow and forearm are passively flexed and supinated, respectively, to place the biceps brachii muscle in a

Numeral	Description
	The patient is able to actively move through:
5	The full available ROM against maximal resistance, gravity eliminated or against gravity
4	The full available ROM against moderate resistance, gravity eliminated or against gravity
3	The full available ROM, gravity eliminated or against gravity
2	Part of the available ROM, gravity eliminated or against gravity
1	None of the available ROM, but there is a palpable or observable flicker of a muscle contraction, gravity eliminated or against gravity
0	None of the available ROM, and there is no palpable or observable muscle contraction, gravity eliminated or against gravity

shortened position, thus rendering it more actively insufficient and reducing the contribution of the short head of biceps brachii to flex and adduct the shoulder.

2. To test a two-joint or multijoint muscle at one joint, first place the nontest joint(s) in midposition.

   Example: When testing the strength of the hamstrings to flex the knee, the hip is positioned in flexion.

3. To test a muscle at a joint where a two-joint or multijoint muscle is the antagonist, place the two-joint or multijoint muscle on slack at the nontest joint(s). This avoids stretching the two-joint or multijoint muscle and creating a situation of passive insufficiency during the muscle test thereby decreasing the ability of the prime mover to move the joint through full ROM.

   Example: When testing the strength of the iliopsoas to flex the hip, the knee is positioned in flexion to place the hamstring muscles on slack and prevent tightness of hamstrings limiting hip flexion ROM.

Recording. The inability to test a muscle accurately (ie, due to pain or noncompliance of the patient) is indicated on the recording form using a question mark beside the grade,[90] for example, "3?". The question mark will prompt the therapist to retest the muscle at another time if appropriate. An explanation is given for the questions mark under the comments or remarks section of the recording form.

On a recording form every space should include an entry.[6] If the test was not performed, NT (not tested)

should be entered and a line may be drawn from the first such entry to the end of several adjacent entries so the NT does not have to be recorded in every space.[6]

Noncompliance of the patient, deviations from standard testing procedure, and other factors that may influence the results of a muscle test should be noted on the chart. Ensure that an appropriate legend of the muscle testing grading is noted on the chart.

A grade of 3 does not necessarily indicate a functional grade. Grades of 3 or less for the upper extremity, trunk and neck and grades of less than a 4 for the lower extremity should be recorded so that they can be identified quickly on reading the chart as being nonfunctional grades or areas of major concern. These nonfunctional grades may be highlighted by placing the grade in brackets. Fatigue should be closely monitored and recorded to facilitate the application of strength tests to ADL.

See Appendix C for a sample muscle test recording form.

SUMMARY—MANUAL ASSESSMENT OF MUSCLE STRENGTH

The main steps in the manual assessment of muscle strength (conventional method) are outlined in Figures 1-26, 1-27, and 1-28 using the shoulder extensors as an example.

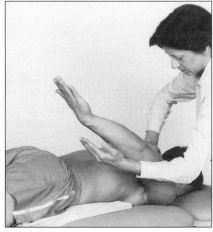

Figure 1-26. Screen test. Palpation of the muscle and observation of the AROM against gravity. If the patient moves through partial ROM the muscle test ends.

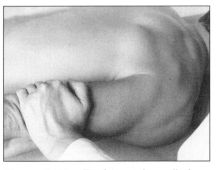

Figure 1-27. Resistance is applied against gravity if the patient is able to move against gravity through the full available PROM in the screen test.

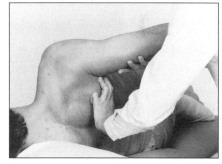

Figure 1-28. Palpation of the muscle and observation of the AROM in a gravity eliminated plane is performed if the patient is unable to move the limb against gravity in the screen test.

▼ FUNCTIONAL APPLICATION OF ASSESSMENT OF JOINT RANGE OF MOTION AND MANUAL MUSCLE TESTING

Evaluation of functional activities, through task analysis and observation of the patient's performance in activities, can guide the therapist in proceeding with a detailed assessment and provide objective and meaningful treatment goals. The therapist may ask the patient about his or her ability to perform activities. It is essential that the therapist observes the patient performing the functional activities.[104] The patient is observed performing functional activities such as dressing, sitting, or walking during the initial assessment.

On completion of the evaluation of ROM and muscle strength the therapist must consider the impact of deficit on the patient's daily life. Knowledge of functional anatomy of the musculoskeletal system is required to integrate the assessment findings into meaningful and practical information. The knowledge of functional anatomy assists the therapist in gaining insight into the effect of joint ROM or strength limitations in the patient's daily life.

REFERENCES

1. Basmajian JV. *Surface Anatomy: An Instructional Manual.* Baltimore: Williams & Wilkins; 1983.
2. Hollis M. *Safer Lifting for Patient Care.* 2nd ed. Oxford, England: Blackwell Scientific Publications; 1985.
3. Kapandji IA. *The Physiology of the Joints.* Vol 1. 5th ed. New York: Churchill Livingstone, 1982.
4. Soames RW, ed. Skeletal system. In: *Gray's Anatomy.* 38th ed. New York: Churchill Livingstone; 1995.
5. Davis BD, McKusick VA, O'Rahilly R (consultants). *Dorland's Pocket Medical Dictionary.* London: WB Saunders; 1968.
6. Duesterhaus Minor MA, Duesterhaus Minor S. *Patient Evaluation Methods for the Health Professional.* Reston, VA: Reston Publishing; 1985.
7. Kendall FP, McCreary EK, Provance PG. *Muscles Testing and Function.* 4th ed. Baltimore: Williams & Wilkins; 1993.
8. Gowitzke BA, Milner M. *Understanding the Scientific Bases of Human Movement.* 2nd ed. Baltimore: Williams & Wilkins; 1980.
9. Lundon K, Hampson D. Acquired ectopic ossification of soft tissues: implications for physical therapy. *Can J Rehabil.* 1997;10:231–246.
10. Cyriax J. *Textbook of Orthopaedic Medicine: vol 1. Diagnosis of Soft Tissue Lesions.* 8th ed. London: Bailliere Tindall; 1982.
11. Norkin CC, White DJ. *Measurement of Joint Motion: A Guide to Goniometry.* 2nd ed. Philadelphia: FA Davis; 1995.
12. Magee DJ. *Orthopedic Physical Assessment.* 3rd ed. Philadelphia: WB Saunders; 1997.
13. Norkin CC, Levangie PK. *Joint Structure & Function: A Comprehensive Analysis.* 2nd ed. Philadelphia: FA Davis; 1992.
14. Woodburne RT. *Essentials to Human Anatomy.* 5th ed. London: Oxford University Press; 1973.
15. Hertling D, Kessler RM. Assessment of musculoskeletal disorders and concepts of management. In: Kessler RM, Hertling D. *Management of Common Musculoskeletal Disorders: Physical Therapy Principles and Methods.* 3rd ed. Philadelphia: Lippincott-Raven Publishers; 1996.
16. Kapandji IA. *The Physiology of the Joints.* Vol 2. 2nd ed. New York: Churchill Livingstone: 1970.
17. Currier DP. *Elements of Research in Physical Therapy* 3rd ed. Baltimore: Williams & Wilkins; 1990.
18. Miller PJ. Assessment of joint motion. In: Rothstein JM, ed. *Measurement in Physical Therapy.* New York: Churchill Livingstone; 1985.
19. Gogia PP, Braatz JH, Rose SJ, Norton BJ. Reliability and validity of goniometric measurements at the knee. *Phys Ther.* 1987;67: 192–195.
20. Enwemeka CS. Radiographic verification of knee goniometry. *Scand J Rehabil Med.* 1986;18:47–49.
21. Fish DR, Wingate L. Sources of goniometric error at the elbow. *Phys Ther.* 1985;65:1666–1670.
22. Gajdosik RL, Bohannon RW. Clinical measurement of range of motion: review of goniometry emphasizing reliability and validity. *Phys Ther.* 1987;67: 1867–1872.
23. Sim J, Arnell P. Measurement validity in physical therapy research. *Phys Ther.* 1993;73:48–56.
24. Youdas JW, Carey JR, Garrett TR. Reliability of measurements of cervical spine range of motion—comparison of three methods. *Phys Ther.* 1991;71:23–29.
25. Low J. The reliability of joint measurement. *Physiotherapy.* 1976;62:227–229.
26. Baldwin J, Cunningham K. Goniometry under attack: a clinical study involving physiotherapists. *Physiother Can.* 1974;26:74–76.
27. Watkins MA, Riddle DL, Lamb RL, Personius WJ. Reliability of goniometric measurements and visual estimates of knee range of motion obtained in a clinical setting. *Phys Ther.* 1991;71:15–22.
28. Bovens AMPM, van Baak MA, Vrencken JGPM, Wijnen JAG, Verstappen FTJ. Variability and reliability of joint measurements. *Am J Sports Med.* 1990;18: 58–63.
29. Pandya S, Florence JM, King WM, Robison JD, Oxnan M, Province MA. Reliability of goniometric measurements in patients with duchenne muscular dystrophy. *Phys Ther.* 1985;65:1339–1342.
30. Elveru RA, Rothstein JM, Lamb RL. Goniometric reliability in a clinical setting: Subtalar and ankle joint measurements. *Phys Ther.* 1988;68:672–677.
31. Boone DC, Azen SP, Lin C-M, Spence C, Baron C, Lee L.

Reliability of goniometric measurements. *Phys Ther.* 1978;58:1355–1360.

32. Dijkstra PU, deBont LGM, van der Weele LTh, Boering G. Joint mobility measurements: reliability of a standardized method. *Journal of Craniomandibular Practice.* 1994;12:52–57.

33. Youdas JW, Bogard CL, Suman VJ. Reliability of goniometric measurements and visual estimates of ankle joint active range of motion obtained in a clinical setting. *Arch Phys Med Rehabil.* 1993;74:1113–1118.

34. Horger MM. The reliability of goniometric measurements of active and passive wrist motions. *Am J Occup Ther.* 1990;44:342–348.

35. Hellebrant FA, Duvall EN, Moore ML. The measurement of joint motion: part III reliability of goniometry. *Phys Ther Rev.* 1949;29:302–307.

36. Rothstein JM, Miller PJ, Roettger RF. Goniometric reliability in a clinical setting: elbow and knee measurements. *Phys Ther.* 1983;63:1611–1615.

37. Riddle DL, Rothstein JM, Lamb RL. Goniometric reliability in a clinical setting: shoulder measurements. *Phys Ther.* 1987;67:668–673.

38. Watkins B, Darrah J, Pain K. Reliability of passive ankle dorsiflexion measurements in children: comparison of universal and biplane goniometers. *Pediatr Phys Ther.* 1995;7:3–8.

39. Stuberg WA, Fuchs RH, Miedaner JA. Reliability of goniometric measurements of children with cerebral palsy. *Develop Med Child Neurol.* 1988;30:657–666.

40. Ashton B, Pickles B, Roll JW. Reliability of goniometric measurements of hip motion in spastic cerebral palsy. *Develop Med Child Neurol.* 1978;20:87–94.

41. Harris SR, Smith LH, Krukowski L. Goniometric reliability for a child with spastic quadriplegia. *J Pediatr Orthop.* 1985;5:348–351.

42. American Academy of Orthopaedic Surgeons. *Joint Motion: Method of Measuring and Recording.* Chicago: Author; 1965.

43. Moore ML. Clinical assessment of joint motion. In: Basmajian JV, ed. *Therapeutic Exercise.* 4th ed. Baltimore: Williams & Wilkins; 1984.

44. Stratford P, Agostino V, Brazeau C, Gowitzke BA. Reliability of joint angle measurement: a discussion of methodology issues. *Physiother Can.* 1984; 36:5–9.

45. Wintz MM. Variations in current manual muscle testing. *Phys Ther Rev.* 1959;39:466–475.

46. Williams M. Manual muscle testing, development and current use. *Phys Ther Rev.* 1956;36:797–805.

47. Rothstein JM. Commentary. *Phys Ther.* 1989;69:61–66. In response to: Bohannon RW. Is the measurement of muscle strength appropriate in patients with brain lesions? A special communication. *Phys Ther.* 1989;69:56–61. (Author's response: 66–67).

48. Fox EL, Mathews DK. *The Physiological Basis of Physical Education and Athletics.* 3rd ed. Philadelphia: Saunders College Publishing; 1981.

49. Knuttgen HG, ed. *Neuromuscular Mechanisms for Therapeutic and Conditioning Exercise.* Baltimore: University Park Press; 1976.

50. Lieber RL, Bodine-Fowler SC. Skeletal muscle mechanics: implications for rehabilitation. *Phys Ther.* 1993;73:25–37.

51. Kisner C, Colby LA. *Therapeutic Exercise: Foundations and Techniques.* 3rd ed. Philadelphia: FA Davis; 1996.

52. Hollis M. *Practical Exercise Therapy.* 3rd ed. Oxford, England: Blackwell Scientific Publications; 1989.

53. Kroemer KHE. Human strength: terminology, measurement, and interpretation of data. *Hum Factors.* 1970;12:297–313.

54. Smith LK, Weiss EL, Lehmkuhl LD. *Brunnstrom's Clinical Kinesiology.* 5th ed. Philadelphia: FA Davis; 1996.

55. Brooks GA, Fahey TD. *Exercise Physiology: Human Bioenergetics and Its Application.* New York: John Wiley & Sons; 1984.

56. Laubach LL. Comparative muscular strength of men and women: a review of the literature. *Aviat Space Environ Med.* 1976;47:534–542.

57. Williams M, Stutzman L. Strength variation through the range of joint motion. *Phys Ther Rev.* 1959;39: 145–152.

58. Kulig K, Andrews JG, Hay JG. Human strength curves. *Exerc Sport Sci Rev.* 1984;12:417–466.

59. Williams M, Tomberlin JA, Robertson KJ. Muscle force curves of school children. *J Am Phys Ther Assoc.* 1965;45:539–549.

60. Wyse JP, Mercer TH, Gleeson NP. Time-of-day dependence of isokinetic leg strength and associated interday variability. *Br J Sports Med.* 1994;28:167–170.

61. Gauthier A, Davenne D, Martin A, Cometti G, Van Hoecke J. Diurnal rhythm of the muscular performance of elbow flexors during isometric contractions. *Chronobiol Int.* 1996;13:135–146.

62. Holewijn M, Heus R. Effects of temperature on electromyogram and muscle function. *Eur J Appl Physiol.* 1992;65:541–545.

63. Kaltenborn FM. *Mobilization of the Extremity Joints.* 3rd ed. Oslo: Olaf Norlis Bokhandel; 1985.

64. MacConaill MA, Basmajian JV. *Muscles and Movements: A Basis for Human Kinesiology.* 2nd ed. New York: Robert E. Krieger; 1977.

65. O'Connor P, Sforzo GA, Frye P. Effect of breathing instruction on blood pressure responses during isometric exercise. *Phys Ther.* 1989;69:55–59.

66. Bohannon RW. Manual muscle test scores and dynamometer test scores of knee extension strength. *Arch Phys Med Rehabil.* 1986;67:390–392.

67. Schwartz S, Cohen ME, Herbison GJ, Shah A. Relationship between two measures of upper extremity strength: manual muscle test compared to hand-held myometry. *Arch Phys Med Rehabil.* 1992;73:1063–1068.

68. Aitkens S, Lord J, Bernauer E, Fowler WM, Lieberman JS, Berck P. Relationship of manual muscle testing to objective strength measurements. *Muscle Nerve.* 1989;12: 173–177.

69. Lamb RL. Manual muscle testing. In: Rothstein JM, ed. *Measurement in Physical Therapy.* New York: Churchill Livingstone; 1985.

70. Silver M, McElroy A, Morrow L, Heafner BK. Further standardization of manual muscle test for clinical study: applied in chronic renal disease. *Phys Ther.* 1970;50: 1456–1464.

71. Lilienfeld AM, Jacobs M, Willis M. A study of the reproducibility of muscle testing and certain other aspects of muscle scoring. *Phys Ther Rev.* 1954;34: 279–289.

72. Iddings DM, Smith LK, Spencer WA. Muscle testing: part 2. Reliability in clinical use. *Phys Ther Rev.* 1961;41:249–256.

73. Frese E, Brown M, Norton BJ. Clinical reliability of manual muscle testing. Middle trapezius and gluteus medius muscles. *Phys Ther.* 1987;67:1072–1076.

74. Florence JM, Pandya S, King WM, et al. Clinical trials in duchenne dystrophy: standardization and reliability of evaluation procedures. *Phys Ther.* 1984;64: 41–45.

75. Beasley WC. Influence of method on estimates of normal knee extensor force among normal and post-polio children. *Phys Ther Rev.* 1956;36:21–41.

76. Beasley WC. Quantitative muscle testing: principles and applications to research and clinical services. *Arch Phys Med Rehabil.* 1961;42:398–425.

77. Hayes KW, Falconer J. Reliability of hand-held dynamometry and its relationship with manual muscle testing in patients with osteoarthritis in the knee. *J Orthop Sports Phys Ther.* 1992;16:145–149.

78. Bohannon RW. Nature, implications, and measurement of limb muscle strength in patients with orthopedic or neurological disorders. *Physical Therapy Practice.* 1992;2:22–31.

79. Dvir Z. Grade 4 in manual muscle testing: the problem with submaximal strength assessment. *Clin Rehabil.* 1997;11:36–41.

80. Griffin JW, McClure MH, Bertorini TE. Sequential isokinetic and manual muscle testing in patients with neuromuscular disease. *Phys Ther.* 1986;66:32–35.

81. Rabin SI, Post M. A comparative study of clinical muscle testing and Cybex evaluation after shoulder operations. *Clin Orthop Rel Res.* 1990;258:147–156.

82. Wadsworth CT, Krishnan R, Sear M, Harrold J, Nielsen DH. Intrarater reliability of manual muscle testing and hand-held dynametric muscle testing. *Phys Ther.* 1987;67:1342–1347.

83. Donaldson R. The importance of position in the examination of muscles and in exercise. *Physiother Rev.* 1927;7:22–24.

84. Chaffin DB. Ergonomics guide for the assessment of human static strength. *Am Ind Hyg Assoc J.* 1975;36:505–511.

85. Brown T, Galea V, McComas A. Loss of twitch torque following muscle compression. *Muscle Nerve* 1997;20:167–171.

86. Wynn Parry CB. Vicarious motions (trick movements). In: Basmajian JV, ed. *Therapeutic Exercise.* 4th ed. Baltimore: Williams & Wilkins; 1984.

87. Daniels L, Worthingham C. *Muscle Testing: Techniques of Manual Examination.* 5th ed. Philadelphia: WB Saunders; 1986.

88. Wright WG. Muscle training in the treatment of infantile paralysis. *Boston Med Surg J.* 1912;167:567–574.

89. Brunnstrom S. Muscle group testing. *Physiother Rev.* 1941;21:3–22.

90. Smith LK, Iddings DM, Spencer WA, Harrington PR. Muscle testing: Part 1. Description of a numerical index for clinical research. *Phys Ther Rev.* 1961;41:99–105.

91. Hines TF. Manual muscle examination. In: Licht S, ed. *Therapeutic Exercise.* 2ne ed. Baltimore: Waverly Press; 1965.

92. Kendall HO, Kendall FP. *Muscles Testing and Function.* Baltimore: Williams & Wilkins; 1949.

93. Kendall FP, McCreary EK. *Muscles Testing and Function.* 3rd ed. Baltimore: Williams & Wilkins; 1983.

94. Christ CB, Boileau RA, Slaughter MH, Stillman RJ, Cameron J. The effect of test protocol instructions on measurement of muscle function in adult men. *J Orthop Sports Phys Ther.* 1993;18:502–510.

95. Johansson CA, Kent BE, Shepard KF. Relationship between verbal command volume and magnitude of muscle contraction. *Phys Ther.* 1983;63:1260–1265.

96. McNair PJ, Depledge J, Brettkelly M, Stanley SN. Verbal encouragement: effects on maximum effort voluntary muscle action. *Br J Sports Med.* 1996;30:243–245.

97. Hislop HJ, Montgomery J. *Daniels and Worthingham's Muscle Testing: Techniques of Manual Examination.* 6th ed. Philadelphia: WB Saunders; 1995.

98. Nicholas JA, Sapega A, Kraus H, Webb JN. Factors influencing manual muscle tests in physical therapy: the magnitude and duration of the force applied. *J Bone Joint Surg [Am].* 1978;60:186–190.

99. Wright WG. Muscle training in the treatment of infantile paralysis. *Boston Med Surg J.* 1912;167:567–574.

100. Lamb DW. A review of manual therapy for spinal pain. In: Boyling JD, Palastanga N. *Grieve's Modern Manual Therapy: The Vertebral Column.* 2nd ed. London: Churchill Livingstone; 1994.

101. Bohannon RW. Make tests and break tests of elbow flexor muscle strength. *Phys Ther.* 1988;68:193–194.

102. Velsher E. Factors affecting higher force readings: a survey of the literature on isometric exercise. *Physiother Can.* 1977;29:141–147.

103. Wilson GJ, Murphy AJ. The use of isometric tests of muscular function in athletic Assessment. *Sports Med.* 1996;22:19–37.

104. McGarvey SR, Morrey BF, Askew LJ, Kai-Nan A. Reliability of isometric strength testing: temporal factors and strength variation. *Clin Orthop.* 1984;185:301–305.

105. Smith LK. Functional tests. *Phys Ther Rev.* 1954;34:19–21.

CHAPTER 2

HEAD, NECK, AND TRUNK

▼ SURFACE ANATOMY: HEAD AND NECK (Figs. 2-1 and 2-2)

Structure	Location
1. Suprasternal (jugular) notch	The rounded depression at the superior border of the sternum and between the medial ends of each clavicle.
2. Thyroid cartilage	The most prominent laryngeal cartilage located at the level of the fourth and fifth cervical vertebrae; subcutaneous projection (Adam's apple).
3. Hyoid bone	A submandibular U-shaped bone located above the thyroid cartilage at the level of the third cervical vertebra; the body is felt in the midline below the chin at the angle formed between the floor of the mouth and the front of the neck.
4. Angle of the mandible	The angle of the jaw located medially and distally to the earlobe.
5. Angle of the mouth	The lateral angle formed by the upper and lower lips.
6. Nasolabial fold	The fold of skin extending from the nose to the angle of the mouth.
7. Temporomandibular joint	The joint may be palpated anterior to the tragus of the external ear during opening and closing of the mouth.
8. Mastoid process	Bony prominence of the skull located behind the ear.
9. Acromion process	Lateral aspect of the spine of the scapula at the tip or point of the shoulder.

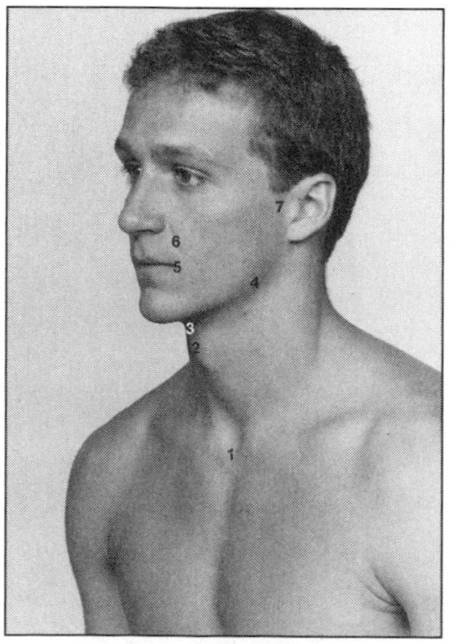

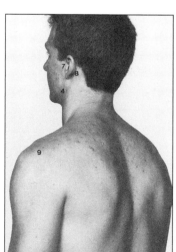

Figure 2-1. Anterolateral aspect of the head and neck.

Figure 2-2. Posterolateral aspect of the head and neck.

▼ ASSESSMENT PROCESS: THE FACE AND NECK

1. The therapist observes:
   a. Head and neck posture, shoulder levels, atrophy, facial expression, facial symmetry, and crossbite or overbite of teeth
   b. Active movements at the shoulders
2. The therapist assesses the *active range of motion* (AROM) of the cervical spine and temporomandibular joint:
   a. Estimating joint ranges of motion
   b. Establishing the presence or absence of pain
   End feels and capsular patterns for the cervical spine, assessed using passive movements, are beyond the scope of this text.
3. The therapist measures the functional range of motion (ROM) of the temporomandibular joint.
4. The therapist measures AROM of the cervical spine through goniometry and tape measure.
5. The therapist assesses muscle strength through manual muscle testing.

TABLE

2-1

▼ **JOINT STRUCTURE: JAW MOVEMENTS**

	Opening of the Mouth (Depression of the Mandible)	Closing of the Mouth (Occlusion)	Protrusion	Retrusion	Lateral Deviation
Articulation[1,2]	Temporomandibular (TM)	TM	TM	TM	TM
Plane	Sagittal	Sagittal	Horizontal	Horizontal	Horizontal
Axis	Frontal	Frontal			
Normal limiting factors[3]	Tension in the sphenomandibular and stylomandibular ligaments	Occlusion or contact of the teeth			
Capsular pattern[4,5]	Limitation of mouth opening				

▼ RANGE OF MOTION ASSESSMENT AND MEASUREMENT

The articulations and joint axes of the temporomandibular joint and cervical spine are illustrated in Figures 2-3, 2-4, and 2-5 and the joint structure is described in Tables 2-1 and 2-2.

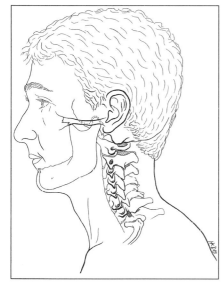

Figure 2-3. Temporomandibular joint and cervical spine articulations.

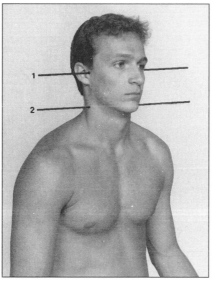

Figure 2-4. (*1*) Temporomandibular joint axis: elevation–depression. (*2*) Cervical spine axis; flexion-extension.

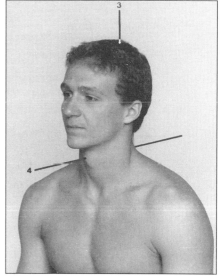

Figure 2-5. Cervical spine axes: (*3*) rotation. (*4*) lateral flexion.

TABLE 2-2

▼ JOINT STRUCTURE: CERVICAL SPINE MOVEMENTS

	Flexion Extension		Lateral Flexion Rotation	
Articulation[1,2]	Atlanto-occipital, atlantoaxial, intervertebral	Atlanto-occipital, atlantoaxial, intervertebral	Atlanto-occipital, intervertebral (with rotation)	Atlanto-occipital,[2] atlantoaxial, intrvertebral (with lateral flexion)[2]
Plane	Sagittal	Sagittal	Frontal	Transverse
Axis	Frontal	Frontal	Sagittal	Vertical
Normal limiting factors[6,7]	Tension in the tectorial membrane, posterior antlantoaxial ligament, posterior longitudinal ligament, ligamentum nuchae, ligamentum flavum, posterior neck muscles; posterior fibers of annulus	Tension in the anterior longitudinal ligament and anterior atlantoaxial ligament; anterior neck muscles; anterior fibers of annulus; bony contact between the spinous processes	Tension in the alar ligament limits lateral flexion to the contralateral side; lateral fibers of annulus; facet joints	Tension in the alar ligament limits rotation to the ipsilateral side; tension in the annulus fibrosis
Normal active range of motion[8]	0–45°	0–45°	0–45°	0–60°

TEMPOROMANDIBULAR JOINT MOVEMENTS (SEE TABLE 2-1)

• **Start Position.** The patient assumes a resting position of the temporomandibular joint. In this position there is minimal muscle action potential in the mandibular muscles; there is no occlused contact between the maxillary and mandibular teeth.[3] The head and neck are in the anatomical position and remain in this position throughout the test movements. From the rest position, the patient is asked to occlude the teeth and depress, protrude, and laterally deviate the jaw to both sides.

• **Occlusion of the Teeth.** The patient closes the jaw to a position where the teeth are fully occluded (Fig. 2-6).

• **Depression of the Mandible.** The patient is asked to open the mouth (Fig. 2-7). On active opening of the mouth the therapist observes for deviation of the mandible from the midline. In normal mouth opening, the mandible moves in a straight line. Deviation of the mandible to the left in the form of a "C"-type curve indicates hypomobility of the temporomandibular joint situated on the convex/closed side of the "C" curve, or hypermobility of the joint on the concave/open side of the curve.[4] Deviation in the shape of an "S"-type curve, may indicate a muscular imbalance or displacement of the condyle.[4] Functional range of movement is determined by placing two or three flexed fingers[4] between the upper and lower central incisor teeth. The fingers represent a distance of 35 to 40 mm.[9] Using a ruler and the upper and lower central incisor teeth for reference, a measure of opening can be obtained[10] for recording change.

• **Protrusion of the Mandible.** The patient protrudes (forward gliding) the lower jaw (Fig. 2-8). The lower jaw should protrude far enough for the patient to place the lower teeth beyond the upper teeth.[9] A ruler measurement may be obtained by measuring the distance between the upper and lower central incisor teeth.[10] Normal protrusion from resting position is 3 to 7 mm.[11]

• **Lateral Deviation of the Mandible.** The patient deviates the lower jaw to one side and then the other (Fig. 2-9). A measure[4] can be obtained for recording purposes by measuring the distance between two selected points that are level, one on the upper teeth and one on the lower teeth, such as the space between the central incisors. The normal ROM is 5 to 12 mm.[11]

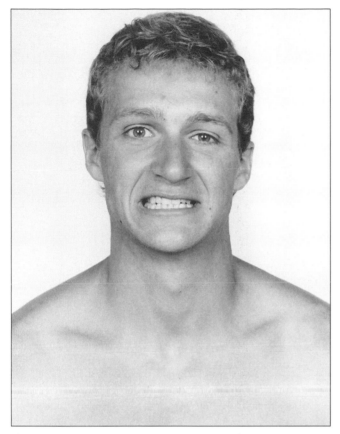

Figure 2-6.   Occlusion of the teeth.

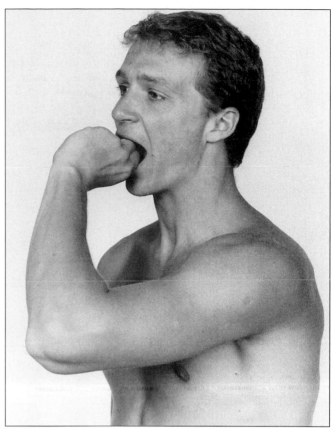

Figure 2-7.   Opening of the mouth (depression of the mandible).

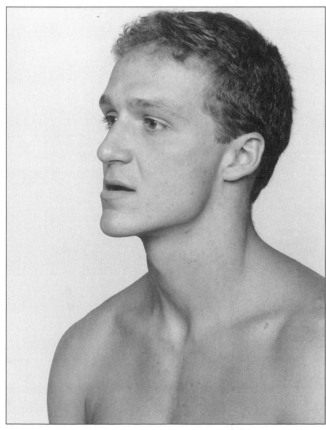

Figure 2-8.   Protrusion of the mandible.

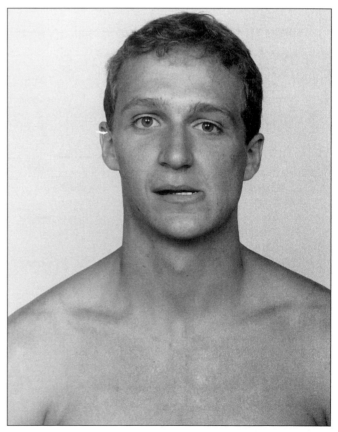

Figure 2-9.   Lateral deviation of the mandible.

NECK MOVEMENTS
(SEE TABLE 2-2)

Note: **Tests of head and neck movement are contraindicated in some instances. Contraindications include pathology that may result in spinal instability and pathology of the vertebral artery. In the absence of contraindications, cervical spine AROM is assessed using a tape measure.** The OB goniometer, presented in Appendix A, is another useful tool for the assessment of neck AROM.

Measurement: Tape Measure. A linear measure is obtained through the use of a tape measure for cervical spine movements. The start position and stabilization are the same for each measurement.

• **Start Position.** The patient is sitting on a chair with a back support. The head and neck are in the anatomical position (Fig. 2-10).

• **Stabilization.** The back of the chair provides support for the thoracic and lumbar spine. Stabilization by the therapist is not practical in this measurement process. The patient is instructed and shown how to stabilize the shoulder girdle to prevent thoracic and lumbar spine movements.

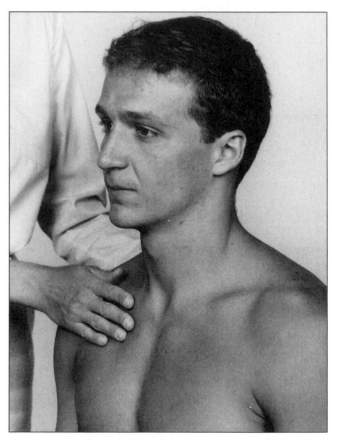

Figure 2-10.   Start position for all movements of the neck.

NECK FLEXION—EXTENSION

• **End Position.** The patient flexes the neck to the limit of the motion. The patient extends the neck to the limit of motion.

• **Measurement.** *Flexion.* A tape measure is used to measure the distance between the tip of the chin and the suprasternal notch. Full ROM is illustrated in Figure 2-11. The patient is able to touch his chin to his chest. Limited range is illustrated in Figure 2-12. The linear measure reflects decreased ROM.

Extension. The same reference points are used. A measure is taken in the anatomical position and in the extended position (Fig. 2-13). The difference between these measures reflects the range of neck extension.

• **Substitution/Trick Movement.** Mouth opening.

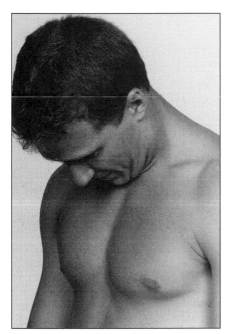

Figure 2-11. Neck flexion: full AROM.

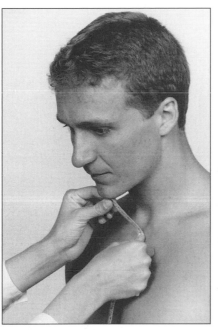

Figure 2-12. Neck flexion: limited AROM.

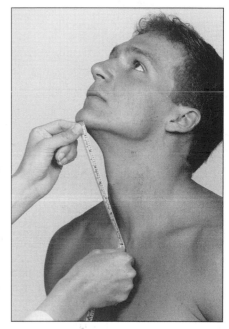

Figure 2-13. Neck extension: full AROM.

NECK LATERAL FLEXION

• **End Position.** The patient flexes the neck to the side (without rotation) to the limit of motion (Fig. 2-14).

• **Measurement.** A tape measure is used to measure the distance between the mastoid process of the skull and the acromion process. A measure is taken in the anatomical position and at the limit of motion of lateral flexion.

• **Substitution/Trick Movement.** Elevation of the shoulder girdle to approximate the ear.

NECK ROTATION

• **End Position.** The patient rotates the head (without flexing or extending) to the limit of motion (Fig. 2-15).

• **Measurement.** A tape measure is used to measure the distance between the tip of the chin and the acromion process. A measure is taken in the anatomical position and at the limit of motion of rotation.

• **Substitution/Trick Motion.** Elevation and/or protrusion of the shoulder girdle to approximate the chin.

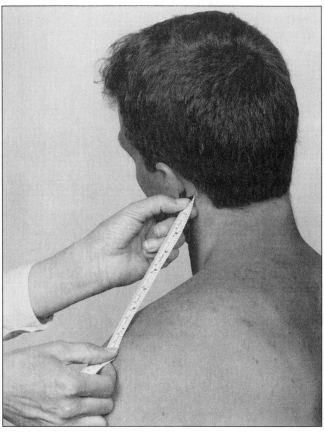

Figure 2-14. Neck lateral flexion.

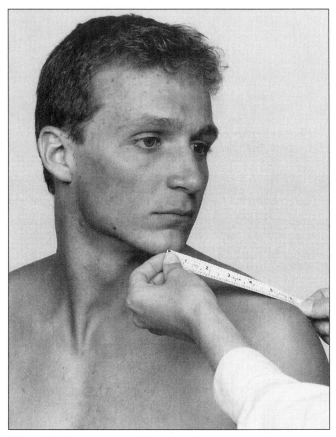

Figure 2-15. Neck rotation.

TABLE 2-3 ▼ MUSCLE ACTIONS, ATTACHMENTS, AND NERVE SUPPLY: THE FACE AND EYES[2]

Muscle	Primary Muscle Action	Muscle Origin	Muscle Insertion	Cranial Nerve
Levator palpebrae superioris	Elevation of upper eyelid	Inferior surface of the small wing of the sphenoid, superior and anterior to the optic canal	Skin of the upper eyelid; anterior surface of the superior tarsus; the superior conjunctival fornix; tubercle on the zygomatic bone; superior aspect of the orbital septum	III
Rectus superior	Elevates the abducted eye	Common annular tendon (fibrous ring surrounding the superior, medial and inferior margins of the optic canal)	The sclera superiorly, posterior to the margin of the cornea	III
Rectus inferior	Depresses the abducted eye	Common annular tendon	The sclera inferiorly, posterior to the margin of the cornea	III
Obliquus superior	Depresses the adducted eye	Body of the sphenoid superomedial to the optic canal; the tendinous attachment of the rectus superior	The tendon passes through the trochlea (a fibrocartilaginous loop attached to the fossa of the frontal bone) and then passes posteriorly, laterally and downward to insert into the sclera posterior to the equator on the superolateral aspect of the eyeball	IV
Obliquus inferior	Elevates the adducted eye	Orbital surface of the maxilla lateral to the nasolacrimal groove	Lateral part of the sclera, posterior to the equator of the eyeball	III
Rectus lateralis	Abducts the eye	Common annular tendon; the orbital surface of the greater wing of the sphenoid bone	The sclera laterally, posterior to the margin of the cornea	VI
Rectus medialis	Adducts the eye	Common annular tendon	The sclera medially, posterior to the margin of the cornea	III
Temporalis	Elevation of the mandible; side-to-side grinding movements of the mandible	Temporal fossa; deep surface of the temporal fascia	The coronoid process of the mandible; anterior border of the ramus of the mandible nearly as far as the last molar	V

TABLE
6-3

▼ MUSCLE ACTIONS, ATTACHMENTS, AND NERVE SUPPLY: THE FACE AND EYES[2] *Continued*

Muscle	Primary Muscle Action	Muscle Origin	Muscle Insertion	Cranial Nerve
Masseter	Elevation of the mandible; small effect in side-to-side movements, protraction, and retraction of the mandible	a. Superficial layer: maxillary process of the zygomatic bone; anterior two thirds of the zygomatic arch b. Middle layer: medial aspect of the anterior two thirds of the zygomatic arch; lower border of the posterior third of the mandibular ramus c. Deep layer: deep surface of the zygomatic arch	a. Superficial layer: angle and inferior half of the lateral surface of the mandibular ramus b. Middle layer: central part of the mandibular ramus c. Deep layer: upper part of the ramus of the mandible; the coronoid process of the mandible	V
Medial pterygoid	Elevation of the mandible; protrusion of the mandible (with the lateral pterygoid); side-to-side movements of the jaw	Medial aspect of the lateral pterygoid plate; pyramidal process of the palatine bone; tuberosity of the maxilla	Posteroinferior part of the medial surfaces of the ramus and angle of the mandible	V
Lateral pterygoid	Protrusion of the mandible (with the medial pterygoid); opening of the mouth; control of the posterior movement of the articular disc of the temporomandibular joint and condyle of the mandible during mouth closing; side-to-side movements of the mandible	a. Upper head: inferior part and lateral surface of the great wing of the sphenoid bone b. Lower head: the lateral surface of the lateral pterygoid plate	Depression on the anterior aspect of the neck of the mandible; articular capsule and disc of the temporomandibular articulation	V

Suprahyoid Muscles (diagastric, stylohyoid, mylohyoid, geniohyoid)

Muscle	Primary Muscle Action	Muscle Origin	Muscle Insertion	Cranial Nerve
Digastric	Depression of the mandible; elevation of the hyoid bone (swallowing, chewing)	Posterior belly: mastoid process of the temporal bone Anterior belly: diagastric fossa on the base of the mandible near the midline	The course of the muscle changes direction as it passes through a fibrous loop attached to the hyoid bone	V, VII
Stylohyoid	Elevation and retraction of the hyoid bone (swallowing)	Posterior aspect of the styloid process of the temporal bone	The body of the hyoid bone as its junction with the greater cornu	VII

TABLE
2-3

▼ **MUSCLE ACTIONS, ATTACHMENTS, AND NERVE SUPPLY: THE FACE AND EYES[2]** *Continued*

Muscle	Primary Muscle Action	Muscle Origin	Muscle Insertion	Cranial Nerve
Mylohoid	Elevation of the floor of the mouth (swallowing); elevation of the hyoid bone; depression of the mandible	The entire mylohyoid line of the mandible	Body of the hyoid bone; median fibrous raphe from the symphysis menti of the mandible to the hyoid bone	V
Geniohyoid	Elevation and protraction of the hyoid bone; depression of the mandible	Inferior mental spine on the posterior aspect of the symphysis menti	Anterior aspect of the body of the hyoid bone	XII
Epicranius occipitofrontalis	Elevation of the eyebrows and skin over the root of the nose, resulting in transverse wrinkling of the forehead	Frontal part: epicranial aponeurosis anterior to the coronal suture	Fibers are continuous with procerus, corrugator supercilii and orbicularis oculi; the skin of the eyebrows and the root of the nose	VII
Corrugator supercilii	Draws the eyebrows together, resulting in vertical wrinkles on the supranasal strip of the forehead	Medial end of the superciliary arch	The skin above the supraorbital margin	VII
Procerus	Draws the medial angle of the eyebrow inferiorly to wrinkle the skin transversely over the bridge of nose	Fascia covering the inferior portion of the nasal bone; superior portion of the lateral nasal cartilage	Skin over the inferior aspect of the forehead between the eyebrows	VII
Orbicularis oculi	a. Orbital part: closes the eyelids tightly drawing the skin of forehead, temple and cheek medially towards the nose b. Palpebral part: closes the eyelids gently	a. Orbital part: nasal part of the frontal bone; frontal process of the maxilla; medial palpebral ligament b. Palpebral part: the medial palpebral ligament and bone immediately above and below the ligament c. Lacrimal part: the lacrimal fascia; the upper part of the crest and adjacent part of the lacrimal bone	The fibers sweep around the circumference of the orbit; skin and subcutaneous tissues of the eyebrow; tarsi of the eyelids; the lateral palpebral raphe	VII
Nasalis				
1. Alar portion	Widens the nasal opening	Maxilla superior to the lateral incisor tooth	Alar cartilage of the nose	VII
2. Transverse portion	Narrows the nasal opening	Maxilla lateral to the nasal notch	By an aponeurosis that merges on the bridge of the nose with the muscle of the contralateral side; the aponeurosis of the procerus muscle	VII

TABLE 2-3

▼ MUSCLE ACTIONS, ATTACHMENTS, AND NERVE SUPPLY: THE FACE AND EYES[2] Continued

Muscle	Primary Muscle Action	Muscle Origin	Muscle Insertion	Cranial Nerve
Depressor septi	Widens the nasal opening	Maxilla superior to the central incisor tooth	The nasal septum	VII
Orbicularis oris	Closure of the lips; protrusion of the lips	The modiolus at the lateralangle of the mouth; several strata of muscle fibers of other facial muscles that insert into the lips, principally buccinator	The majority of fibers, into the deep surface of the skin and mucous membrane	VII
Buccinator	Compression of the cheeks against the teeth	The alveolar processes of the mandible and maxilla, opposite the three molar teeth; the anterior border of the pterygomandibular raphe	The skin and mucosa of the lips blending with orbicularis oris; the modiolus	VII
Levator anguli oris	Elevation of the angle of the mouth; produces the nasolabial furrow	Canine fossa of the maxilla just inferior to the infraorbital foramen	The modiolus at the lateral angle of the mouth blends with orbicularis oris, depressor anguli oris; the dermal floor of the lower part of the nasolabial furrow	VII
Risorius	Retraction of the angle of the mouth	The parotid fascia over the masseter; parotid fascia; zygomatic arch; fascia enclosing pars modiolaris of platysma; fascia over mastoid process	The modiolus at the lateral angle of the mouth	VII
Zygomaticus major	Draws the angle of the mouth superiorly and laterally	Zygomatic bone anterior to the zygomaticotemporal suture	The modiolus at the lateral angle of the mouth blending with levator anguli oris, and orbicularis oris	VII
Platysma	Depression of the corner of the mouth and lower lip; depression of the jaw; tenses skin over the neck	The fascia covering the superior portion of the pectoralis major and deltoid muscles	Inferior border of the mandible; the skin and subcutaneous tissues of the inferior aspect of the face and corner of the mouth into the modiolus; blends with the contralateral platysma medially; lateral half of the lower lip	VII
Depressor anguli oris	Depression of the angle of the mouth	Oblique line of the mandible	The modiolus at the lateral angle of the mouth	VII

TABLE 2-3

▼ MUSCLE ACTIONS, ATTACHMENTS, AND NERVE SUPPLY: THE FACE AND EYES[2] *Continued*

Muscle	Primary Muscle Action	Muscle Origin	Muscle Insertion	Cranial Nerve
Depressor labii inferioris	Depression and lateral movement of the lower lip	Oblique line of the mandible, between the mental foramen and the symphysis menti	Skin of the lower lip blending with the contralateral depressor labii inferioris and orbicularis oris	VII
Levator labii superioris	Elevation and eversion of the upper lip	Inferior margin of the orbital opening immediately superior to the infraorbital foramen, from the maxilla and zygomatic bones	The muscular substance of the lateral half of the upper lip	VII
Zygomaticus minor	Elevation of the upper lip	Lateral aspect of the zygomatic bone immediately posterior to the zygomaticomaxillary suture	The muscular substance of the lateral aspect of the upper lip	VII
Levator labii superioris alaeque-nasi	Elevation of the upper lip; dilation of the nostril	Superior aspect of the frontal process of the maxilla	Ala of the nose; skin and muscular substance on the lateral aspect of the upper lip	VII
Mentalis	Elevation and protrusion of the lower lip	Incisive fossa of the mandible	Skin of the chin	VII
Genioglossus	Tongue protrusion; depression of the middle region of the tongue	Upper genial tubercle on the inner surface of the symphysis of the mandible	Under surface of the tongue from the root to the apex of the tongue; via an aponeurosis to the superior aspect of the anterior surface of the hyoid bone	XII

The muscles of the face and eyes (Figs. 2-16 through 2-19) are innervated by the cranial nerves (CN). The motor functions of CN III, IV, V, VI, VII, and XII are tested as a component part of a neurological examination. The objectives of testing are to determine the presence or absence of dysfunction and the functional implications of weakness or paralysis to the patient. The muscles are tested in groups according to their CN supply and common function.

Conventional grading is not applied to the results of the tests as it is not always practical or possible to palpate the muscle, apply resistance, or position the patient. The results of the tests can be descriptive or recorded according to a defined set of parameters as follows: normal (N, 5) for completion of the test movement with ease and control, fair (F, 3) for performance of test movement with difficulty, trace (T, 1) for minimal muscle contraction, and zero (0) when no contraction can be elicited.[7] Observation of asymmetrical movement is documented.[12]

A description of the test for the infrahyoid muscles is included with the facial muscles due to the functional significance of these muscles in mastication and swallowing. Swallowing is a complex process that involves the participation of the muscles of the jaw, tongue, lips, soft palate, pharynx, larynx, and suprahyoid and infrahyoid muscle groups. Weakness or paralysis in any of these muscles can affect the ability of the patient to move food from the tongue to the pharynx and esophagus. Head control is also necessary for swallowing. When testing the facial, submandibular, and neck muscles, the therapist should routinely ask the patient if difficulty is experienced in swallowing or observe the patient as liquid or a bolus of food is swallowed.

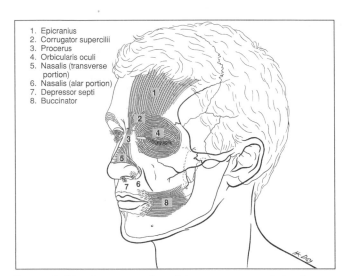

1. Epicranius
2. Corrugator supercilii
3. Procerus
4. Orbicularis oculi
5. Nasalis (transverse portion)
6. Nasalis (alar portion)
7. Depressor septi
8. Buccinator

Figure 2-16.   Deep muscles of the eye, nose, and cheek.

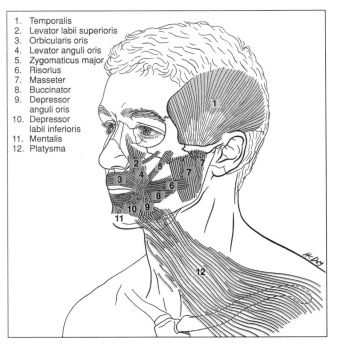

1. Temporalis
2. Levator labii superioris
3. Orbicularis oris
4. Levator anguli oris
5. Zygomaticus major
6. Risorius
7. Masseter
8. Buccinator
9. Depressor anguli oris
10. Depressor labii inferioris
11. Mentalis
12. Platysma

Figure 2-18.   Muscles of the mouth, temporomandibular region, and platysma.

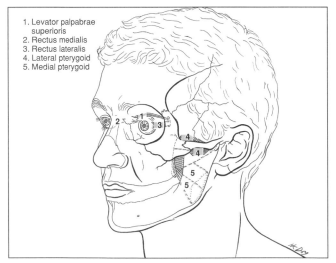

1. Levator palpabrae superioris
2. Rectus medialis
3. Rectus lateralis
4. Lateral pterygoid
5. Medial pterygoid

Figure 2-17.   Muscles of the eye region and temporomandibular region.

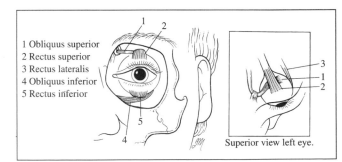

1 Obliquus superior
2 Rectus superior
3 Rectus lateralis
4 Obliquus inferior
5 Rectus inferior

Superior view left eye.

Figure 2-19.   Muscles controlling eye movements.

OCULOMOTOR, TROCHLEAR, AND ABDUCENS NERVES (CN III, IV, AND VI)

Motor Function. Motor functions are opening of the eyelid (levator palpebrae superioris) (see Fig. 2-17) and control of eye movements (the six extraocular muscles) (see Figs. 2-17 and 2-19).

Component Movements Tested. Component movements are elevation of the upper eyelids and elevation, abduction, depression, and adduction of the eyeballs.

ELEVATION OF THE UPPER EYELID (LEVATOR PALPEBRAE SUPERIORIS)

Test. The patient elevates or raises the upper eyelid (Fig. 2-20). The clinical term used to describe the inability to perform this movement is ptosis.

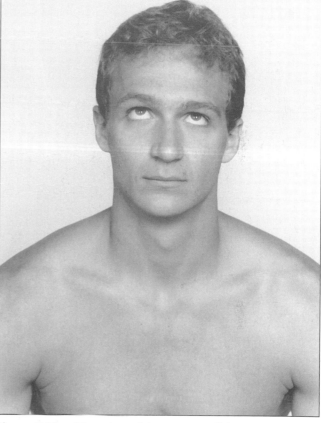

Figure 2-20. Elevation of the upper eyelid.

MOVEMENTS OF THE EYEBALL (RECTUS SUPERIOR, RECTUS INFERIOR, OBLIQUUS SUPERIOR, OBLIQUUS INFERIOR, RECTUS LATERALIS, RECTUS MEDIALIS)

Each extraocular muscle can be tested by examining the muscle in its position of greatest efficiency. This position is when the action of the muscle is at a right angle to the axis around which it is moving the eyeball.[13] The start position is with the patient looking straight ahead. The patient is asked to look in various directions. The presence of diplopia (double vision) should be determined in conjunction with individual muscle tests.[13–15] All test movements described pertain to the *right eye* of the patient (Figs. 2-21 through 2-26). Simultaneous observation of specific movements of both eyes combines muscle tests and may be preferred. The muscle combinations are:

1. Right rectus superior and left obliquus inferior (see Fig. 2-21)
2. Left obliquus superior and right rectus inferior (see Fig. 2-22)
3. Right obliquus superior and left rectus inferior (see Fig. 2-23)
4. Left rectus superior and right obliquus inferior (see Fig. 2-24)
5. Left rectus medialis and right rectus lateralis (see Fig. 2-25)
6. Right rectus medialis and left rectus lateralis (see Fig. 2-26)

Observe whether the movement is normal (ie, smooth through the full ROM) or abnormal.[7]

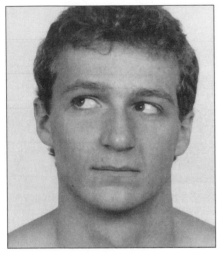

Figure 2-21.   Rectus superior is tested by asking the patient to look upward and outward. Observe for limitation in elevation.

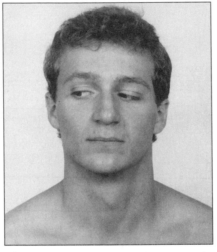

Figure 2-22.   Rectus inferior is tested by asking the patient to look down and out. Observe for limitation in depression.

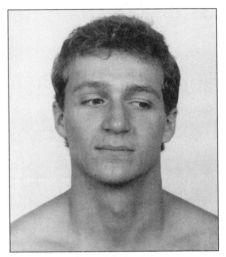

Figure 2-23.   Obliquus superior is tested by asking the patient to look downward and inward. Observe for limitation in depression.

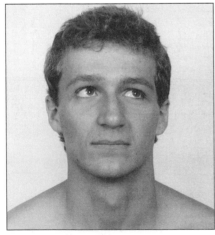

Figure 2-24.   Obliquus inferior is tested by asking the patient to look upward and inward. Observe for limitation in elevation.

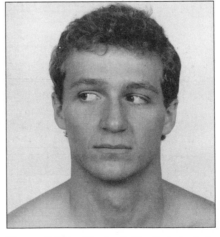

Figure 2-25.   Rectus lateralis is tested by asking the patient to look outward (abduction). Observe the limitation in abduction.

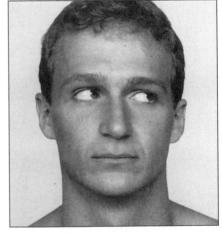

Figure 2-26.   Rectus medialis is tested by asking the patient to look inward (adduction). Observe for limitation in adduction.

TRIGEMINAL NERVE (CN V)

Motor Function. Motor function is mastication.

Component Movements Tested. Component movements are elevation, depression, protrusion, and retrusion of the mandible.

ELEVATION AND RETRUSION OF THE MANDIBLE (TEMPORALIS, MASSETER, MEDIAL PTERYGOID, LATERAL PTERYGOID [SUPERIOR HEAD])

Test. The patient closes the jaw and firmly clenches the teeth (Fig. 2-27). The force of contraction and muscle bulk of temporalis and masseter may be determined by palpation. Temporalis may be palpated over the temporal bone. Masseter may be palpated over the angle of the mandible.

DEPRESSION OF THE MANDIBLE (LATERAL PTERYGOID, SUPRAHYOIDS [MYLOHYOID, DIGASTRIC, STYLOHYOID, GENIOHYOID])

Test. The patient opens the mouth by depressing the mandible (Fig. 2-28). Lateral pterygoid is active throughout the total range and the digastric is active in complete or forceful depression.[16] The anterior portion of digastric can be palpated inferiorly to the mandible. The hyoid bone is fixed by the infrahyoid muscles when the suprahyoid muscles contract.[3,12,17]

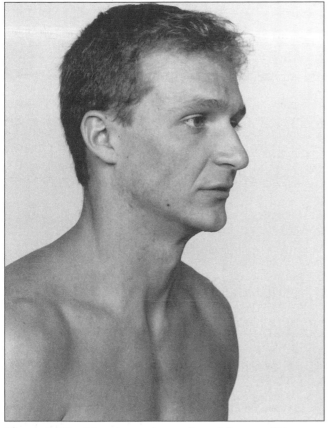

Figure 2-27. Elevation and retrusion of the mandible.

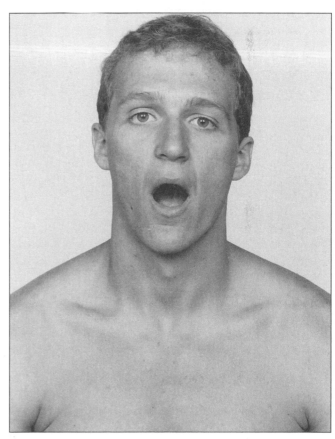

Figure 2-28. Depression of the mandible.

PROTRUSION OF THE MANDIBLE (MEDIAL AND LATERAL PTERYGOIDS)

Test. With the mouth partially open, the patient protrudes the mandible (Fig. 2-29).

LATERAL DEVIATION OF THE MANDIBLE (TEMPORALIS, MEDIAL AND LATERAL PTERYGOIDS, MASSETER)

Test. With the mouth slightly open, the patient deviates the lower jaw to one side and then the other (Fig. 2-30).

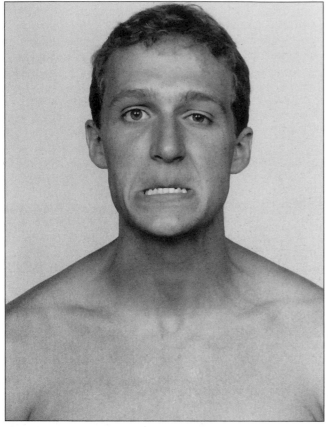

Figure 2-29.   Protrusion of the mandible.

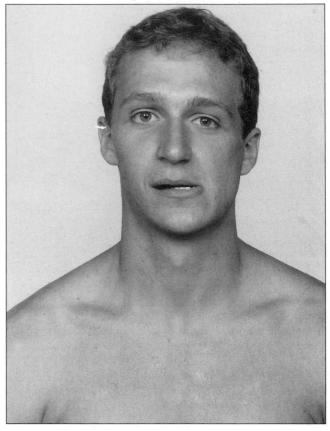

Figure 2-30.   Contraction of the left temporalis and right medial and lateral pterygoids produces left lateral deviation of the mandible.

FACIAL NERVE (CN VII)

Motor Function. Motor functions are facial expression and control of the musculature of the eyebrows, eyelids, nose, and mouth.

Component Movements Tested. Component movements are (1) eyebrows: elevation, adduction and depression; (2) eyelids: closure; (3) nose: dilation and constriction of the nasal opening; and (4) mouth: closure and protrusion of the lips; compression of the cheeks; elevation, retraction, and depression of the angle of the mouth; elevation of the upper lip; and elevation and protrusion of the lower lip.

ELEVATION OF THE EYEBROWS (EPICRANIUS [OCCIPITOFRONTALIS])

Test. The patient elevates the eyebrows (Fig. 2-31). The action forms transverse wrinkles of the skin of the forehead and the expression of surprise.

ADDUCTION OF THE EYEBROWS (CORRUGATOR SUPERCILLI)

Test. The patient pulls the medial aspect of the eyebrows together (Fig. 2-32). This action forms vertical wrinkles between the eyebrows and the expression of frowning.

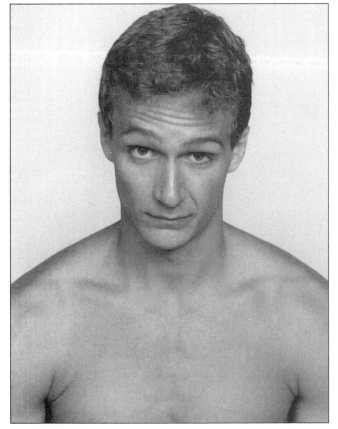

Figure 2-31.   Elevation of the eyebrows.

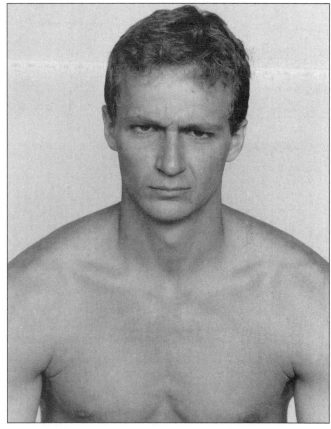

Figure 2-32.   Adduction and depression of the eyebrows.

DEPRESSION OF THE MEDIAL ANGLE OF THE EYEBROW (PROCERUS)

Test. The patient draws the medial angle of the eyebrows down and elevates the skin of the nose (Fig. 2-33). This action produces transverse wrinkles over the bridge of the nose. The patient may be asked to wrinkle the skin over the bridge of the nose as in the expression of distaste.

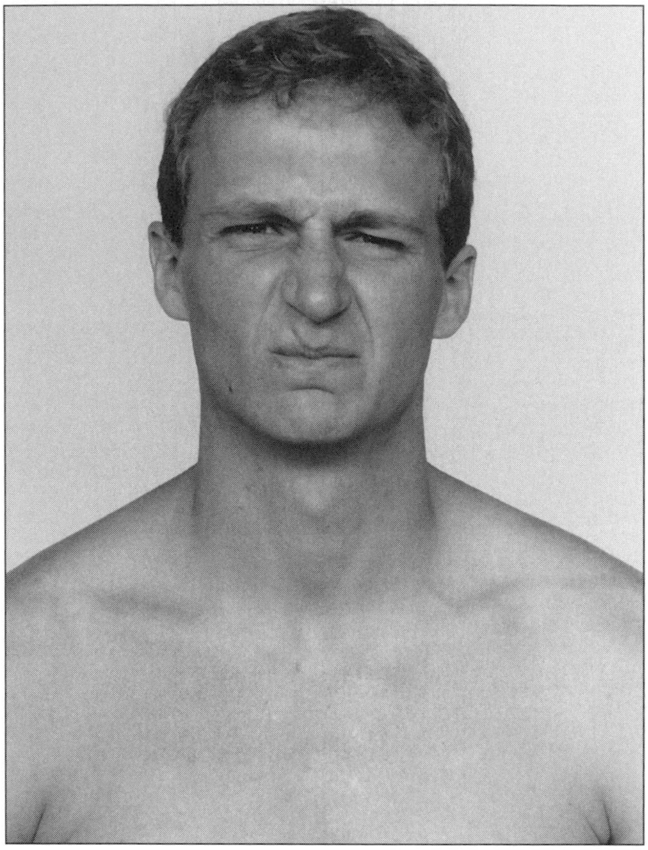

CLOSURE OF THE EYELIDS (ORBICULARIS OCULI)

Test. The patient closes the eyelids tightly (Fig. 2-34). This action pulls the skin of the forehead, temple, and cheek medially toward the nose.

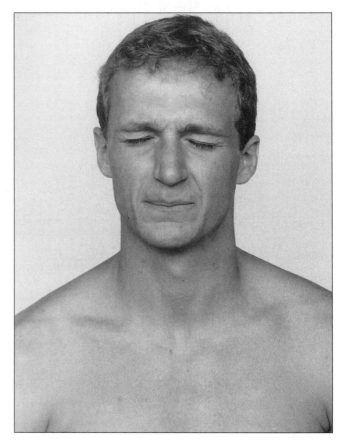

Figure 2-33. Depression of the medial angle of the eyebrow.

Figure 2-34. Closure of the eyelids.

DILATION OF THE NASAL APERTURE (NASALIS [ALAR PORTION] DEPRESSOR SEPTI)

Test. The patient dilates or widens the nostrils (Fig. 2-35). To accomplish the movement, the patient may be asked to take a deep breath.

CONSTRICTION OF THE NASAL APERTURE (NASALIS [TRANSVERSE PORTION])

Test. The patient compresses the nostrils together (Fig. 2-36).

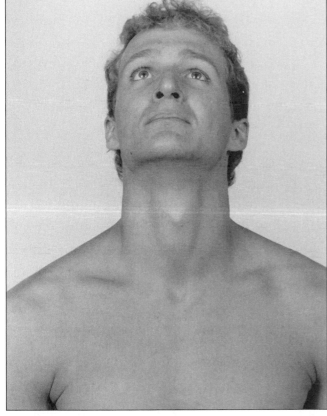

Figure 2-35.   Dilation of the nasal aperture.

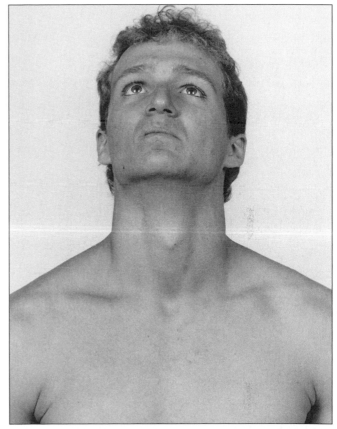

Figure 2-36.   Constriction of the nasal aperture.

CLOSURE AND PROTRUSION OF THE LIPS (ORBICULARIS ORIS)

Test. The patient closes and protrudes the lips (Fig. 2-37). The patient may be asked to simulate whistling by pursing the lips.

COMPRESSION OF THE CHEEKS (BUCCINATOR)

Test. The patient compresses the cheeks against the teeth (Fig. 2-38). The patient may be asked to simulate the blowing action of playing a wind instrument. Buccinator may be palpated in the cheek during the movement.

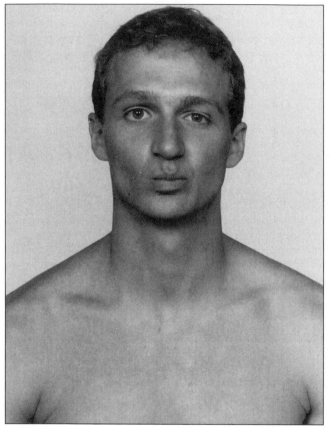

Figure 2-37.   Closure and protrusion of the lips.

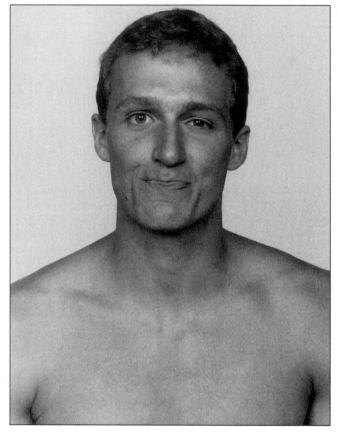

Figure 2-38.   Compression of the cheeks against the teeth.

ELEVATION OF THE ANGLE OF THE MOUTH (LEVATOR ANGULI ORIS)

Test. The patient raises the angle or corner of the mouth (Fig. 2-39). This action deepens the nasolabial fold.

ELEVATION AND RETRACTION OF THE ANGLE OF THE MOUTH (ZYGOMATICUS MAJOR)

Test. The patient draws the angle of the mouth upward and laterally (Fig. 2-40). This action forms the facial expression of smiling. The muscle can be palpated above and lateral to the angle of the mouth.

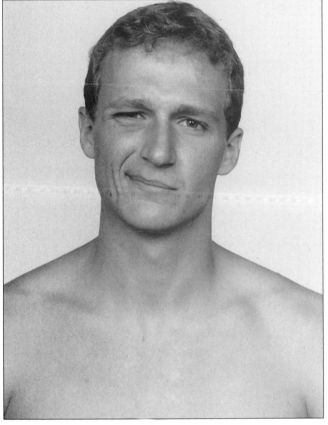

Figure 2-39. Elevation of the angle of the mouth.

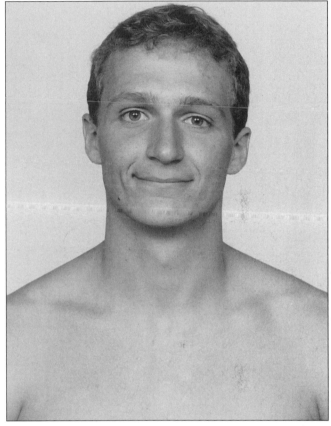

Figure 2-40. Elevation and retraction of the angle of the mouth.

RETRACTION OF THE ANGLE OF THE MOUTH (RISORIUS)

Test. The patient retracts or draws the angle of the mouth in a posterior direction (Fig. 2-41). This action forms the facial expression of a grimace.

DEPRESSION OF THE ANGLE OF THE MOUTH AND LOWER LIP (PLATYSMA, DEPRESSOR ANGULI ORIS, DEPRESSOR LABII INFERIORIS)

Test. The patient depresses the lower lip and angles of the mouth by drawing down the corners of the mouth and tensing the skin between the chin and the clavicle (Fig. 2-42). The patient may be asked to simulate the movement of easing the pressure of a tight shirt collar.

ELEVATION OF THE UPPER LIP (LEVATOR LABII SUPERIORIS, ZYGOMATICUS MINOR)

Test. The patient elevates and protrudes (everts) the upper lip (Fig. 2-43) as in showing the incisor teeth or upper gums.

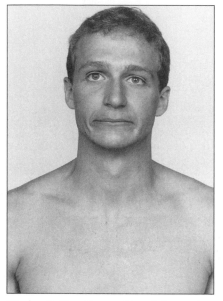

Figure 2-41.   Retraction of the angle of the mouth.

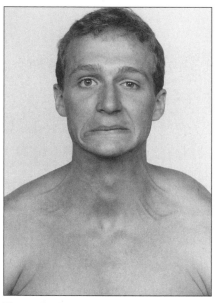

Figure 2-42.   Depression of the angle of the mouth.

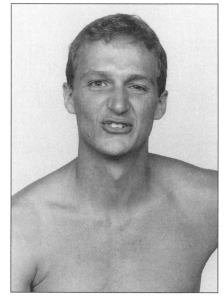

Figure 2-43.   Elevation of the upper lip.

ELEVATION AND PROTRUSION OF THE LOWER LIP (MENTALIS)

Test. The patient elevates the skin of the chin and protrudes the lower lip (Fig. 2-44). This action forms the facial expression of pouting.

HYPOGLOSSAL NERVE (CN XII)

Motor Function. The muscles supplied by the hypoglossal nerve act to produce tongue movements for the functions of mastication, taste, deglutition, speech, and oral hygiene.

Component Movements Tested. Tongue protrusion is the only movement tested.

PROTRUSION OF THE TONGUE (GENIOGLOSSUS)

Test. The mouth is open and the tongue is resting on the floor of the mouth. A wooden tongue depressor is placed on the midline of the chin to obtain a reference line for the midline of the tongue.[14] The patient is asked to protrude the tongue so that the tip of the tongue touches the tongue depressor (Fig. 2-45). Note any deviation to the side of the lesion by observing the line formed by the lingual septum line and the edge of the tongue blade. During tongue movement, the genioglossus muscle pulls the hyoid bone in an anterosuperior direction. The movement of the hyoid bone may be palpated. The tongue is inspected for atrophy on the side of the lesion.

Note: Should there be risk of infection or contact with body fluids, the therapist must use universal precautions and be gloved, masked, and gowned as required.

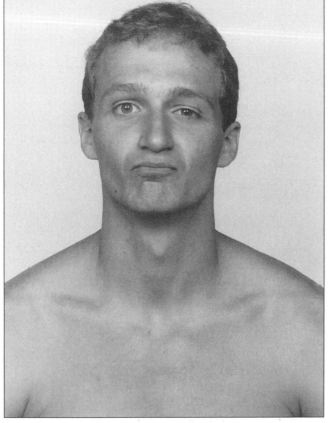

Figure 2-44. Elevation and protrusion of the lower lip.

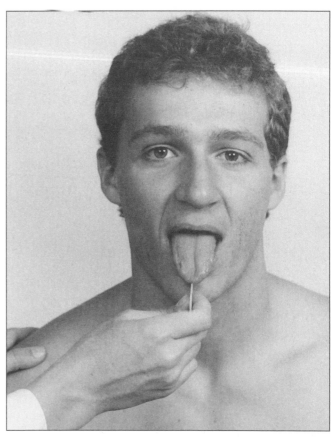

Figure 2-45. Protrusion of the tongue.

INFRAHYOID (STRAP) MUSCLES: STERNOHYOID, THYROHYOID, OMOHYOID

Motor Function. The primary function of the infrahyoid muscles is to depress the hyoid bone during swallowing and speaking.

Component Movements Tested. Depression of the hyoid bone (infrahyoid muscles) with depression of the tongue (hyoglossus muscle).

Test. The patient is asked to depress the root of the tongue as in swallowing (Figs. 2-46 and 2-47). The therapist may palpate the contraction of the infrahyoid muscles inferiorly to the hyoid bone.

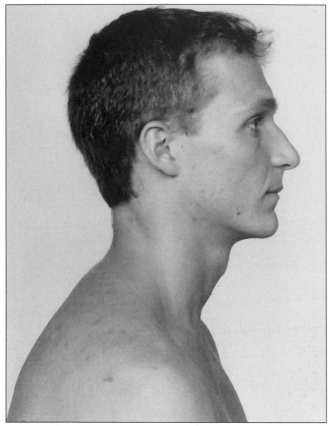

Figure 2-46.   Relaxed position of the hyoid bone.

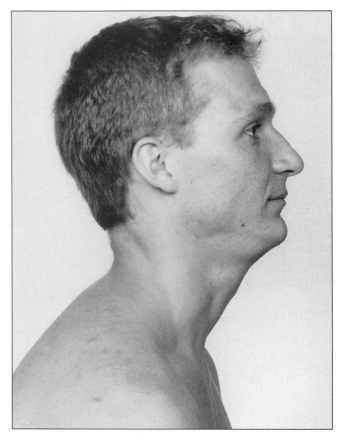

Figure 2-47.   Depression of the hyoid bone.

▼ MUSCLE STRENGTH ASSESSMENT: MUSCLES OF THE HEAD AND NECK (TABLE 2-4)

Note: **Manual muscle testing of the head and neck is contraindicated in some instances. Contraindications include pathology that may result in spinal instability and pathology of the vertebral artery. In the absence of** **contraindications to resisted head and neck movements, resistance is applied with care not to apply too much resistance for the muscles being tested.**

TABLE 2-4 ▼ MUSCLE ACTIONS, ATTACHMENTS, AND NERVE SUPPLY: THE HEAD AND NECK[2]

Muscle	Primary Muscle Action	Muscle Origin	Muscle Insertion	Peripheral (Cranial) Nerve	Nerve Root
Infrahyoid Muscles (sternohyoid, sternothyroid, thyrohyoid)					
Sternohyoid	Depression of the hyoid bone	Posterior aspect of the medial end of the clavicle; posterior sternoclavicular ligament; superior and posterior aspect of the manubrium	Inferior aspect of the body of the hyoid bone	Ansa cervicalis	C123
Sternothyroid	Depression of the larynx	Posterior aspect of the manubrium below the origin of the sternohyoid and from the edge of the first costal cartilage	Oblique line on the lamina of the thyroid cartilage	Ansa cervicalis	C123
Thyrohyoid	Depression of the hyoid bone; elevation of the larynx	Oblique line on the lamina of the thyroid cartilage	Inferior border of the greater cornu and the adjacent part of the body of the hyoid bone	(Hypoglossal CN XII)	C1
Omohyoid	Depression of the hyoid bone	Superior border of the scapula near the scapular notch; superior transverse scapular ligament	A band of deep cervical fascia holds the intermediate portion of the muscle down towards the clavicle and first rib and the course of the muscle changes direction at this point; lower border of the body of the hyoid bone	Ansa cervicalis	C123
Sternomastoid	Neck extension; neck flexion; contralateral neck rotation; ipsilateral neck side flexion	a. Sternal head: superior aspect of the manubrium b. Clavicular head: superior surface of the medial third of the clavicle	Lateral aspect of the mastoid process; lateral half of the superior nuchal line	(CN XI)	C234

Muscle	Primary Muscle Action	Muscle Origin	Muscle Insertion	Peripheral (Cranial) Nerve	Nerve Root
Longus colli	Neck flexion; contralateral neck rotation (inferior oblique fibers); neck side flexion (oblique fibers)	a. Inferior oblique part: anterior aspect of the bodies T1 to T3 b. Superior oblique part: the anterior tubercles of the transverse processes of C3 to C5 c. Vertical part: anterior aspect of the bodies of T1 to T3 and C5 to C7	a. Inferior oblique part: the anterior tubercles of the transverse processes of C5 and C6 b. Superior oblique part: anterolateral surface of the tubercle on the anterior arch of the atlas c. Vertical part: anterior aspects of the bodies of C2 to C4		C23456
Longus capitis	Flexes the head	Anterior tubercles of the transverse processes of C3 to C6	Inferior surface of the basilar aspect of the occipital bone		C123
Rectus capitis anterior	Flexes the head	Anterior aspect of the lateral mass of the atlas; root of the transverse process of the atlas	Inferior surface of the basilar aspect of the occipital bone anterior to the occipital condyle		C12
Rectus capitis lateralis	Ipsilateral lateral flexion of the head	Superior aspect of the transverse process of the atlas	Inferior aspect of the jugular process of the occipital bone		C12
Scalenus anterior	Neck flexion and ipsilateral neck lateral flexion Contralateral neck rotation	Anterior tubercles of the transverse processes of C3 to C6	Scalene tubercle on the inner border of the first rib and the ridge on the upper surface of the rib anterior to the groove for the subclavian artery		C456
Scalenus medius	Ipsilateral neck lateral flexion	Transverse process of the axis; anterior aspect of the posterior tubercles of the transverse processes of C3 to C7	Superior aspect of the first rib between the tubercle of the rib and the groove for the subclavian artery		C3–8
Scalenus posterior	Ipsilateral neck lateral flexion	Posterior tubercles of the transverse processes of C4 to C6	Lateral surface of the second rib		C678
Upper fibers of trapezius	Head and neck extension	Medial third of the superior nuchal line of the occipital bone; external occipital protuberance; ligamentum nuchae	Posterior border of the lateral one third of the clavicle	(CN XI)	

TABLE
2-4

MUSCLE ACTIONS, ATTACHMENTS, AND NERVE SUPPLY: THE HEAD AND NECK[2] *Continued*

Muscle	Primary Muscle Action	Muscle Origin	Muscle Insertion	Peripheral (Cranial) Nerve	Nerve Root
Splenius capitis	Neck extension; ipsilateral neck rotation	Inferior half of the ligamentum nuchae; the spinous processes of C7 and T1 to T4 and the corresponding supraspinous ligaments	Mastoid process of the temporal bone; the occipital bone inferior to the lateral third of the superior nuchal line	Middle cervical spinal nerves	
Splenius cervicis	Neck extension; ipsilateral neck rotation	The spinous processes of T3 to T6	Posterior tubercles of the transverse processes of the upper three cervical vertebrae	Lower cervical spinal nerves	
Rectus capitis posterior major	Head extension and ipsilateral head rotation	Spinous process of the axis	Lateral part of the inferior nuchal line and area of bone just inferior to the line	First cervical spinal nerve	
Rectus capitis posterior minor	Head extension	Tubercle on the posterior arch of the atlas	Medial part of the inferior nuchal line and the area of bone between the line and foramen magnum	First cervical spinal nerve	
Obliquus capitis inferior	Ipsilateral head rotation	Lateral aspect of the spine and adjacent superior aspect of the lamina of the axis	Inferior and posterior aspect of the transverse process of the atlas	First cervical spinal nerve	
Obliquus capitis superior	Head extension and ipsilateral head lateral flexion	Superior surface of the transverse process of the atlas	Occipital bone between the superior and inferior nuchal lines lateral to the semispinalis capitis	First cervical spinal nerve	

Note: See Table 2-6 for other neck extensor muscles.

ANTERIOR HEAD AND NECK FLEXORS: RECTUS CAPITIS ANTERIOR, LONGUS CAPITIS, LONGUS COLLI, SCALENUS ANTERIOR, STERNOMASTOID

Accessory muscles: Scalenus medius, scalenus posterior, suprahyoids, infrahyoids, and rectus capitis lateralis.

The head and neck flexors (Fig. 2-48) are tested in the against gravity position. The anterior head and neck flexors are tested as a group; followed by isolation of the sternomastoid muscles.

• **Start Position.** The patient is supine (Fig. 2-49). The arms are over the head resting on the plinth. The elbows are flexed.

• **Stabilization.** The trunk is stabilized by the plinth. The anterior abdominal muscles must be strong enough to provide anterior fixation of the thorax on the pelvis.[17] In a patient with weak abdominals, stabilization is provided by downward pressure of the therapist's hand on the thorax (Fig. 2-50).

• **Movement.** The patient flexes the head and neck through partial (grade 2) or full range (grade 3) (Fig. 2-51). The patient is instructed to keep the chin depressed.

• **Palpation.** Longus capitis, longus colli, and rectus capitis anterior are too deep to palpate. The sternomastoid muscle may be palpated proximal to the clavicle or sternum. The muscle is more easily palpated in the isolated

test involving rotation. The scalenus anterior may be palpated above the clavicle and behind the sternomastoid.

• **Resistance Location.** Applied on the forehead (Fig. 2-52).

• **Resistance Direction.** Head and neck extension.

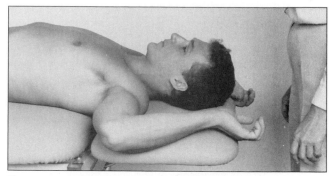

Figure 2-49. Start position for head and neck flexion.

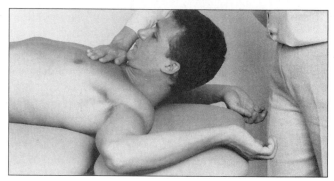

Figure 2-50. Screen position: head and neck flexion with stabilization.

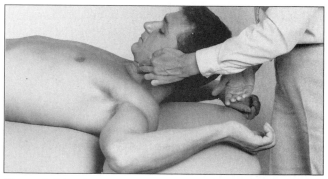

Figure 2-51. Screen position: head and neck flexion.

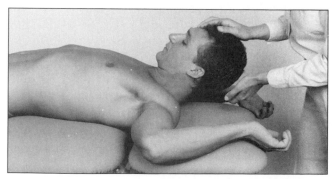

Figure 2-52. Resistance: head and neck flexors.

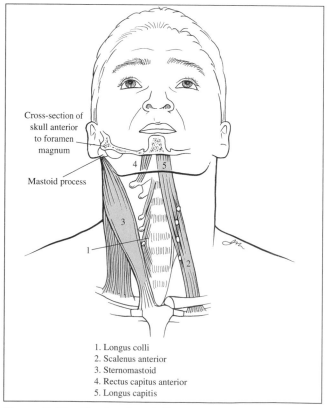

Cross-section of skull anterior to foramen magnum

Mastoid process

1. Longus colli
2. Scalenus anterior
3. Sternomastoid
4. Rectus capitus anterior
5. Longus capitis

Figure 2-48. Head and neck flexor muscles.

ANTEROLATERAL NECK FLEXOR: STERNOMASTOID

• Start Position. The patient is supine (Fig. 2-53). The arms are over the head resting on the plinth. The elbows are flexed.

• Stabilization. The trunk is stabilized by the plinth. With abdominal muscle weakness stabilization of the thorax is required.[18]

• Movement. The patient laterally flexes on the test side and rotates the neck to the opposite side (Fig. 2-54). Each side is tested.

• Palpation. Each sternomastoid muscle can be palpated at any point along the oblique ridge of the muscle from the mastoid process to the sternum or clavicle.

• Resistance Location. The therapist's fingers are used to apply resistance on the temporal region of the head (Figs. 2-55 and 2-56).

• Resistance Direction. Oblique posterior direction and ipsilateral rotation.

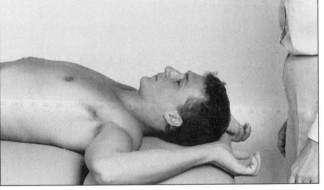

Figure 2-53. Start position: sternomastoid.

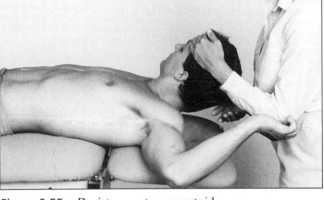

Figure 2-55. Resistance: sternomastoid.

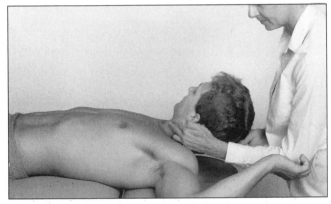

Figure 2-54. Screen position: sternomastoid.

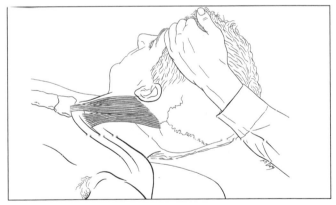

Figure 2-56. Sternomastoid.

HEAD AND NECK EXTENSORS

The head and neck extensors are tested as a group in the against gravity position. The muscles include semispinalis capitis, rectus capitis posterior (major and minor), obliquus capitis (inferior and superior), splenius capitis, semispinalis cervicis, longissimus capitis and cervicis, splenius cervicis, spinalis capitis and cervicis, and iliocostalis cervicis.

The strength of upper trapezius is tested as an elevator of the scapula.

- **Start Position.** The patient is prone (Fig. 2-57). The arms are over the head resting on the side of the plinth. The elbows are flexed.

- **Stabilization.** The patient grasps the end of the plinth for stabilization. The therapist may stabilize the upper thoracic region to prevent trunk extension.

- **Movement.** The patient extends and rotates the head and neck (Fig. 2-58).

- **Palpation.** The extensor muscles (Fig. 2-60) are palpated as a group paravertebrally.

- **Resistance Location.** Applied on the head just proximal to the occiput (Fig. 2-59).

- **Resistance Direction.** Head and neck flexion and rotation.

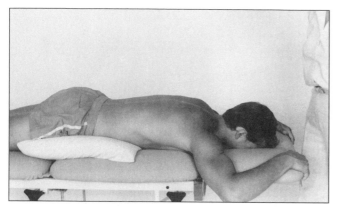

Figure 2-57. Start position: head and neck extensors.

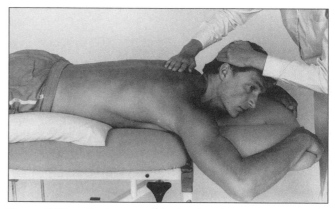

Figure 2-59. Resistance: right head and neck extensors.

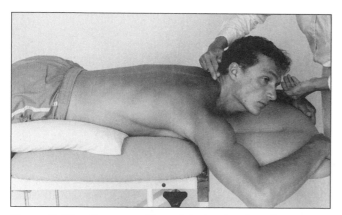

Figure 2-58. Screen position: right head and neck extensors.

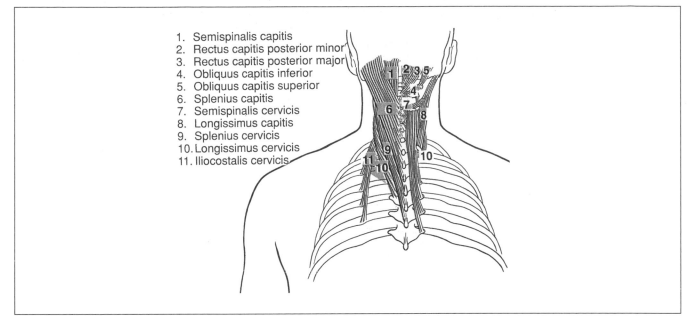

1. Semispinalis capitis
2. Rectus capitis posterior minor
3. Rectus capitis posterior major
4. Obliquus capitis inferior
5. Obliquus capitis superior
6. Splenius capitis
7. Semispinalis cervicis
8. Longissimus capitis
9. Splenius cervicis
10. Longissimus cervicis
11. Iliocostalis cervicis

Figure 2-60.   Head and neck extensors.

Structure	Location
1. Suprasternal (jugular) notch	The rounded depression at the superior border of the sternum, between the medial ends of each clavicle.
2. Xiphoid process	The lower end of the body of the sternum.
3. Anterior superior iliac spine (ASIS)	Round bony prominence at the anterior end of the iliac crest.
4. Iliac crest	Upper border of the ilium; a convex bony ridge, the top of which is level with the space between the spines of L4 and L5.
5. Posterior superior iliac spine (PSIS)	Round bony prominence at the posterior end of the iliac crest, felt subcutaneously at the dimples on the proximal aspect of the buttocks.
6. S2 spinous process	At the midpoint of a line drawn between each PSIS.
7. Inferior angle of the scapula	At the inferior aspect of the vertebral border of the scapula.
8. Spine of the scapula	The bony ridge running obliquely across the upper four-fifths of the scapula.
9. T7 spinous process	Midline of the body at the level of the inferior angle of the scapula with the body in the anatomical position.
10. T3 spinous process	With the body in the anatomical position it is at the midpoint of a line drawn between the roots of the spines of each scapula.
11. C7 spinous process	Often the most prominent spinous process at the base of the neck.

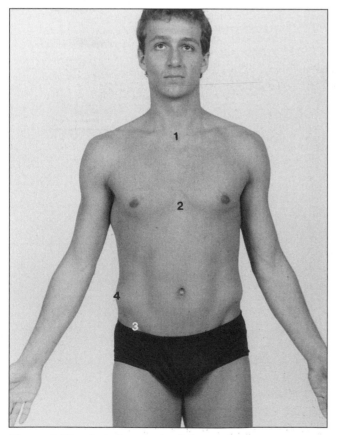

Figure 2-61. Anterior aspect of the trunk.

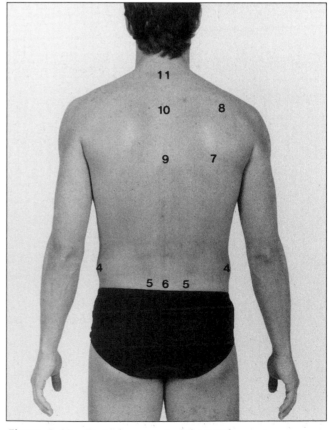

Figure 2-62. Posterior aspect of the trunk.

▼ RANGE OF MOTION ASSESSMENT

The articulations and joint axes of the trunk are illustrated in Figures 2-63, 2-64, and 2-65.

Assessment Process: The Trunk

1. The therapist observes:
   a. Function
   b. Trunk posture, chest contour, and the levels of the shoulders, scapulae, and pelvis
   c. Active movements at the hip, chest, and shoulder joints
2. The therapist assesses *active range of motion* (AROM):
   a. To estimate the joint ranges of motion (ROM).
   b. To establish the presence or absence of pain.
3. The therapist measures AROM through goniometry and using a tape measure.
4. The therapist assesses muscle strength through manual muscle testing.

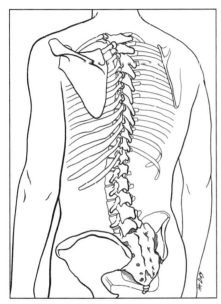

Figure 2-63. Trunk articulations.

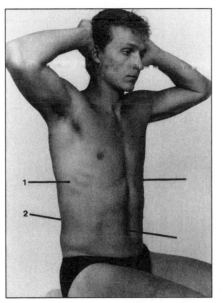

Figure 2-64. Trunk axes: (*1*) flexion-extension; (*2*) lateral flexion.

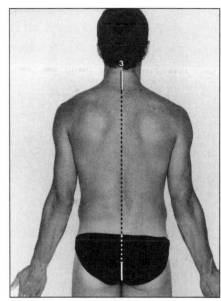

Figure 2-65. Trunk axis: (*3*) rotation.

RANGE OF MOTION ASSESSMENT AND MEASUREMENT

TRUNK MOVEMENTS (TABLE 2-5)

Objective measures of spinal mobility are described using a tape measure. These are often deleted from the assessment procedure in the clinic. The therapist may prefer to observe the patient to assess spinal movements, any deviations from normal, and the presence or absence of a rib hump. The OB goniometer, presented in Appendix A, is another useful tool for the measurement of trunk movements.

TABLE 2-5 ▼ JOINT STRUCTURE: TRUNK MOVEMENTS

	Flexion Extension	Lateral Flexion Rotation		
Articulation[19]	Lumbar spine, thoracic spine (mainly T6–12)	Lumbar spine, thoracic spine (mainly T6–12)	Lumbar spine, thoracic spine	Thoracic spine, lumbosacral articulation
Plane	Sagittal	Sagittal	Frontal	Horizontal
Axis	Frontal	Frontal	Sagittal	Vertical
Normal limiting factors[6,7]	Tension in the posterior longitudinal supraspinous, and interspinous ligaments, the ligamentum flavum, facet joint capsules and spinal extensor muscles; apposition of the anterior margins of the vertebral bodies, compression of the intervertebral discs anteriorly and tension in the posterior fibers of the annulus	Tension in the anterior longitudinal ligament, abdominal muscles, facet joint capsules and the anterior fibers of the annulus; contact between adjacent spinous processes; compression of the intervertebral discs posteriorly	Contact between the iliac crest and thorax; tension in the contralateral trunk side flexors and spinal ligaments; tension in the contralateral fibers of the annulus; compression of the intervertebral discs ipsilaterally	Tension in the costovertebral ligaments and annulus fibrosus of the intervertebral discs; tension in the ipsilateral external and contralateral internal abdominal oblique muscles; apposition of the articular facets
Normal active range of motion[8]	0–80° 10 cm (4 in)	0–20–30°	0–35°	0–45°
Capsular pattern:	It is difficult to perform passive movements of the trunk due to its size and weight. It is difficult to determine the capsular pattern for the trunk.[5]			

TRUNK FLEXION AND EXTENSION– THORACOLUMBAR SPINE

Measurement: Tape Measure

• **Start Position.** The patient is standing with feet shoulder width apart (Fig. 2-66). For thoracolumbar extension, the patient's hands are placed on the iliac crests and into the small of the back (not shown).

• **End Position.** The patient flexes the trunk forward to the limit of motion for thoracolumbar flexion (Fig. 2-67). The patient extends the trunk backward to the limit of motion for thoracolumbar extension (not shown).

• **Measurement.** A tape measure is used to measure the distance between the spinous processes of C7 and S2. A measure is taken in the start position and at the limit of motion. The difference between the two measures is the thoracolumbar spinal flexion ROM (about 10 cm) or the thoracolumbar spinal extension ROM (2.5 cm).[4]

• **Substitution/Trick Movement.** None.

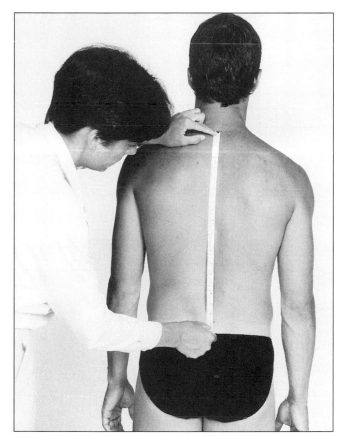

Figure 2-66.   Start position: thoracolumbar spinal flexion.

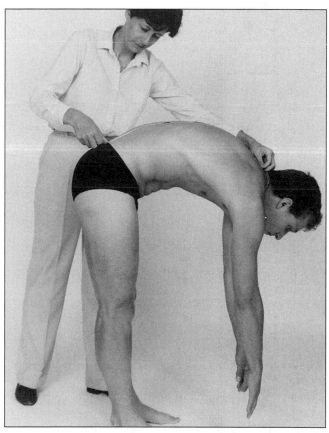

Figure 2-67.   End position: thoracolumbar spinal flexion.

TRUNK FLEXION AND EXTENSION–LUMBAR SPINE

Measurement: Tape Measure

• Start Position. The patient is standing with feet shoulder width apart (Fig. 2-68).

• End Position. The patient flexes the trunk forward to the limit of motion (Fig. 2-69).

• Measurement. A tape measure is used to measure a distance and mark a point 10 cm above the spinous process of S2. A measure is taken in the start position and at the limit of motion. The difference between the two measures is the lumbar spinal flexion ROM. This method of measurement is referred to as the modified Schober test.[20]

This technique can also be used to assess lumbar extension ROM in standing with the patient's hands placed on the iliac crests and into the small of the back (not shown). The patient extends the trunk backward to the limit of motion for lumbar extension and the difference between the two measures is the lumbar spinal extension ROM.

• Substitution/Trick Movement. None.

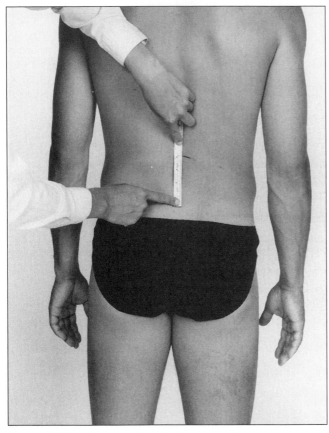

Figure 2-68.   Start position: lumbar spinal flexion.

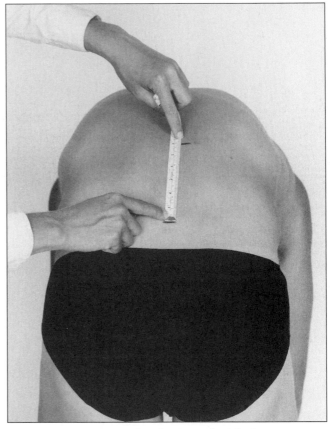

Figure 2-69.   End position: lumbar spinal flexion.

TRUNK EXTENSION– THORACOLUMBAR SPINE

Measurement: Tape Measure

• **Start Position.** The patient is prone with a pillow under the abdomen (Fig. 2-70). The hands are positioned on the plinth at shoulder level.

• **Stabilization.** A strap is placed over the pelvis.

• **End Position.** The patient extends the elbows to raise the trunk and extends the thoracolumbar spine (Fig. 2-71).

• **Measurement.** A tape measure is used to measure the distance between the suprasternal notch and the plinth at the limit of motion.

• **Substitution/Trick Movement.** Lifting of the pelvis from the plinth. This method is unsuitable for patients who have upper extremity muscle weakness or find the prone position uncomfortable. In these cases spinal extension is assessed in standing using the OB goniometer (see Appendix A) or a tape measure.

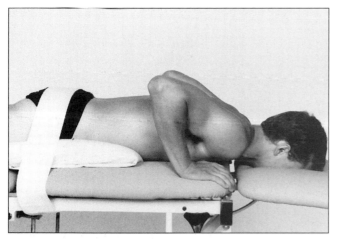

Figure 2-70.   Start position: thoracolumbar spinal extension.

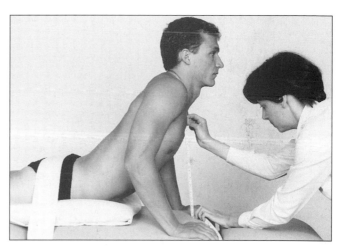

Figure 2-71.   End position: thoracolumbar spinal extension.

TRUNK LATERAL FLEXION

Measurement: Tape Measure

• **Start Position.** The patient is standing with the feet shoulder width apart (Fig. 2-72).

• **Stabilization.** None.

• **End Position.** The patient laterally flexes the trunk to the limit of motion (Fig. 2-73).

• **Measurement.** A tape measure is used to measure the distance between the tip of the third digit and the floor.

• **Substitution/Trick Movement.** Trunk flexion, trunk extension, ipsilateral hip and knee flexion, and raising the contralateral or ipsilateral foot from the floor.

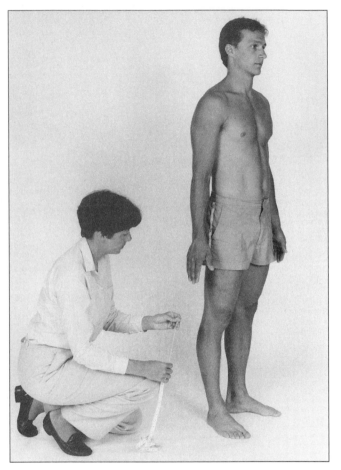

Figure 2-72. Start position: trunk lateral flexion.

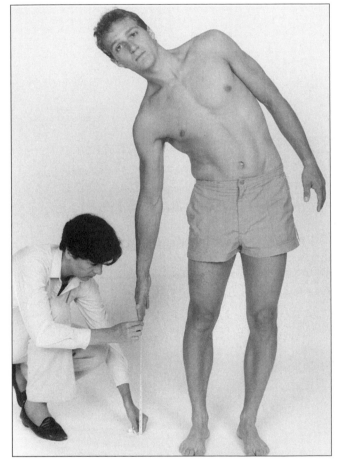

Figure 2-73. End position: trunk lateral flexion.

TRUNK ROTATION

Observation

• **Start Position.** The patient is sitting with the feet supported on a stool and the arms crossed in front of the chest (Fig. 2-74).

• **Stabilization.** The therapist stabilizes the pelvis.

• **End Position.** The patient rotates the trunk to the limit of motion. The therapist visually estimates the trunk rotation ROM (45°) (Fig. 2-75).

• **Substitution/Trick Movement.** Trunk flexion, trunk extension, and shoulder horizontal abduction in the direction of trunk rotation.

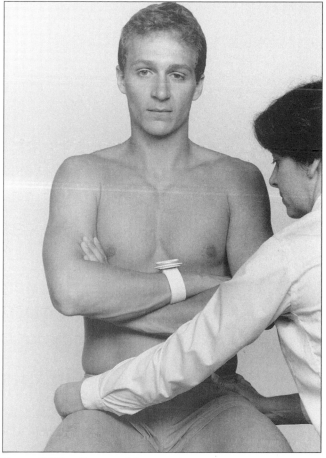

Figure 2-74.   Start position: trunk rotation.

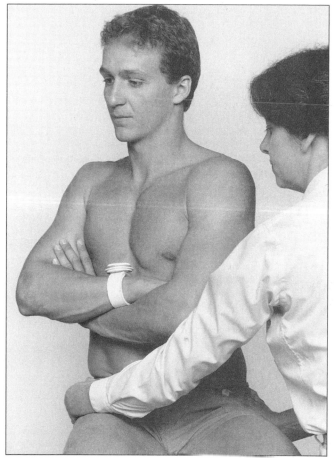

Figure 2-75.   End position: trunk rotation.

CHEST EXPANSION

Measurement: Tape Measure

• **Start Position.** The patient is sitting. The patient makes a full expiration (Fig. 2-76).

• **End Position.** The patient makes a full inspiration (Fig. 2-77).

• **Measurement.** A tape measure is used to measure the circumference of the chest at the level of the xiphisternal joint. Measures are taken at full expiration and at full inspiration. The difference between the two measures is the chest expansion. The chest expansion may also be measured at the levels of the nipple line and anterior axillary fold. The chest expansion measured at the latter points is slightly less than that at the xiphisternal joint. It is recommended[21] that two measurement sites, specifically the xiphoid and axilla, and a consistent patient position be used to provide a thorough evaluation of pulmonary status. A wide range of normal values exists for normal chest expansion and beginning in the late thirties chest expansion gradually decreases with increasing age.[22] Decreased chest expansion may indicate costovertebral joint involvement in certain pathological conditions[23] or may occur with chronic obstructive pulmonary disease (eg, emphysema).

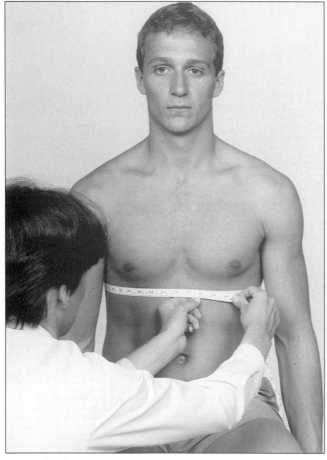

Figure 2-76. Start position: full expiration measured at the level of the xiphisternal joint.

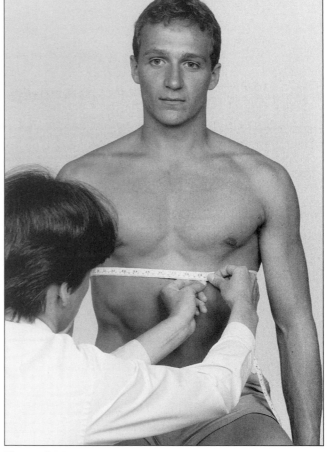

Figure 2-77. End position: full inspiration measured at the level of the xiphisternal joint.

MEASUREMENT OF MUSCLE LENGTH: TRUNK EXTENSORS AND HAMSTRINGS (TOE-TOUCH TEST)

Trunk extensors: erector spinae (iliocostalis thoracis and lumborum, longissimus thoracis, spinalis thoracis, semispinalis thoracis, multifidus); hip extensor and knee flexor muscles: hamstrings (semitendinosus, semimembranosus, biceps femoris).

The toe-touch test provides a composite measure of hip, spine, and shoulder girdle ROM.

• **Start Position.** The patient is standing (Fig. 2-78).

• **Stabilization.** None.

• **End Position.** The patient flexes the trunk and hips and reaches toward the toes to the limit of motion (Fig. 2-79).

• **Measurement.** A tape measure is used to measure the distance between the tip of the great toe and the most distant point reached by both hands. Normal ROM is present if the patient can touch the toes. In the event the patient is able to reach beyond floor level, the test can be carried out with the patient standing on a step or platform to measure reach distance beyond the supporting surface.

• **Substitution/Trick Movement.** Knee flexion.

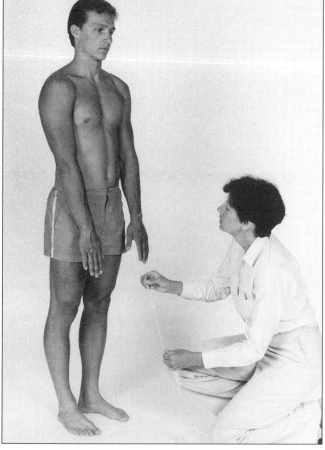

Figure 2-78.   Start position: toe-touch test.

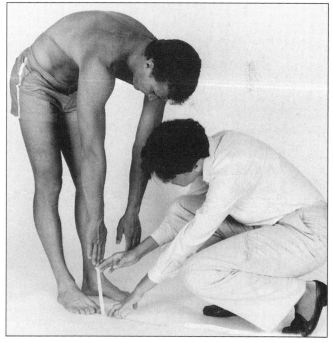

Figure 2-79.   End position: trunk extensor and hamstring muscle length.

TABLE 2-6 ▼ MUSCLE ACTIONS, ATTACHMENTS, AND NERVE SUPPLY: THE TRUNK, HEAD, AND NECK[2]

Muscle	Primary Muscle Action	Muscle Origin	Muscle Insertion	Peripheral Nerve	Nerve Root
Rectus abdominis	Trunk flexion	Crest and superior ramus of the pubis; ligaments covering the anterior surface of the symphysis pubis	Fifth, sixth, and seventh costal cartilages	Lower six or seven thoracic spinal nerves	T5–12
External abdominal oblique	Trunk rotation; trunk flexion	Eight digitations from the external and inferior surfaces of the lower eight ribs	Anterior half of the outer lip of the iliac crest; by an aponeurosis to merge with a similar aponeurosis from the opposite side into the linea alba from the xiphoid process to the symphysis pubis; as the inguinal ligament into the anterior superior iliac spine and the pubic tubercle	Lower six thoracic spinal nerves	T6–12
Internal abdominal oblique	Trunk rotation; trunk flexion	Lateral two thirds of the inguinal ligament; anterior two thirds of the iliac crest; the thoracolumbar fascia	Inferior borders of the lower three or four ribs; pubic crest and medial aspect of the pecten pubis; by an aponeurosis that splits around the rectus abdominus and inserts into the linea alba and the cartilages of ribs seven, eight, and nine	Lower six thoracic and first lumbar spinal nerves	T6–12, L1

TABLE 2-6

▼ MUSCLE ACTIONS, ATTACHMENTS, AND NERVE SUPPLY: THE TRUNK, HEAD, AND NECK[2] *Continued*

Muscle	Primary Muscle Action	Muscle Origin	Muscle Insertion	Peripheral Nerve	Nerve Root
Transversus abdominus	Compresses the abdominal contents	Lateral third of the inguinal ligament; anterior two thirds of the inner lip of the iliac crest; the thoracolumbar fascia between the iliac crest and rib twelve; the internal aspects of the costal cartilages of the lower six ribs	By an aponeurosis into the crest and pecten of the pubis and linea alba	Lower six thoracic and first lumbar spinal nerves	T6–12, L1
Quadratus lumborum	Elevation of the pelvis; trunk side flexion	The iliolumbar ligament and the adjacent posterior aspect of the iliac crest	Medial half of the inferior border of the twelfth rib; by four small tendons into the tips of the transverse processes of the upper four lumbar vertebrae	Twelfth thoracic and upper three or four lumbar spinal nerves	T12, L1–4
Erector spinae	The erector spinae lies along the sides of the vertebral column. The muscle is composed of three major columns of muscle mass (from lateral to medial: iliocostalis, longissimus and spinalis) all having a common origin: The posterior aspects of the sacrum and iliac crest; the sacrotuberous and dorsal sacroiliac ligaments; the L1 to L5 and T11 and T12 spinous processes, and corresponding supraspinous ligament.				C1–8 T1–12 L1–5

The three columns have origins of attachment in addition to the common origin. The three columns become identifiable at different levels of the lumbar region. Each column is composed of three smaller parts that span from six to ten segments of the vertebral column.

Muscle	Primary Muscle Action	Muscle Origin	Muscle Insertion	Peripheral Nerve	Nerve Root
a. Iliocostalis 1. Iliocostalis lumborum	Trunk extension; trunk side flexion		Inferior borders of the angles of ribs five to twelve	Lower cervical, thoracic and upper lumbar spinal nerves	

TABLE C-6

▼ MUSCLE ACTIONS, ATTACHMENTS, AND NERVE SUPPLY: THE TRUNK, HEAD, AND NECK[2] *Continued*

Muscle	Primary Muscle Action	Muscle Origin	Muscle Insertion	Peripheral Nerve	Nerve Root
2. Iliocostalis thoracis	Trunk extension; trunk side flexion	The superior borders of the angles of ribs six to twelve	Superior borders of the angles of ribs one to six; posterior aspect of the C7 transverse process		
3. Iliocostalis cervicis	Neck extension; neck side flexion	The angles of ribs three to six	Posterior tubercles of the transverse processes of C4 to C6		
b. Longissimus					
1. Longissimus thoracis	Trunk extension	The posterior aspects of the transverse processes and accessory process of L1 to L5; the middle layer of the thoracolumbar fascia	The tips of the transverse processes of T1 to T12; between the tubercles and angles of the lower nine to ten ribs	Lower cervical, thoracic and lumbar spinal nerves	
2. Longissimus cervicis	Neck extension	Transverse processes of T1 to T5	Posterior tubercles of the transverse processes of C2 to C6		
3. Longissimus capitis	Head and neck extension Head and neck rotation (ipsilateral)	Transverse processes of T1 to T5; articular processes of C3 to C7	Mastoid process		
c. Spinalis					
1. Spinalis thoracis	Trunk extension	Spinous processes of L1, L2, T11, and T12	Spinous processes of T1 to T4 or T8	Lower cervical and thoracic spinal nerves	
2. Spinalis cervicis	Neck extension	Inferior aspect of the ligamentum nuchae, spinous processes of C7, T1, and T2	The spinous processes of C1 to C3		
3. Spinalis capitis	Head extension	Tips of the transverse processes of C7 and T1 to T7; articular processes of C5 to C7	Region between the superior and inferior nuchal lines of the occiput		

TABLE
2-6

▼ **MUSCLE ACTIONS, ATTACHMENTS, AND NERVE SUPPLY: THE TRUNK, HEAD, AND NECK[2]** *Continued*

Muscle	Primary Muscle Action	Muscle Origin	Muscle Insertion	Peripheral Nerve	Nerve Root
Transversospinalis a. Semispinalis					
1. Semispinalis thoracis	Trunk extension; contralateral trunk rotation	Transverse processes of T6 to T10	Spinous processes of C6, C7 and T1 to T4	Cervical and thoracic spinal nerves	
2. Semispinalis cervicis	Neck extension; contralateral neck rotation	Transverse processes of T1 to T6	Spinous processes of C2 to C5		
3. Semispinalis capitis	Head extension; contralateral rotation of head	Tips of the transverse processes of C7 and T1 to T7; articular processes of C4 to C6	Medial aspect of the region between the superior and inferior nuchal lines of the occipital bone		
b. Multifidus	Trunk extension; trunk side flexion; trunk rotation (control of posture)	Posterior aspect of the sacrum; aponeurosis of erector spinae; posterior superior iliac spine; dorsal sacroiliac ligament; transverse processes of C4 through L5	Into the spinous processes of from one to four of the vertebrae above	Dorsal rami of the spinal nerves	
Rotatores	Trunk rotation (control of posture)	Superior and posterior aspect of the transverse processes of the vertebrae in the cervical, thoracic and lumbar regions	Inferior and lateral aspect of the lamina of the vertebra above in the cervical, thoracic and lumbar regions	Dorsal rami of the spinal nerves	
Interspinales	Trunk extension (control of posture)	Short muscular fasciculi between the spines of contiguous vertebrae lateral to the interspinous ligament bilaterally in the cervical, thoracic and lumbar regions		Dorsal rami of the spinal nerves	
Intertransversarii	Trunk side flexion (control of posture)	Short muscles between the transverse processes of contiguous vertebrae in the cervical, thoracic and lumbar regions		Dorsal and ventral rami of the spinal nerves	

TRUNK FLEXION

The strength of the neck and hip flexors should be tested before testing the strength of the abdominal muscles.[17] If the neck flexors are weak, the head will have to be supported during the testing.

A half curl-up is performed to assess abdominal muscle strength. The movement begins from a position of crook lying with the feet unsupported. The patient initially tilts the pelvis posteriorly to flex the lumbar spine, flexes the cervical spine, and then flexes the thoracic spine to lift the head and scapulae off the plinth.

Using the curl-up movement with the feet unsupported is more effective in activating the rectus abdominus muscle than performing the full sit-up from the supine position with the feet supported.[24] The first phase of the curl-up, start position to 45°, is primarily performed by the rectus abdominis, whereas the second phase, from 45° to the sitting position, is primarily performed by the iliacus muscle.[25] Therefore, a half curl-up is used to test abdominal muscle strength.

Rectus Abdominis

Accessory muscles: iliopsoas, rectus femoris, internal abdominal oblique, and external abdominal oblique.

The rectus abdominis muscle (Fig. 2-85) is tested in the against gravity position for all grades.

• **Start Position.** The patient is crook-lying.

• **Stabilization.** Flexion of the cervical spine serves to fix the thorax and when combined with a posterior pelvic tilt provides the optimal posture for decreasing the lumbar lordosis, reducing the stress on the low back, and activating the abdominal muscles[26] in performing the curl-up. If the patient is unable to perform a posterior pelvic tilt and maintain the lumbar spine in a flexed

position when being tested for abdominal muscle strength, the test is discontinued.

To prevent contraction of the iliopsoas muscle and greater hyperextension of the lumbar spine, the therapist should not stabilize the feet.[27]

• **Movement.** The patient attempts to tilt the pelvis posteriorly to flex the lumbar spine (Fig. 2-80). Grade 1: No movement is possible but a flicker of a muscle contraction may be palpated as the patient attempts to lift the head or cough. Grade 0: No palpable contraction is evident.

• **Palpation.** Lateral to the midline on the anterior abdominal wall midway between the sternum and the pubis.

• **Movement.** Grade 2 (Fig. 2-81): The patient initially tilts the pelvis posteriorly to flex the lumbar spine, flexes the cervical spine, and then flexes the thoracic spine. The patient lifts the head and scapulae off the plinth, with the arms by the side.

• **Movement.** Grade 3 (Fig. 2-82): The patient initially tilts the pelvis posteriorly to flex the lumbar spine, flexes the cervical spine, and then flexes the thoracic spine with the arms held in front of the trunk. The patient performs the movement slowly.

• **Substitution/Trick Movement.** Hip flexors (lumbar lordosis).[17]

• **Resistance.** Resistance is not applied manually by the therapist but is provided through positioning of the arms. The resistance of the head, trunk, and upper limbs decreases as the upper limbs are moved caudally.[16] Accordingly, the arms are positioned across the chest (Fig. 2-83) or with the hands beside the ears (Fig. 2-84) throughout the movement, for grades of 4 and 5, respectively.

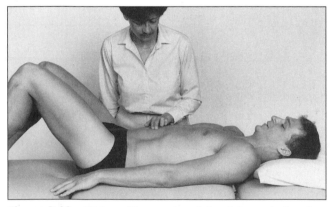

Figure 2-80. Test position: rectus abdominis, grade 0 or 1.

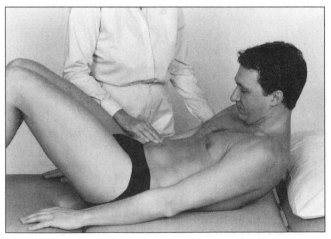

Figure 2-81. Test position: rectus abdominis, grade 2.

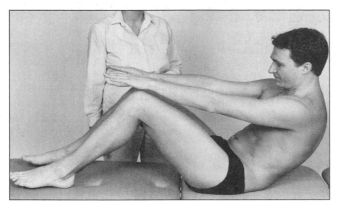

Figure 2-82.   Screen position: rectus abdominis.

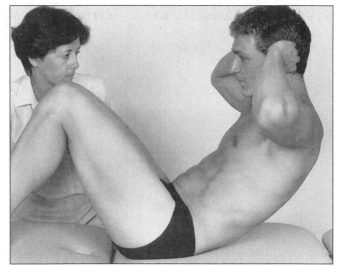

Figure 2-84.   Test position: rectus abdominis, grade 5.

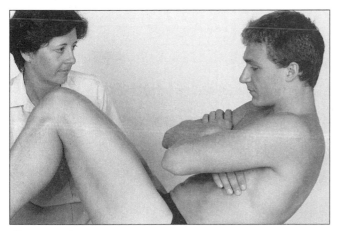

Figure 2-83.   Test position: rectus abdominis, grade 4.

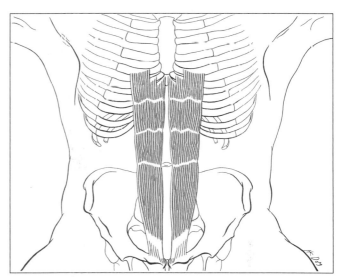

Figure 2-85.   Rectus abdominis.

TRUNK ROTATION

Against Gravity: External Abdominal Oblique, Internal Abdominal Oblique

Accessory muscles: rectus abdominus, semispinalis thoracis, multifidus, rotatores, and latissimus dorsi.

- **Start Position.** The patient is crook-lying (see Fig. 2-80).

- **Stabilization.** None.

- **Movement.** With the arms held in front of the trunk the patient flexes and rotates the trunk to perform a half curl-up with rotation (Fig. 2-86). The patient performs the movement slowly.

- **Palpation.** External abdominal oblique, at the lower edge of the rib cage. Internal abdominal oblique, medial to and above the anterior superior iliac spine.

- **Substitution/Trick Movement.** None.

- **Resistance.** Resistance is not applied manually by the therapist. Resistance is provided through positioning of the arms[18] and increases as the arms are moved cranially. The arms are positioned across the chest (Fig. 2-87) or with the hands beside the ears (Fig. 2-88) throughout the movement, for grades of 4 and 5, respectively.

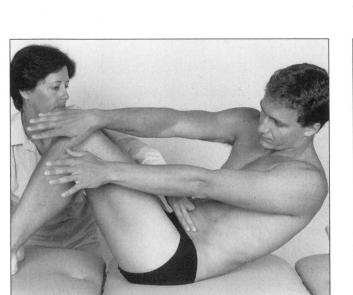

Figure 2-86. Screen position: right external abdominal oblique and left internal abdominal oblique.

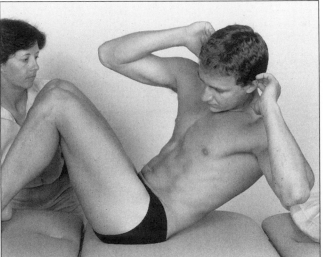

Figure 2-88. Test position: right external abdominal oblique and left internal abdominal oblique, grade 5.

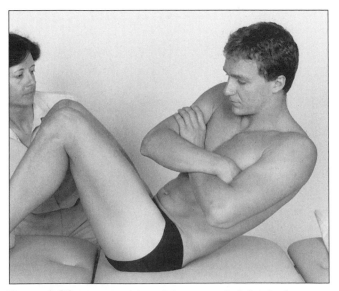

Figure 2-87. Test position: right external abdominal oblique and left internal abdominal oblique, grade 4.

Gravity Eliminated: External Abdominal Oblique, Internal Abdominal Oblique

• **Start Position.** The patient is sitting with the hands off the plinth and the feet supported (Fig. 2-89).

• **Stabilization.** The pelvis is stabilized by the patient's body weight.

• **End Position.** The patient rotates the thorax with slight flexion (Figs. 2-90 and 2-91).

• **Substitution/Trick Movement.** None.
   Deviation of the umbilicus[17]: With marked weakness of the abdominal muscles deviation of the umbilicus can occur during testing. The umbilicus will be pulled toward the stronger muscle(s) and away from the weaker muscle(s). The umbilicus may also be pulled by and deviate toward a muscle that is shortened and being stretched. Palpation of the muscles can be used to confirm the presence of deviation of the umbilicus due to muscle imbalance.

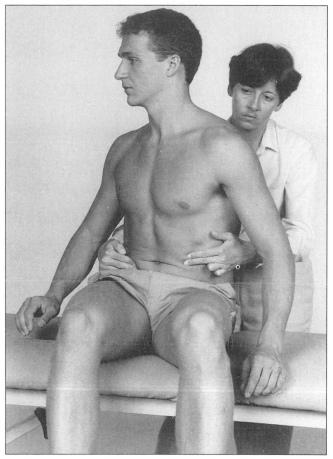

Figure 2-90. End position: left external abdominal oblique, right internal abdominal oblique.

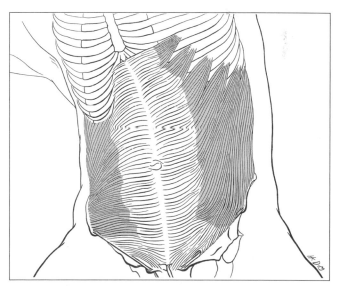

Figure 2-91. Left external abdominal oblique, right internal abdominal oblique.

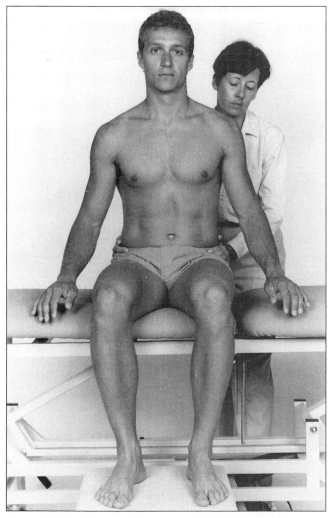

Figure 2-89. Start position: external abdominal oblique, internal abdominal oblique.

DOUBLE STRAIGHT LEG LOWERING (EXTERNAL ABDOMINAL OBLIQUE, INTERNAL ABDOMINAL OBLIQUE, RECTUS ABDOMINIS)[28]

• **Start Position.** The patient is lying supine, the therapist raises the legs to a position of 90° hip flexion (Fig. 2-92). The patient posteriorly tilts the pelvis, to flex the lumbar spine and flatten the small of the back onto the plinth.

• **Stabilization.** None.

• **Movement.** The therapist places one hand touching the posterolateral aspect of the ilium to ensure the posterior pelvic tilt is maintained while the patient slowly lowers the legs to the plinth.

Movement is stopped when the patient can no longer maintain the posterior pelvic tilt. When the therapist feels the pelvis begin to anteriorly rotate, the therapist supports the legs and notes the angle between the legs and the plinth before lowering the legs to the plinth.

• **Measurement.** A visual estimate or a universal goniometer is used to measure the angle of hip flexion at the limit of motion. The goniometer alignment is the same as for hip flexion or straight leg raise (SLR) ROM.

• **Grading.**[17] Angles of hip flexion are translated into grades as follows: grade 3 is 90° to 75°; grade 3+ is 74° to 60° (Fig. 2-93); grade 4- is 59° to 45°; grade 4 is 44° to 30°; grade 4+ is 29° to 15° (Fig. 2-94); grade 5 is 14° to 0°.

• **Palpation.** External abdominal oblique, at the lower edge of the rib cage. Internal abdominal oblique, medial to and above the anterior superior iliac spine. Rectus abdominus, lateral to the midline on the anterior abdominal wall midway between the sternum and the pubis.

• **Substitution/Trick Movement.** Increased lumbar lordosis due to anterior tilting of the pelvis.

• **Resistance.** Resistance is not applied manually by the therapist but is provided through the increased torque created by the lower extremities as the limbs are moved from 90° hip flexion to the surface of the plinth.

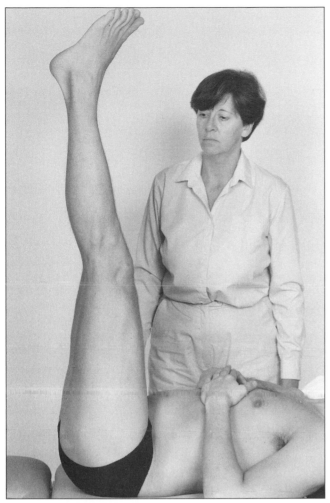

Figure 2-92.   Start position: double straight leg lowering.

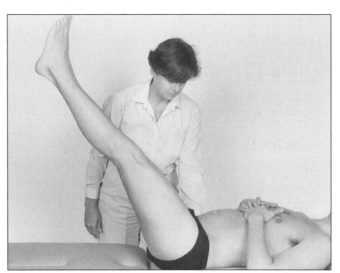

Figure 2-93.   Test position: hip flexion 60° grade 3+.

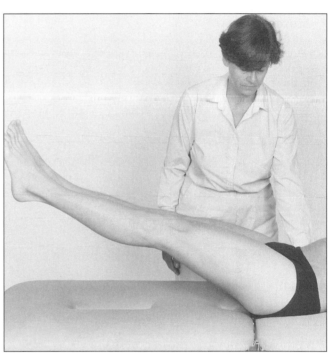

Figure 2-94.   Test position: hip flexion 20° grade 4+.

TRUNK EXTENSION (ERECTOR SPINAE: ILIOCOSTALIS THORACIS AND LUMBORUM, LONGISSIMUS THORACIS, SPINALIS THORACIS, SEMISPINALIS THORACIS AND MULTIFIDUS)

Accessory muscles: interspinales, quadratus lumborum, and latissimus dorsi. The strength of the neck and hip extensors should be tested before testing the strength of the trunk extensor muscles.[18] If the neck extensors are weak, the head will have to be supported during testing. If the hip extensors are weak or paralyzed, the pelvis cannot be adequately fixed in an extended position on the thigh as the patient attempts trunk extension and the patient will be unable to extend the trunk.[17]

The trunk extensors are tested as a group in the against gravity position.

• **Start Position.** The patient is prone lying with the feet over the end of the plinth and a pillow under the abdomen (Fig. 2-95).

• **Stabilization.** A strap is placed over the pelvis to isolate the lumbar extensor muscles[29] and the therapist stabilizes the legs proximal to the ankles.

• **Movement.** Grade 1: No movement is possible but a flicker of a muscle contraction can be palpated or observed as the patient attempts to lift the head. Grade 0: There is no palpable or observable muscle contraction.

• **Palpation.** The trunk extensor muscles (Fig. 2-100) are palpated as a group paravertebral to the lumbar or thoracic spines.

• **Movement.** Grade 2: With the arms by the sides, the patient lifts the head and upper portion of the sternum off the plinth (Fig. 2-96).

• **Movement.** Grade 3: With the hands held behind the back, the patient extends the trunk and lifts the head and the sternum, so that the xiphoid process is off the plinth (Fig. 2-97).

• **Substitution/Trick Movement.** None.

• **Resistance.** Resistance is not applied manually by the therapist. Resistance is provided through positioning of the arms and increases as the upper limbs are positioned toward the head. The hands are positioned behind the low back (Fig. 2-98) or behind the head (Fig. 2-99) to test for grades 4 and 5, respectively.[18]

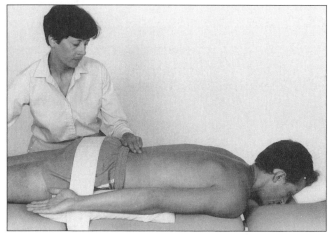

Figure 2-95.　Test position: trunk extensors, grade 0 or 1.

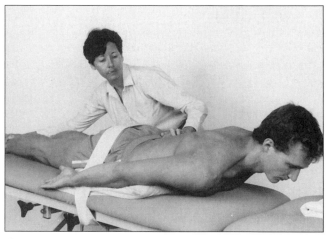

Figure 2-96.　Test position: trunk extensors, grade 2.

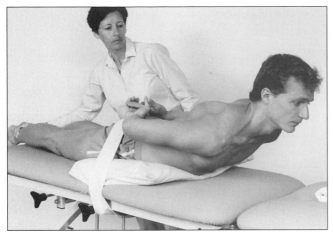

Figure 2-97.   Screen position: trunk extensors.

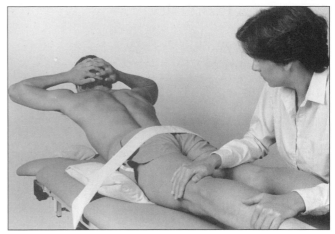

Figure 2-99.   Test position: trunk extensors, grade 5.

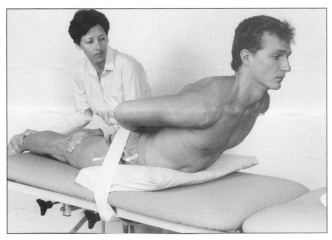

Figure 2-98.   Test position: trunk extensors, grade 4.

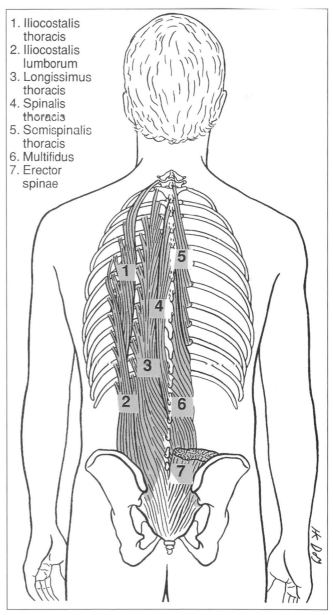

1. Iliocostalis
   thoracis
2. Iliocostalis
   lumborum
3. Longissimus
   thoracis
4. Spinalis
   thoracis
5. Semispinalis
   thoracis
6. Multifidus
7. Erector
   spinae

Figure 2-100.   Trunk extensors.

PELVIC ELEVATION

Gravity Eliminated: Quadratus Lumborum

Accessory muscles: latissimus dorsi, contralateral hip abductors, internal abdominal oblique, external abdominal oblique, and erector spinae.

The quadratus lumborum muscle is tested in the gravity eliminated position.

• **Start Position.** The patient lies prone with the feet off the end of the plinth, the hip in abduction, and slight extension (Fig. 2-101).

• **Stabilization.** The weight of the trunk; the patient holds the edges of the plinth.

• **Palpation.** Above the crest of the ilium, lateral to the paravertebral extensor muscle mass.

• **Movement.** The patient elevates the iliac crest toward the ribs through the full ROM (Fig. 2-102).

• **Substitution/Trick Movement.** Lateral fibers of the external abdominal oblique and internal abdominal oblique, latissimus dorsi, and erector spinae.

Resisted Gravity Eliminated: Quadratus Lumborum

• **Start Position.** The patient lies prone with the feet off the end of the plinth, with the hip in abduction and slight extension (see Fig. 2-101).

• **Stabilization.** The weight of the trunk; the patient holds the edges of the plinth.

• **Movement.** The patient elevates the iliac crest toward the ribs through the full ROM.

• **Resistance Location.** Anterior aspect of the distal end of the femur (Fig. 2-103). Alternatively, resistance can be applied on the posterolateral aspect of the iliac crest if hip pathology is present (Fig. 2-104).

• **Resistance Direction.** A traction force equal to the weight of the leg is applied to the femur when performing a screen test and additional resistance is applied for grades 4 and 5.

Alternatively, quadratus lumborum may be tested against gravity in standing. The therapist must ensure the contralateral hip abductors do not contract to depress the ipsilateral pelvis and elevate the iliac crest on the test side for quadratus lumborum.[18]

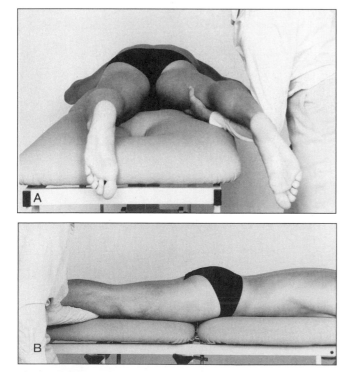

Figure 2-101.   Start position: quadratus lumborum.

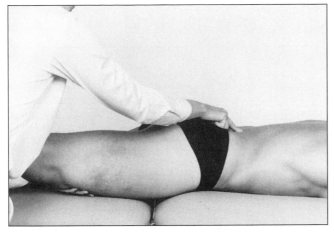

Figure 2-102. End position: quadratus lumborum.

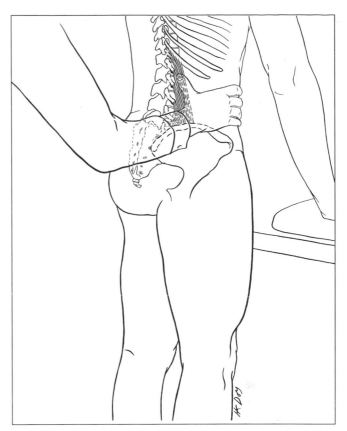

Figure 2-104. Quadratus lumborum.

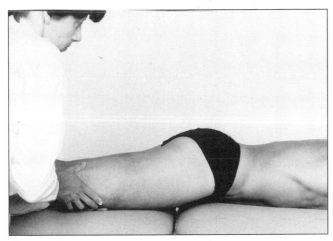

Figure 2-103. Resistance: quadratus lumborum.

JOINT FUNCTION

The trunk complex consists of the vertebral column, thorax, sternum, ribs, sacrum, and coccyx. The vertebral column and its system of linkages has particular significance in functional application of ROM and strength. The stability function of the spine includes resisting compressive forces; supporting the major portion of the body weight; supporting the head, arms, and trunk against the force of gravity; shock absorption; protection of the spinal cord; and providing a stable structure for movement of the extremities.[6,30]

The articulations at the intervertebral and facet joints of the vertebral column permit movement in flexion, extension, lateral flexion, and rotation to allow neck and back mobility. The functional range of the spine is increased by the tilt of the pelvis. The total motion of the spine is the result of the collective movements of the articulations of the various segments of the vertebral column[6,31,32] and functional ranges vary between individuals.[32] Restriction of motion at any level may result in increased motion at another level.[32] Mobility in all planes is the greatest at the cervical spine segment. The thoracic spine has limited mobility in all planes due to the limitations imposed by the thorax.[1,6,31] Through movements of the thoracic wall, intrathoracic volume is increased or decreased for inspiration and expiration. The lumbar spine is most mobile in the sagittal plane. Functional ROM is described for the cervical and the thoracic and lumbar spines.

FUNCTIONAL RANGE OF MOTION

Cervical Spine

The movement components of the cervical spine allow movement for functioning of the sense organs within the head[33] and expression of nonverbal communication, including affirmative (nodding) or negative responses. Maintenance of ROM in flexion, extension, lateral flexion, and rotation is of particular importance to the individual for interacting with the environment through the sense of vision. The significance of the interdependence between vision and neck movements is demonstrated in many self-care, leisure, and occupational tasks. Full ROM in all planes is not required for most self-care activities (Figs. 2-105 and 2-106). Ranges approximating full values may be required for such activities as shoulder checking in driving (lateral flexion and rotation) as illustrated in Figure 2-107, painting a ceiling, placing an object on a high shelf (Fig. 2-108), gazing at the stars (extension), and many specific leisure and occupational tasks linking vision and neck movements. When eye mobility is restricted greater cervical spine ROM may be required[34] or head posture may be affected[35] to accommodate for the restricted field of gaze.

Thoracic and Lumbar Spine

Rotation of the trunk is achieved through the movement components of the thoracic and lumbar spine and is coupled with slight lateral flexion.[16,30,32] Rotation is a movement that is most free in the upper spinal segments and progressively diminishes in the lower segments.[16] Rotation of the trunk extends the reach of the hands beyond the contralateral side of the body and permits the individual to face different directions without foot movement (Fig. 2-109).

The major contribution of the mobility in the lumbar spine to daily functioning is through flexion and extension movements. When combined with the thoracic and cervical segments, the individual is able to reach the more distal parts of the lower extremities and objects in the environment (Figs. 2-110 and 2-111). The final degrees of functional range are achieved through the interaction of the pelvis and hip.[6,31]

Coordination of movement in the lumbar and pelvic regions provides smooth movement and a large excursion of movement for the lower extremity and trunk. This special instance of coordinated pattern of movement between the lumbar spine and pelvis is called lumbar-pelvic rhythm[36] and occurs when forward flexing to touch the toes (see Figs. 2-78 and 2-79). The first part of the motion consists of lumbar flexion. This is followed by anterior tilting of the pelvis to complete the motion. On return to the upright position the pelvis tilts posteriorly followed by extension of the lumbar spine.

Normal ROM for lumbar spine flexion is about 60°.[37] Sitting to put on a sock (see Fig. 2-111) and squatting to pick up an object from the floor are examples of activities that require almost full lumbar spine flexion, that is, about 90% and 95% of full flexion, respectively.[37] Moving from standing to sitting and returning to standing position require about 56% to 66% of full lumbar flexion ROM.[37]

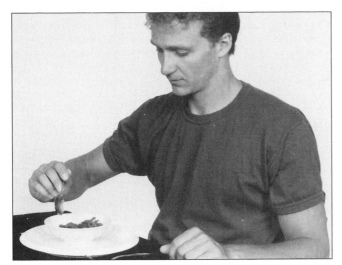

Figure 2-105. Eating: an activity requiring less than full neck flexion ROM.

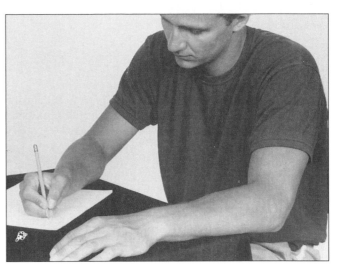

Figure 2-106. Writing at a desk: an activity requiring less than full neck flexion ROM.

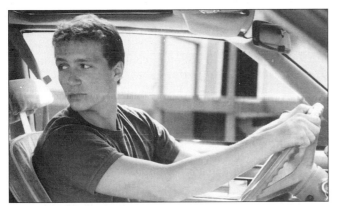

Figure 2-107. An activity requiring full neck rotation ROM.

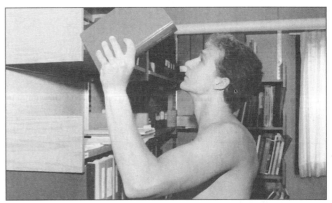

Figure 2-108. An activity requiring full extension ROM.

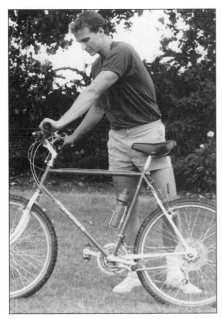

Figure 2-109. Trunk rotation.

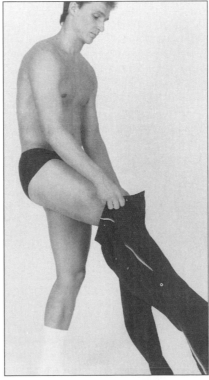

Figure 2-110. Trunk flexion.

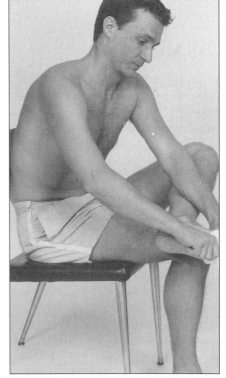

Figure 2-111. Lumbar flexion.

MUSCLE FUNCTION

Head and Neck

The muscles of the head and neck maintain the posture of the head, position the head to accommodate vision and feeding, and assist with breathing and coughing. Group muscle actions and some individual muscle actions of the head and neck are described relative to function.

Head and Neck Flexors. The longus colli, longus capitis, sternocleidomastoid, and scalenus anterior, medius, and posterior contracting bilaterally are the head and neck flexors. The sternocleidomastoids contracting bilaterally flex the cervical spine relative to the thoracic spine and flex the head if the prevertebral muscles contract to flatten the cervical spine and keep it rigid.[1] The scaleni muscles contracting bilaterally also flex the cervical spine on the thoracic spine when the prevertebral muscles hold the cervical spine rigid.[1] Chewing, swallowing and speaking are the main functions of the infrahyoid and suprahyoid muscles as these muscles act on the hyoid bone, mandible, and thyroid cartilage.[30] These muscles also flex the cervical spine when the masseter and temporalis muscles contract to keep the mandible closed.[1] The rectus capitis anterior and lateralis muscles contracting bilaterally, flex the head on the cervical spine.[1]

The head and neck flexors contract when flexion occurs against a resistance, such as the weight of the head. The flexors flex the head and neck and hold this position when the head is lifted off the supporting surface in the supine position, as illustrated in getting out of bed (Fig. 2-112). The flexors control neck extension when the head is lowered back onto the supporting surface when lying down supine. In upright postures, the head and neck flexors contract when flexion is full and forced. This combined action of the flexors occurs when one looks down to manipulate buttons at the top of a shirt and when doing up the clasp of a necklace at the back of the neck.

When eating, bilateral contraction of the sternoclei-domastoid pulls the head forward and assists the longus colli to flex the cervical spine.[2] Electromyographic study has demonstrated sufficient bilateral activity in the longus colli and sternocleidomastoid muscles on anterior protrusion of the head to maintain the head in this position[38] (Fig. 2-113).

Head and Neck Extensors. The extensor muscles of the head and neck include the semispinalis capitis and cervicis, splenius capitis and cervicis, rectus capitis posterior major and minor, obliquus capitis inferior and superior, and the erector spinae (ie, iliocostalis cervicis, longissimus capitis and cervicis, and spinalis capitis and cervicis muscles). The levator scapulae, sternocleidomastoid, and upper fibers of trapezius also act to extend the head and neck. The sternocleidomastoid contracting bilaterally acts as an extensor of the head and flexes the cervical spine on the thoracic spine when the cervical spine is flexible and not flattened and held rigid by the prevertebral muscles.[1] Unilateral contraction of sternocleidomastoid produces neck extension with lateral flexion to the same side and rotation to the opposite side.[1] The obliquus capitis inferior and superior and rectus capitis posterior major and minor, contracting bilaterally, extend the head and upper cervical spine.[1] Bilateral contraction of the head and neck extensor muscles produces neck extension eliminating the actions of lateral flexion and rotation that occur if these muscles contract unilaterally.

The head and neck extensors contract when extension is forced at the end of the ROM or occurs against a resistance. Activities carried out overhead require contraction of the extensors at the end of the ROM, such as, reaching for a book on a high shelf (Fig. 2-114). Other activities that require contraction at the end of the range of motion include drinking from a glass (see Fig. 5-174) and looking down the bowling lane as the bowling ball is released from the hand. The neck extensors contract and work against resistance to lift the head off the supporting surface when lying prone and control neck flexion when the head is lowered to the surface again. The ex-

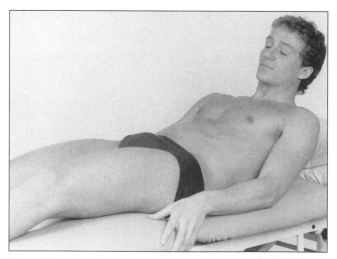

Figure 2-112.   Neck flexor and abdominal muscle function.

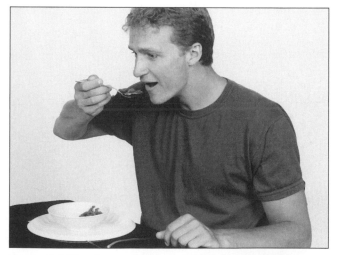

Figure 2-113.   Sternocleidomastoid and longus colli function to anteriorly protrude the head.

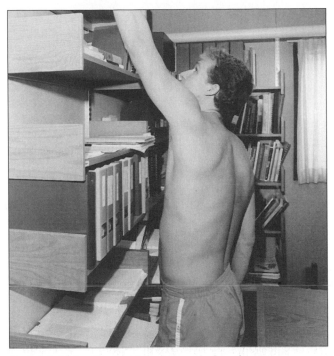

Figure 2-114.   Neck extensor muscle function.

that require placement of the hand at the back of the head, the cervical spine and head may be rotated.

Breathing.[30] Some of the muscles of the neck assist with breathing. Scalenus anterior, medius, and posterior are primary muscles of inspiration and elevate the first and second ribs when the cervical spine is fixed. Sternocleidomastoid, suprahyoid, and infrahyoid muscles act as accessory muscles of inspiration, being recruited on forceful breathing, for example, when exercising. Coughing requires contraction from the primary, accessory, and stabilizing muscles of respiration.

Posture. The position of the line of gravity anterior to the atlantooccipital joint of the neck produces a flexion moment that tends to cause the head to fall forward. Forward flexion of the head in sitting and standing is prevented by the contraction of the head and neck extensors. The weight of the head and the force of contraction of the neck extensors increases cervical lordosis.[39] The contraction of longus colli stabilizes and counteracts the forces tending to increase lordosis, thus maintaining the cervical lordosis.[39]

Trunk

The trunk muscles stabilize the thorax, pelvis, and spine for movements of the head and extremities, maintain posture, and assist with breathing, coughing, and straining. The abdominals support and protect the abdominal viscera. The trunk muscles contribute to a normal walking pattern and contract to protect the spine in lifting activities.

Trunk Flexion. The psoas major muscle and the abdominal and erector spinae muscle groups are responsible for trunk flexion. The abdominal muscles contract when trunk flexion is performed against a resistance, such as, body weight. The abdominal muscles are therefore the prime movers when one rises from the supine position to get out of bed (see Fig. 2-112). In the supine position the rectus abdominis is the most active abdominal muscle when the head is raised,[40] contracting to stabilize the thorax. The abdominal muscles contract isometrically and function to stabilize the thorax and pelvis when performing pushing, pulling, or lifting activities.[6]

Flexion of the trunk in standing position occurs as one picks up an object from the floor or ties a shoelace. Trunk flexion is initiated by contraction of the abdominals and the vertebral portion of the psoas major muscle.[32] Once the trunk is inclined forward gravity takes over to flex the trunk. Flexion of the trunk is then controlled through contraction of the erector spinae muscle until a "critical position" is reached when the erector spinae muscle relaxes and further flexion occurs through hip flexion.[41] The posterior layer of the thoracolumbar fascia,[42] elastic forces generated in the extensor musculature as a result of the passive stretch on the muscles,[43] and the posterior intervertebral ligaments support the trunk in the fully flexed position when the erector spinae is relaxed. Wolf and coworkers[44] identify the critical

tensors contract in activities where the head is inclined forward, such as writing (see Fig. 2-106) and reading.[30] Activity in the neck extensors ceases when the neck becomes fully flexed and the tension in the ligamentum nuchae maintains the position of the head.[30]

Head and Neck Lateral Flexors. Unilateral contraction of the head and neck extensors and many of the head and neck flexors laterally flex the head and neck to the same side. Functionally these muscles contract to laterally flex the cervical spine and position and control the tilt of the head so that one can correctly see objects that are not level. The lateral flexors can contract to position the head and assist in realigning the body in the upright posture from either a recumbent or inverted posture. The lateral flexors contract to hold the head in position when one moves from a side-lying position to a sitting position to get out of bed.

Head and Neck Rotators. The rectus capitis major and minor, obliquus capitis superior and inferior, sternocleidomastoid, scalenus anterior, medius and posterior, upper fibers of trapezius, semispinalis cervicis, splenius capitis and cervicis, multifidus, rotatores and the erector spinae (ie, iliocostalis cervicis and longissimus capitis and cervicis) muscles rotate the head and neck when contraction occurs unilaterally. The main function of the rotators is to rotate the head and neck to look from side to side as one would do to shoulder check when driving (see Fig. 2-107) or track the ball during a tennis match. In rolling from supine to side lie or prone lie positions the movement of the trunk may be initiated by rotating the head and neck in the direction of the move. The rotators contract when indicating a negative response to a question. When performing activities, such as combing the hair, position to be at greater than 70° of trunk flexion, most often between 80° and 90°. If further trunk flexion is required at the end of the movement, the abdominal muscles must contract to force the movement.[45]

Trunk Extension. The erector spinae muscle contracts to initiate trunk extension in the standing position and once started gravity pulls the trunk into further extension and the movement is controlled by the contraction of the abdominal muscles.[32] The erector spinae contracts again, if required, to force extension at the end of the ROM.[32] When extension is performed against resistance, the erector spinae muscle contracts to perform the entire movement. This is illustrated when in the prone position the trunk is extended to reach for a light switch located at the head of the bed.

When lifting objects off the floor from a forward flexed position, the pattern of muscle activity is the reverse of that required to flex forward in standing. There is no contraction of the erector spinae muscles at the beginning of the lift, the thoracolumbar fascia, elastic forces generated in the extensor musculature, and the posterior intervertebral ligaments take the load and the movement to extend occurs initially at the hip joints, as the pelvis rotates posteriorly. As the movement continues the erector spinae muscle contracts close to the critical position and the contraction continues until the erect position is reached.[41] Great forces are placed on the trunk when lifting in the forward flexed position; therefore, this position should be discouraged and the lift performed with the back straight and the knees flexed[46] with the object being lifted positioned as close to the body as possible. When heavy weights are lifted and large forces are placed on the spine, the abdominal (primarily the transversus abdominus[47]), diaphragm, and intercostal muscles contract to increase the intra-abdominal and intrathoracic pressures so that the thorax and abdomen become semirigid cylinders.[48] This results in some of the force from the weight being transmitted through the arms to the thorax and abdomen and then to the pelvis, taking some of the load off the spine.[48] This also results in additional trunk stabilization and an extensor moment is applied to the lumbar spine[47] through activation of the transversus abdominus and subsequent increased tension in the thoracolumbar fascia.

Trunk Lateral Flexion. The erector spinae, intertransversarii, and posterolateral fibers of the external abdominal oblique, quadratus lumborum, and iliopsoas muscles contribute to lateral flexion of the trunk. Lateral flexion is not used often in activities unless to pick an object up from a low table at one's side or when moving from a side-lying position to sitting on the edge of a bed or sitting to a side-lying position. The lateral flexors contract on the ipsilateral side to initiate movement and contract on the contralateral side to modify the movement in the upright position.[32]

Trunk Rotation. The trunk rotator muscles include the erector spinae, multifidus, rotatores, and internal and external abdominal oblique muscles. The internal and ex-ternal abdominal obliques are the prime rotators of the trunk.[49] The extensor muscles function to counteract the flexion torque created by the oblique abdominal muscles during trunk rotation.[49] The muscles contract to rotate the trunk to change position while recumbent and when one turns to look in a posterior direction.

Posture. Electromyographic studies report slight activity in the erector spinae muscle[41] and slight contraction in the internal abdominal oblique muscle[40] in standing. The erector spinae contracts during unsupported upright sitting but is relaxed when sitting in the "slumped" position with the spine in full flexion.[41]

Breathing. The erector spinae is active during inspiration when ventilatory demand is increased.[50] With an increased inspiratory effort, forces are transmitted to the spine through the costovertebral and costotransverse articulations encouraging flexion of the spine. Spinal flexion will cause a deflationary effect on the rib cage. This deflationary effect is counteracted by the erector spinae contracting to stiffen and extend the vertebral column.

The abdominal muscles are inactive during expiration at rest. When ventilatory demands increase, the abdominal muscles (rectus abdominus, external abdominal oblique, internal abdominal oblique, transversus abdominus) contract to pull the rib cage down and increase the intra-abdominal pressure, thus pushing the abdominal contents and diaphragm upward into the thoracic cavity, decreasing the lung volume to expel air.[51]

Gait.[6] As the pelvis rotates forward on the side of the advancing leg the upper trunk rotates forward on the opposite side to decrease the motion of the body during the gait cycle. The erector spinae muscles contract on the contralateral side to the supporting leg to prevent the trunk falling forward due to the hip flexion moment created on the stance leg. The erector spinae muscles contract at initial contact and preswing. The abdominal muscles do not normally contract when walking on the level.[52]

REFERENCES

1. Kapandji IA. *The Physiology of the Joints.* Vol 3. 2nd ed. London: Churchill Livingstone; 1974.
2. Soames RW, ed. Skeletal system. Salmons S, ed. Muscle. *Gray's Anatomy.* 38th ed. New York: Churchill Livingstone; 1995.
3. Hertling D. The temporomandibular joint. In: Hertling D, Kessler RM. *Management of Common Musculoskeletal Disorders: Physical Therapy Principles and Methods.* 3rd ed. Philadelphia: Harper & Row: 1996.
4. Magee DJ. *Orthopedic Physical Assessment.* 3rd ed. Philadelphia: WB Saunders; 1997.
5. Cyriax J. *Textbook of Orthopaedic Medicine, Vol 1. Diagnosis of Soft Tissue Lesions.* 8th ed. London: Bailliere Tindall; 1982.
6. Norkin CC, Levangie PK. *Joint Structure & Function: A Comprehensive Analysis.* 2nd ed. Philadelphia: FA Davis; 1992.
7. Daniels L, Worthingham C. *Muscle Testing: Technique of Manual Examination.* 5th ed. Philadelphia: WB Saunders; 1986.

8. Hoppenfeld S. *Physical Examination of the Spine and Extremities.* New York: Appelton-Century-Crofts; 1976.
9. Norkin CC, White DJ. *Measurement of Joint Motion: A Guide to Goniometry.* 2nd ed. Philadelphia: FA Davis; 1995.
10. Thurnwald PA. The effect of age and gender on normal temporomandibular joint movement. *Physiotherapy Theory and Practice.* 1991;7:209–221.
11. American Academy of Orthopaedic Surgeons. *Joint Motion: Method of Measuring and Recording.* Chicago: Author; 1965.
12. Hislop HJ, Montgomery J. *Daniels and Worthingham's Muscle Testing: Techniques of Manual Examination.* 6th ed. Philadelphia: WB Saunders; 1995.
13. Moore KL. *Clinically Oriented Anatomy.* Baltimore: Williams & Wilkins; 1980.
14. Gilroy J, Holliday PL. *Basic Neurology.* New York: MacMillan, 1982.
15. Mancall EL. *Alpers and Mancall's Essentials of the Neurologic Examination.* 2nd ed. Philadelphia: FA Davis; 1981.
16. MacConaill MA, Basmajian JV. *Muscles and Movements: A Basis for Human Kinesiology.* Huntington, NY: RE Krieger; 1977.
17. Kendall FP, McCreary EK, Provance PG. *Muscles Testing and Function.* 4th ed. Baltimore: Williams & Wilkins; 1993.
18. Kendall FP, McCreary EK. *Muscles Testing and Function.* 3rd ed. Baltimore: Williams & Wilkins; 1983.
19. White AA, Panjabi MM. *Clinical Biomechanics of the Spine.* Philadelphia: JB Lippincott; 1978.
20. Rodnan GP, Schumacher HR, eds. *Primer on the Rheumatic Diseases.* 8th ed. Atlanta, GA: Arthritis Foundation; 1983.
21. Harris J, Johansen J, Pedersen S, LaPier TK. Site of measurement and subject position affect chest expansion measurements. *Cardiopulmonary Physical Therapy.* 1997; 8:12–17.
22. Moll JMH, Wright V. An objective clinical study of chest expansion. *Ann Rheum Dis.* 1972;31:1–8.
23. Neustadt DH. Ankylosing spondylitis. *Postgrad Med.* 1977;61:124–135.
24. Beim GM, Giraldo JL, Pincivero DM, Borror MJ, Fu FH. Abdominal strengthening exercises: a comparative EMG study. *J Sport Rehabil.* 1997;6:11–20.
25. Flint MM. An electromyographic comparison of the function of the iliacus and the rectus abdominis muscles. *J Am Phys Ther Assoc.* 1965;45:248–253.
26. Shirado O, Toshikazu I, Kaneda K, Strax TE. Electromyographic analysis of four techniques for isometric trunk muscle exercises. *Arch Phys Med Rehabil.* 1995;76: 225–229.
27. Norris CM. Abdominal muscle training in sport. *Br J Sports Med.* 1993;27:19–27.
28. Gilleard WL, Brown JMM. An electromyographic validation of an abdominal muscle test. *Arch Phys Med Rehabil.* 1994;75:1002–1007.
29. Graves JE, Webb DC, Pollock ML, et al. Pelvic stabilization during resistance training: its effect on the development of lumbar extension strength. *Arch Phys Med Rehabil.* 1994;75:210–215.
30. Smith LK, Weiss EL, Lemkuhl LD. *Brunnstrom's Clinical Kinesiology.* 5th ed. Philadelphia: FA Davis; 1996.
31. Soderberg GL. *Kinesiology: Application to Pathological Motion.* 2nd ed. Baltimore: Williams & Wilkins; 1997.
32. Lindh M. Biomechanics of the lumbar spine. In: Nordin M, Frankel VH. *Basic Biomechanics of the Musculoskeletal System.* 2nd ed. Philadelphia: Lea & Febiger; 1989.
33. Cailliet R. *Neck and Arm Pain.* 3rd ed. Philadelphia: FA Davis; 1991.
34. Hutton JT, Shapiro I, Christians B. Functional significance of restricted gaze. *Arch Phys Med Rehabil.* 1982; 63:617–619.
35. Muñoz M. Congenital absence of the Inferior rectus muscle. *Am J Opthalmol.* 1992;121:327–329.
36. Cailliet R. *Low Back Pain Syndrome.* 5th ed. Philadelphia: FA Davis; 1995.
37. Hsieh CJ, Pringle RK. Range of motion of the lumbar spine required for four activities of daily living. *J Manipulative Physiol Therap.* 1994;17:353–358.
38. Vitti M, Fujiwara M, Basmajian JV, Iida M. The integrated roles of longus colli and sternomastoid muscles: an electromyographic study. *Anat Rec.* 1973;177:471–484.
39. Mayoux-Benhamou MA, Revel M, Vallée C, Roudier R, Barbet JP, Bargy F. Longus colli has a postural function on cervical curvature. *Surg Radiol Anat.* 1994;16: 367–371.
40. Carman DJ, Blanton PL, Biggs NL. Electromyographic study of the anterolateral abdominal musculature utilizing indwelling electrodes. *Am J Phys Med.* 1972;51: 113 129.
41. Floyd WF, Silver PHS. The function of the erectores spinae muscles in certain movements and postures in man. *J Physiol.* 1955;129:184–203.
42. Bogduk N, MacIntosh JE. The applied anatomy of the thoracolumbar fascia. *Spine.* 1984;9:164–170.
43. McGill SM, Kippers V. Transfer of loads between lumbar tissues during the flexion-relaxation phenomenon. *Spine.* 1994;19:2190–2196.
44. Wolf SL, Basmajian JV, Russe TC, Kutner M. Normative data on low back mobility and activity levels. *Am J Phys Med.* 1979;58:217–229.
45. Basmajian JV, DeLuca CJ. *Muscles Alive: Their Functions Revealed by Electromyography.* 5th ed. Baltimore: Williams & Wilkins; 1985.
46. Davis PR, Troup JDG, Burnard JH. Movements of the thoracic and lumbar spine when lifting: a chrono-cyclophotographic study. *J Anat (Lond).* 1965;99:13–26.
47. Cresswell AG, Thorstensson A. Changes in intra-abdominal pressure, trunk muscle activation and force during isokinetic lifting and lowering. *Eur J Appl Physiol.* 1994;68:315–321.
48. Morris JM, Lucas DB, Bresler B. Role of the trunk in stability of the spine. *J Bone Jt Surg.* 1961;43A:327–351.
49. MacIntosh JE, Pearcy MJ, Bogduk N. The axial torque of the lumbar back muscles: torsion strength of the back muscles. *Aust N Z J Surg.* 1993;63:205–212.
50. Cala SJ, Edyvean J, Engel LA. Chest wall and trunk muscle activity during inspiratory loading. *J Appl Physiol.* 1992;73:2373–2381.
51. Epstein SK. An overview of respiratory muscle function. *Clin Chest Med.* 1994;15:619–639.
52. Sheffield FJ. Electromyographic study of the abdominal muscles in walking and other movements. *Am J Phys Med.* 1962;41:142–147.

SHOULDER COMPLEX

▼ SURFACE ANATOMY (Figs. 3-1, 3-2, and 3-3)

Structure	Location
1. Inion	Dome-shaped process that marks the center of the superior nuchal line.
2. Vertebral border of the scapula	Approximately 5 to 6 cm lateral to the thoracic spinous processes covering ribs 2 to 7.
3. Inferior angle of the scapula	At the inferior aspect of the vertebral border of the scapula.
4. Spine of the scapula	The bony ridge running obliquely across the upper four fifths of the scapula.
5. Acromion process	Lateral aspect of the spine of the scapula at the tip of the shoulder.
6. Clavicle	Prominent S-shaped bone on the anterosuperior aspect of the thorax.
7. Coracoid process	Approximately 2 cm distal to the junction of the middle and lateral thirds of the clavicle in the deltopectoral triangle. Press firmly upward and laterally, deep to the anterior fibers of the deltoid.
8. Brachial pulse	Palpate pulse on the medial, proximal aspect of the upper arm posterior to coracobrachialis.
9. Lateral epicondyle of the humerus	Lateral projection at the distal end of the humerus.
10. Olecranon process of the ulna	Posterior aspect of the elbow at the proximal end of the shaft of the ulna.
11. T12 spinous process	The most distal thoracic spinous process slightly above the level of the olecranon process of the ulna when the body is in the anatomical position.

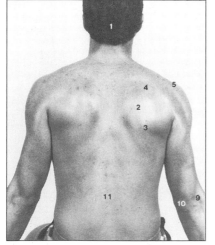

Figure 3-1. Posterior aspect of the shoulder complex.

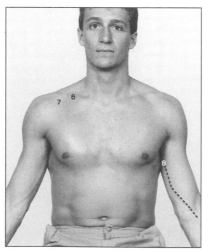

Figure 3-2. Anterior aspect of the shoulder complex.

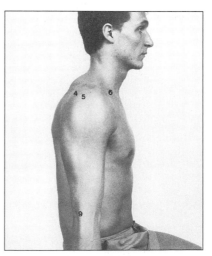

Figure 3-3. Lateral aspect of the shoulder complex.

▼ ASSESSMENT PROCESS: THE SHOULDER COMPLEX

1. The therapist observes:
   a. Function
   b. Posture, body symmetry, atrophy, and skin condition
   c. Active range of movement (AROM) at the scapula, shoulder, and elbow. Restricted motion at the sternoclavicular and acromioclavicular joints will affect motion of the shoulder complex.
2. The therapist assesses passive range of motion (PROM) by:
   a. Estimating joint PROM
   b. Determining the end feels at the joint
   c. Establishing the presence or absence of pain
   d. Determining the presence of a capsular or noncapsular pattern
3. The therapist measures PROM through goniometry.
4. The therapist assesses muscle strength through manual muscle testing.

	Elevation	Depression	Abduction (Protraction)	Adduction (Retraction)
Articulation[1,2]	Scapulothoracic Acromioclavicular Sternoclavicular	Scapulothoracic Acromioclavicular Sternoclavicular	Scapulothoracic Acromioclavicular Sternoclavicular	Scapulothoracic Acromioclavicular Sternoclavicular
Plane	Frontal	Frontal	Horizontal	Horizontal
Axis	Sagittal	Sagittal	Vertical	Vertical
Normal limiting factors[1,3–6]	Tension in the costoclavicular ligament, inferior sternoclavicular joint capsule, lower fibers of trapezius, pectoralis minor, and subclavius	Tension in the interclavicular ligament, sternoclavicular ligament, articular disk, upper fibers of trapezius, and levator scapulae; bony contact between the clavicle and the superior aspect of the first rib	Tension in the trapezoid ligament, posterior sternoclavicular ligament, posterior lamina of the costoclavicular ligament, trapezius, and rhomboids	Tension in the conoid ligament, anterior lamina of the costoclavicular ligament, anterior sternoclavicular ligament, pectoralis minor, and serratus anterior
Normal end feel[3,7,8]	Firm	Firm/hard	Firm	Firm
Normal active range of motion[1]	10–12 cm (total range for elevation—depression)		15 cm (total range for abduction—adduction)	

	Medial Rotation (Downward Rotation)	Lateral Rotation (Upward Rotation)
Articulation[1,2]	Scapulothoracic Acromioclavicular Sternoclavicular	Scapulothoracic Acromioclavicular Sternoclavicular
Plane	Frontal	Frontal
Axis	Sagittal	Sagittal
Normal limiting factors[1,3–6]	Tension in the conoid ligament and serratus anterior	Tension in the trapezoid ligament, the rhomboid muscles, and the levator scapulae
Normal end feel[3,7,8]	Firm	Firm
Normal active range of motion[1]	60° displacement of inferior angle is 10–12 cm (total range for medial–lateral rotation)	

Note: Medial and lateral rotations of the scapula are associated with extension and/or adduction and flexion and/or abduction of the shoulder, respectively.

▼ RANGE OF MOTION ASSESSMENT AND MEASUREMENT

The articulations of the shoulder complex and the joint axes of the scapula and glenohumeral joint are illustrated in Figures 3-4 through 3-7.

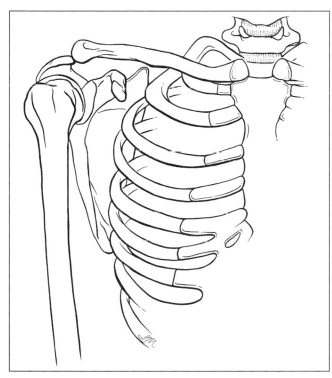

Figure 3-4. Shoulder complex articulations.

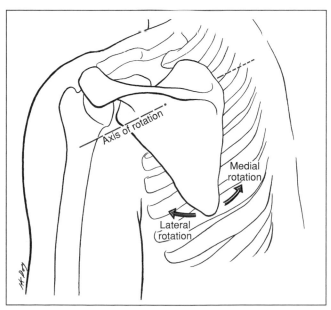

Figure 3-5. Scapular axis of rotation.

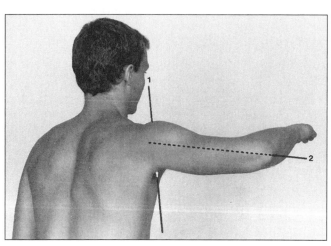

Figure 3-6. Glenohumeral axes: (*1*) horizontal abduction-adduction; (*2*) internal-external rotation.

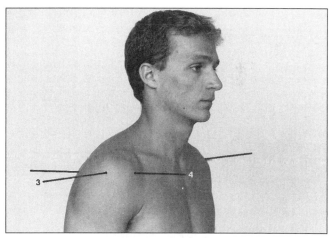

Figure 3-7. Glenohumeral axes: (*3*) flexion-extension; (*4*) abduction-adduction.

GENERAL SCAN: UPPER EXTREMITY ACTIVE RANGE OF MOTION

The AROM of the upper extremity joints is scanned, starting with the patient in the sitting or standing position with the arms at the sides (Fig. 3-8). The patient places the left hand behind the neck, then reaches down the spine to the limit of movement (Fig. 3-9A). The therapist observes the ROM of scapular abduction and lateral rotation, shoulder elevation and external rotation, elbow flexion, forearm supination, wrist radial deviation, and finger extension. The patient places the right hand on the low back, then reaches up the spine to the limit of movement (see Fig. 3-9A). The therapist observes the ROM of scapular adduction and medial rotation, shoulder extension and internal rotation, elbow flexion, forearm pronation, wrist radial deviation, and finger extension. The vertebral levels reached at the levels of the tips of the middle fingers as the patient reaches behind the neck or up the back, may be used as a measure of AROM of the upper extremity joints.

The patient returns to the start position and the scan is carried out as the patient places the right hand behind the neck, then reaches down the spine to the limit of movement and places the left hand on the low back, then reaches up the spine to the limit of movement (Fig. 3-9B). There is often an appreciable difference in the ROM between sides, as shown in Figure 3-9.

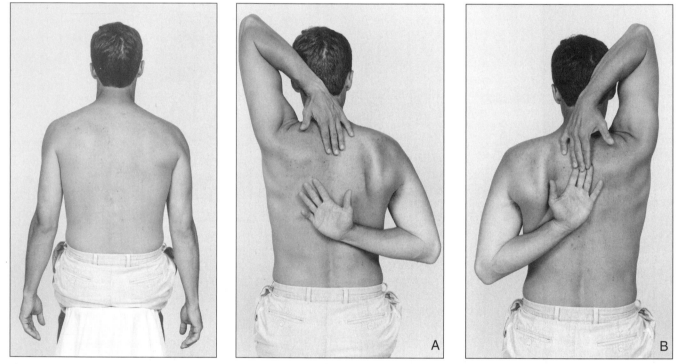

Figure 3-8. Start position: scan of AROM of the upper extremities.

Figure 3-9. End positions: scan of AROM of the upper extremities.

SCAPULAR MOVEMENTS (TABLE 3-1)

Scapular movement is assessed by visual observation of active movement and through passive movement. The ROM is estimated as either "full" or "restricted."

Active Movement

• **Start Position.** The patient is sitting and assumes a relaxed, anatomical posture (Fig. 3-10). The therapist observes the motions from behind the patient.

Active Movement: Scapular Elevation

• **Movement.** The patient moves the shoulders toward the ears in an upward or cranial direction (Fig. 3-11).

Active Movement: Scapular Depression

• **Movement.** The patient moves the shoulders toward the waist in a downward or caudal direction (Fig. 3-12).

Active Movement: Scapular Abduction

• **Movement.** From the start position, the patient flexes the arms to 90°, and scapular abduction is observed as the patient reaches forward (Fig. 3-13). The vertebral borders of the scapulae move away from the vertebral column.

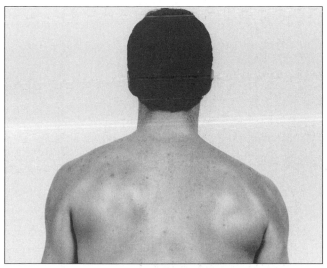

Figure 3-10.   Start position for all active scapular movements.

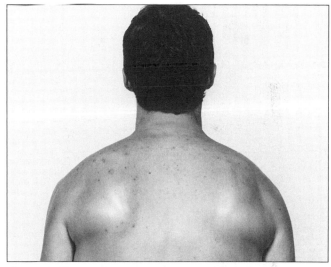

Figure 3-12.   Active movement: scapular depression.

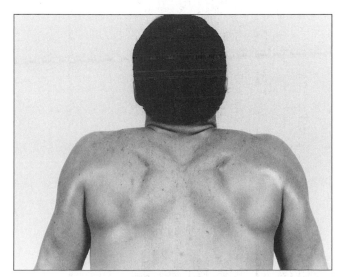

Figure 3-11.   Active movement: scapular elevation.

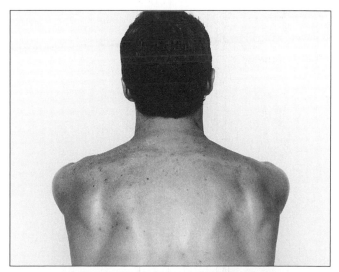

Figure 3-13.   Active movement: scapular abduction.

Active Movement: Scapular Adduction

• **Movement.** The patient moves the scapulae horizontally toward the vertebral column (Fig. 3-14).

Active Movement: Scapular Medial Rotation

• **Movement.** The patient extends and adducts the arm to place the hand across the small of the back and the inferior angle of the scapula moves in a medial direction (Fig. 3-15).

Active Movement: Scapular Lateral Rotation

• **Movement.** The patient elevates the arm through flexion or abduction (Fig. 3-16). During elevation, the inferior angle of the scapula moves in a lateral direction.

Passive Movement

• **Start Position.** The patient is in a side-lying position with the head relaxed and supported on a pillow. This position remains unchanged for all scapular movements.

• **Stabilization.** The weight of the trunk stabilizes the thorax.

Passive Movement: Scapular Elevation

• **Procedure.** The therapist's right hand cups the inferior angle of the scapula and elevates the scapula. The left hand assists in controlling the direction of movement (Fig. 3-17).

• **End Feel.** Firm.

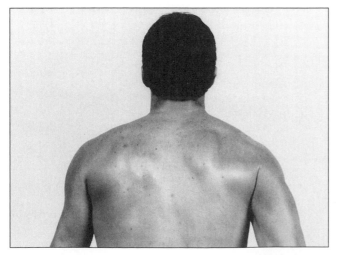

Figure 3-14.   Active movement: scapular adduction.

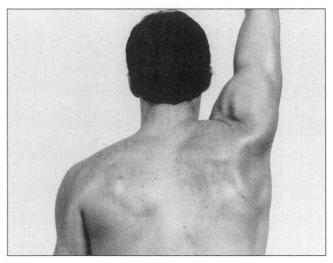

Figure 3-16.   Active movement: scapular lateral rotation.

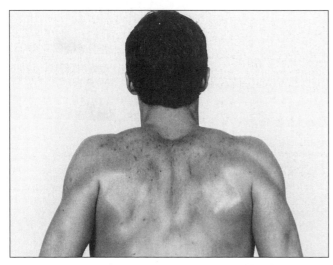

Figure 3-15.   Active movement: scapular medial rotation.

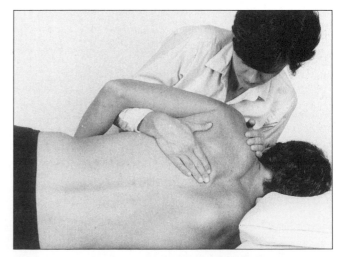

Figure 3-17.   Passive movement: scapular elevation.

Passive Movement: Scapular Depression

- **Procedure.** The therapist's left hand is placed on the top of the shoulder and depresses the scapula. The right hand cups the inferior angle of the scapula to control the direction of movement (Fig. 3-18).

- **End Feel.** Firm/hard.

Passive Movement: Scapular Abduction

- **Procedure.** The therapist uses the thumb and index finger of the right hand to grasp the vertebral border and inferior angle of the scapula and abducts the scapula. The therapist's left hand is placed on top of the shoulder to assist in abduction (Fig. 3-19).

- **End Feel.** Firm.

Passive Movement: Scapular Adduction

- **Procedure.** The therapist uses the thumb and index finger of the right hand to grasp the axillary border and inferior angle of the scapula and adducts the scapula. The therapist's left hand is placed on top of the shoulder to assist in adduction (Fig. 3-20).

- **End Feel.** Firm.

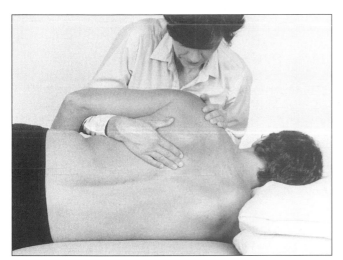

Figure 3-18.　Passive movement: scapular depression.

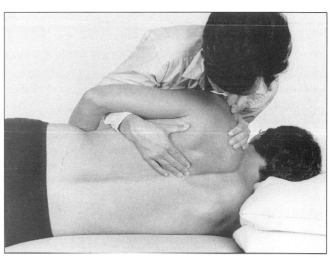

Figure 3-20.　Passive movement: scapular adduction.

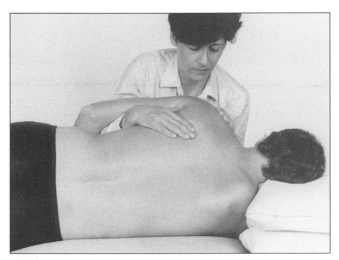

Figure 3-19.　Passive movement: scapular abduction.

SHOULDER COMPLEX— MOVEMENTS (TABLES 3-2 AND 3-3)

The sternoclavicular, acromioclavicular, scapulothoracic, and glenohumeral joints make up the shoulder complex (see Fig. 3-4). The shoulder complex can be divided into two components: (1) the shoulder girdle, which includes the sternoclavicular, acromioclavicular, and scapulothoracic joints, and (2) the glenohumeral joint. Restricted motion at the glenohumeral joint can be compensated for by movements at the shoulder gir-dle. Therefore, when assessing and measuring PROM it is important to differentiate between motion occurring at the shoulder girdle (scapular motion) and motion at the glenohumeral joint. To isolate the glenohumeral joint PROM, the therapist must stabilize the scapula and clavicle. To ensure adequate stabilization of the scapula and clavicle when performing PROM and measuring glenohumeral joint motion, a second therapist may assist to align the goniometer. To assess and measure movements that require motion at all articulations of the shoulder complex the trunk is stabilized.

TABLE 3-2 ▼ JOINT STRUCTURE: GLENOHUMERAL MOVEMENTS

	Extension	Internal Rotation	External Rotation	Horizontal Abduction	Horizontal Adduction
Articulation[1,2]	Glenohumeral	Glenohumeral	Glenohumeral	Glenohumeral	Glenohumeral
Plane	Sagittal	Horizontal	Horizontal	Horizontal	Horizontal
Axis	Frontal	Longitudinal	Longitudinal	Vertical	Vertical
Normal limiting factors[1,3–6]	Tension in the anterior band of the coracohumeral ligament, the anterior joint capsule, and clavicular fibers of pectoralis major	Tension in the posterior joint casule, infraspinatus, and teres minor	Tension in all bands of the glenohumeral ligament, coracohumeral ligament, the anterior joint capsule, subscapularis, pectoralis major, teres major, and latissimus dorsi	Tension in the anterior joint capsule, the glenohumeral ligament, and pectoralis major	Tension in the posterior joint capsule Soft tissue apposition
Normal end feel[3,7,8]	Firm	Firm	Firm	Firm	Firm/soft
Normal active range of motion[9]	0–60°	0–70°	0–90°	0–45°	0–135°

TABLE
3-3 ▼ JOINT STRUCTURE: SHOULDER COMPLEX MOVEMENTS

	Elevation Through Flexion	Elevation Through Abduction
Articulation[1,2]	Glenohumeral Acromioclavicular Sternoclavicular Scapulothoracic	Glenohumeral Acromioclavicular Sternoclavicular Scapulothoracic Subdeltoid[1]
Plane	Sagittal	Frontal
Axis	Frontal	Sagittal
Normal limiting factors[1,3–6]	Tension in the posterior band of the coracohumeral ligament, posterior joint capsule, shoulder extensors, and external rotators; scapular movement limited by tension in rhomboids, levator scapulae, and the trapezoid ligament	Tension in the middle and inferior bands of the glenohumeral ligament, inferior joint capsule, shoulder adductors; greater tuberosity of the humerus contacting the upper portion of the glenoid and glenoid labrum or the lateral surface of the acromion; scapular movement limited by tension in rhomboids, levator scapulae, and the trapezoid ligament
Normal end feel[3,7,8]	Firm	Firm/hard
Normal active range of motion[1,2,9]	0–180° 0–60°, glenohumeral 60–180°, glenohumeral, scapular movement, and trunk movement	0–180° 0–30°, glenohumeral 30–180°, glenohumeral, scapular movement, and trunk movement
Capsular pattern[7,8]	Glenohumeral: external rotation, abduction (only through 90–120° range), internal rotation Sternoclavicular/acromioclavicular: pain at extreme range of motion notably horizontal adduction and full elevation	

SHOULDER COMPLEX

SHOULDER ELEVATION THROUGH FLEXION (GLENOHUMERAL JOINT AND SCAPULAR MOTION)

AROM Assessment

• **Substitution/Trick Movement.** Trunk extension and shoulder abduction.

PROM Assessment

• **Start Position.** The patient is in crook-lying (Fig. 3-21) or a sitting position. The arm is at the side with the palm facing medially.

• **Stabilization.** The weight of the trunk. The therapist stabilizes the thorax.

• **Therapist's Distal Hand Placement.** The therapist grasps the distal humerus.

• **End Position.** The therapist applies slight traction to and moves the humerus anteriorly and upward to the limit of motion for shoulder elevation through flexion (Fig. 3-22). The elbow is maintained in extension to prevent restriction of shoulder flexion ROM due to passive insufficiency of the two-joint triceps muscle.[10]

• **End Feel.** Firm.

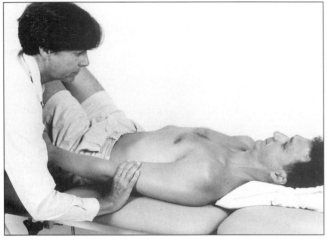

Figure 3-21. Start position for shoulder elevation through flexion.

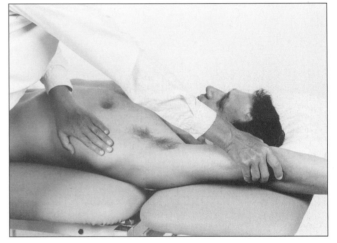

Figure 3-22. Firm end feel at limit of shoulder elevation through flexion.

Measurement: Universal Goniometer

- **Start Position.** The patient is in a crook-lying position (Fig. 3-23) or sitting (see Fig. 3-26). The arm is at the side, with the palm facing medially.

- **Stabilization.** The weight of the trunk. The scapula is left free to move.

- **Goniometer Axis.** The axis is placed at the lateral aspect of the center of the humeral head, about 2.5 cm inferior to the lateral aspect of the acromion process.

- **Stationary Arm.** Parallel to the lateral midline of the trunk.

- **Movable Arm.** Parallel to the longitudinal axis of the humerus.

- **End Position** The humerus is moved in an anterior and upward direction to the limit of motion in elevation (180°). This movement represents scapular and glenohumeral motion (Fig. 3-24).

GLENOHUMERAL JOINT FLEXION

AROM Assessment. The patient is not able to perform isolated glenohumeral joint flexion ROM without the scapula being stabilized.

PROM Assessment

- **Start Position.** The patient is in crook-lying (see Fig. 3-21) or a sitting position. The arm is at the side with the palm facing medially.

- **Stabilization.** The therapist places one hand on the axillary border of the scapula to stabilize the scapula.

- **Therapist's Distal Hand Placement.** The therapist grasps the distal humerus.

- **End Position.** While stabilizing the scapula, the therapist applies slight traction to and moves the humerus anteriorly and upward to the limit of motion to assess glenohumeral joint motion (Fig. 3-25).

- **End Feel.** Firm.

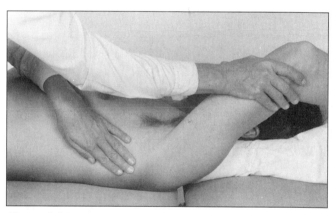

Figure 3-25.   Firm end feel at limit of glenohumeral joint flexion.

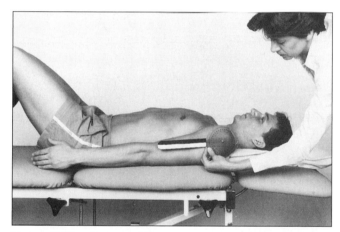

Figure 3-23.   Start position for shoulder elevation through flexion: supine.

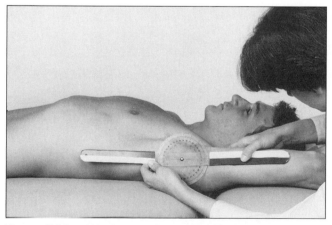

Figure 3-24.   Shoulder elevation through flexion.

Measurement: Universal Goniometer

• **Start Position.** The patient is in sitting (Fig. 3-26) or crook-lying. The arm is at the side, with the palm facing medially.

• **Stabilization.** The therapist stabilizes the scapula and clavicle.

• **Goniometer Axis.** The axis is placed at the lateral aspect of the center of the humeral head, about 2.5 cm inferior to the lateral aspect of the acromion process.

• **Stationary Arm.** Parallel to the lateral midline of the trunk.

• **Movable Arm.** Parallel to the longitudinal axis of the humerus.

• **End Position.** The humerus is moved in an anterior and upward direction to the limit of motion ($120°^5$) to measure glenohumeral joint flexion (Fig. 3-27).

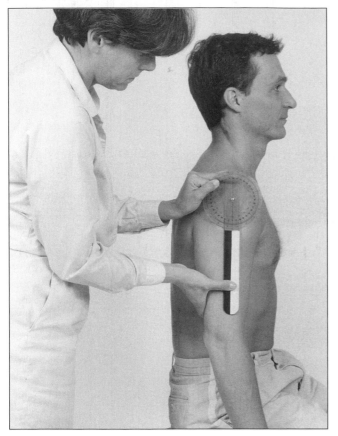

Figure 3-26.   Start position for shoulder elevation through flexion: sitting.

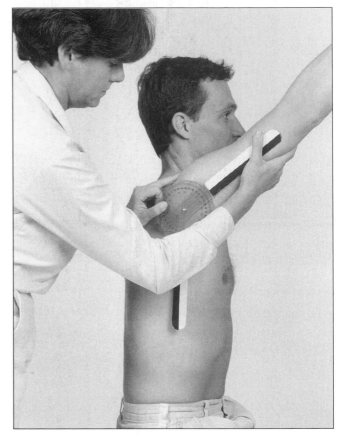

Figure 3-27.   Glenohumeral joint flexion ROM.

SHOULDER EXTENSION

AROM Assessment

• **Substitution/Trick Movement.** Scapular anterior tilting, scapular elevation and shoulder abduction. In sitting, the patient may flex and ipsilaterally rotate the trunk.

PROM Assessment

• **Start Position.** The patient is prone (Fig. 3-28) or sitting. The arm is at the side, with the palm facing medially.

• **Stabilization.** The therapist stabilizes the scapula to isolate and assess glenohumeral joint motion.

• **Therapist's Distal Hand Placement.** The therapist grasps the distal humerus.

• **End Position.** The therapist applies slight traction to and moves the humerus posteriorly until the scapula begins to move (Fig. 3-29). The elbow is flexed to prevent restriction of shoulder extension ROM due to passive insufficiency of the two-joint biceps brachii muscle.[10]

• **End Feel.** Firm.

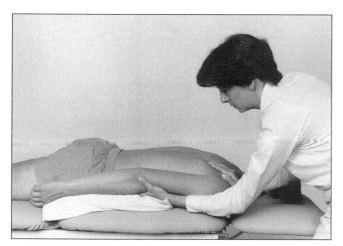

Figure 3-28. Start position for glenohumeral joint extension.

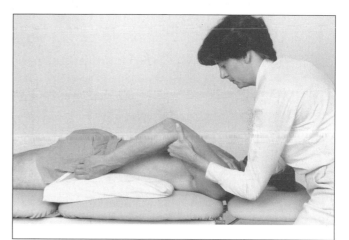

Figure 3-29. Firm end feel at limit of glenohumeral joint extension.

Measurement: Universal Goniometer

- **Start Position.** The patient is prone (Fig. 3-30) or sitting. The arm is at the side, with the palm facing medially.

- **Stabilization.** The therapist's forearm may be used to stabilize the scapula.

- **Goniometer Axis.** The axis is placed at the lateral aspect of the center of the humeral head, about 2.5 cm inferior to the lateral aspect of the acromion process.

- **Stationary Arm.** Parallel to the lateral midline of the trunk.

- **Movable Arm.** Parallel to the longitudinal axis of the humerus, pointing toward the lateral epicondyle of the humerus.

- **End Position.** The humerus is moved posteriorly to the limit of motion (60°) (Figs. 3-31 and 3-32).

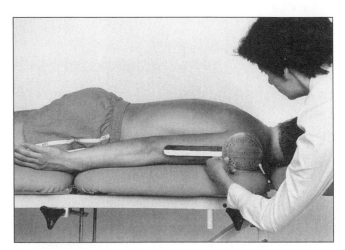

Figure 3-30.   Start position for shoulder extension.

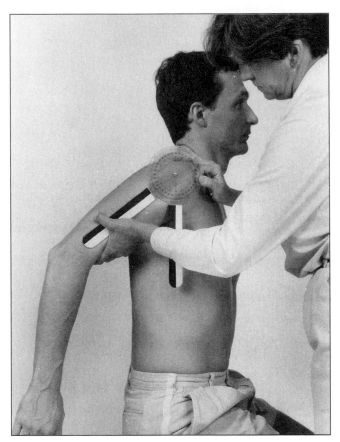

Figure 3-32.   Shoulder extension: sitting.

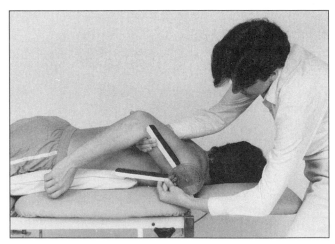

Figure 3-31.   Shoulder extension: prone.

SHOULDER ELEVATION THROUGH ABDUCTION (GLENOHUMERAL JOINT AND SCAPULAR MOTION)

AROM Assessment

• **Substitution/Trick Movement.** Contralateral trunk side flexion, scapular elevation, and shoulder flexion.

PROM Assessment. The humerus is externally rotated when performing shoulder elevation through abduction to allow the greater tuberosity of the humerus to clear the acromion process. Before testing elevation through abduction, ensure the patient is capable of full shoulder external rotation.

• **Start Position.** The patient is sitting (Fig. 3-33) or supine. The arm is at the side with the shoulder in external rotation.

• **Stabilization.** The therapist stabilizes the trunk.

• **Therapist's Distal Hand Placement.** The therapist grasps the distal humerus.

• **End Position** The therapist applies slight traction to and moves the humerus laterally and upward to the limit of motion for elevation through abduction (Fig. 3-34).

• **End Feel.** Firm.

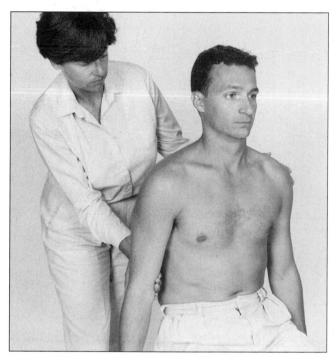

Figure 3-33.   Start position for shoulder elevation through abduction.

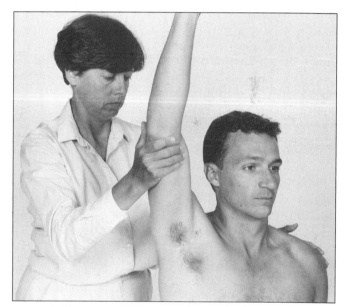

Figure 3-34.   Firm end feel at limit of shoulder elevation through abduction.

Measurement: Universal Goniometer

• **Start Position.** The patient is supine (Fig. 3-35) or sitting. The arm is at the side in adduction and external rotation.

• **Stabilization.** The weight of the trunk.

• **Goniometer Axis.** The axis is placed at the midpoint of the anterior or posterior aspect of the glenohumeral joint, about 1.3 cm inferior and lateral to the coracoid process (Fig. 3-36).The posterior aspect may be preferred for measurement of this range in women because the breast may interfere with the goniometer placement anteriorly (Fig. 3-38).

• **Stationary Arm.** Parallel to the sternum.

• **Movable Arm.** Parallel to the longitudinal axis of the humerus.

• **End Position.** The humerus is moved laterally and upward to the limit of motion in elevation (180°) (Fig. 3-37). This movement represents scapular and glenohumeral movement.

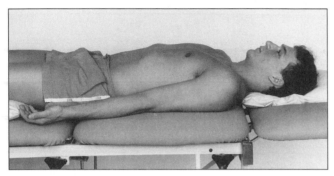

Figure 3-35.   Start position for shoulder elevation through abduction.

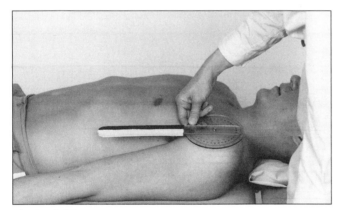

Figure 3-36.   Goniometer placement for shoulder elevation through abduction.

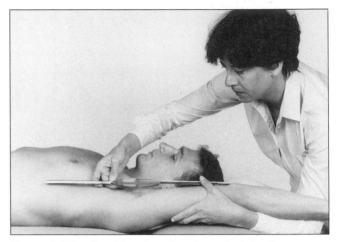

Figure 3-37.   Shoulder elevation through abduction.

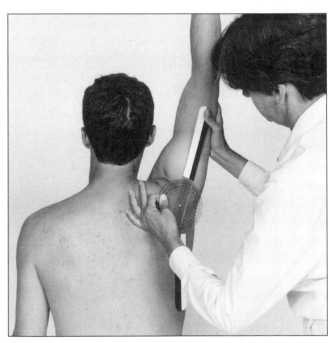

Figure 3-38.   Shoulder elevation through abduction: sitting.

GLENOHUMERAL JOINT ABDUCTION

AROM Assessment. The patient is not able to perform isolated glenohumeral joint abduction ROM without the scapula being stabilized.

PROM Assessment

• Start Position. The patient is supine (Fig. 3-39) or sitting. The arm is at the side with the elbow flexed to 90°.

• Stabilization. The therapist stabilizes the scapula and clavicle.

• Therapist's Distal Hand Placement. The therapist grasps the distal humerus.

• End Position. The therapist applies slight traction to and moves the humerus laterally and upward to the limit of motion of glenohumeral joint abduction (Fig. 3-40).

• End Feel. Firm or hard.

Measurement: Universal Goniometer (not shown)

• Start Position. The patient is supine or sitting. The arm is at the side with the elbow flexed to 90° (see Fig. 3-39).

• Stabilization. The therapist stabilizes the scapula and clavicle to isolate and measure glenohumeral joint abduction.

• Goniometer Axis. The axis is placed at the midpoint of the anterior or posterior aspect of the glenohumeral joint, about 1.3 cm inferior and lateral to the coracoid process (see Fig. 3-36).

• Stationary Arm. Parallel to the sternum.

• Movable Arm. Parallel to the longitudinal axis of the humerus.

• End Position. The humerus is moved laterally and upward to the limit of motion (90–120°[5]) to measure glenohumeral joint abduction.

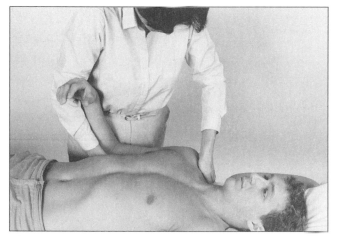

Figure 3-39. Start position for glenohumeral joint abduction.

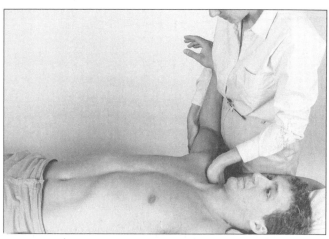

Figure 3-40. Firm or hard end feel at limit of glenohumeral joint abduction.

SHOULDER HORIZONTAL ABDUCTION AND ADDUCTION

AROM Assessment

• **Substitution/Trick Movement.** Trunk rotation.

PROM Assessment

• **Start Position.** The patient is sitting. The shoulder is in 90° of abduction and neutral rotation. The elbow is flexed and the forearm is in midposition (Fig. 3-41).

• **Stabilization.** The therapist stabilizes the trunk and scapula to isolate and assess glenohumeral joint motion.

• **Therapist's Distal Hand Placement.** The therapist supports the arm in abduction and grasps the distal humerus.

• **End Position.** The therapist applies slight traction to and moves the humerus posteriorly to the limit of motion for horizontal abduction (Fig. 3-42) and anteriorly to the limit of motion for horizontal adduction (Fig. 3-43).

• **End Feels.** Horizontal abduction—firm; horizontal adduction—firm/soft.

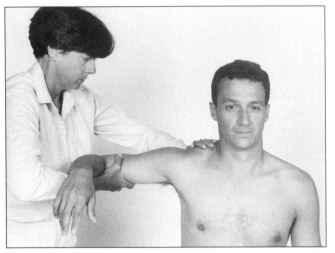

Figure 3-41.   Start position for shoulder horizontal abduction and horizontal adduction.

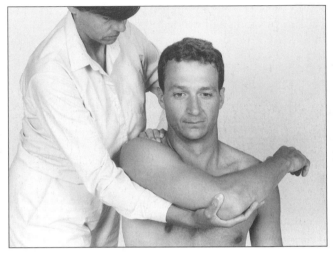

Figure 3-43.   Firm or soft end feel at limit of shoulder horizontal adduction.

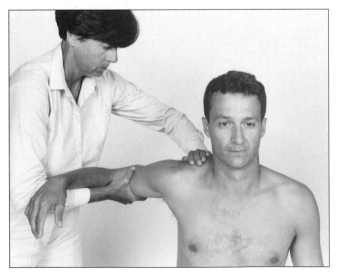

Figure 3-42.   Firm end feel at limit of shoulder horizontal abduction.

Measurement: Universal Goniometer

• **Start Position.** The patient is sitting. The shoulder is in 90° of abduction and neutral rotation. The elbow is flexed and the forearm is in midposition (Fig. 3-44). An alternate start position has the shoulder in 90° of flexion, the elbow is flexed, and the forearm is in midposition (Fig. 3-47). The start position of the shoulder should be recorded.

• **Stabilization.** The therapist stabilizes the trunk and scapula.

• **Goniometer Axis.** The axis is placed on top of the acromion process.

• **Stationary Arm.** Perpendicular to the trunk.

• **Movable Arm.** Parallel to the longitudinal axis of the humerus.

• **End Position.** The therapist supports the arm in abduction. The therapist applies slight traction to and moves the humerus posteriorly to the limit of motion in horizontal abduction (45°) (Fig. 3-45) and anteriorly across the chest to the limit of motion in horizontal adduction (135°) (Fig. 3-46).

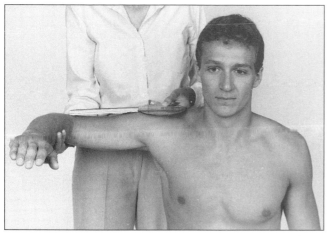

Figure 3-44. Start position for horizontal abduction and adduction.

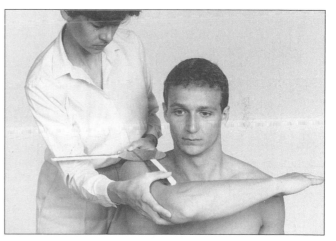

Figure 3-46. Shoulder horizontal adduction.

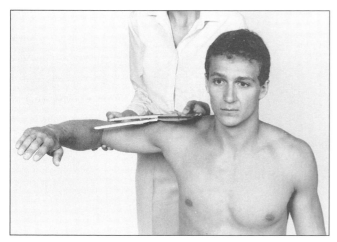

Figure 3-45. Shoulder horizontal abduction.

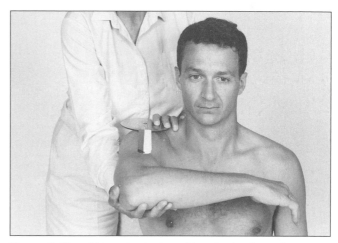

Figure 3-47. Alternate start position for horizontal abduction and adduction.

SHOULDER INTERNAL ROTATION

AROM Assessment

• Substitution/Trick Movement. In prone with the shoulder in 90° abduction: elbow extension, scapular elevation, and shoulder abduction. In sitting with the arm at the side: scapular elevation, shoulder abduction and trunk rotation.

PROM Assessment

• Start Position. The patient is prone or supine. In prone, the shoulder is in 90° of abduction, the elbow is flexed to 90°, and the forearm is in midposition (Fig. 3-48). A towel is placed under the humerus to achieve the abducted position. This start position is contraindicated if the patient has a history of posterior dislocation of the glenohumeral joint.

• Stabilization. The therapist stabilizes the scapula and maintains the position of the humerus, without restricting movement.

• Therapist's Distal Hand Placement. The therapist grasps the distal radius and ulna.

• End Position. The therapist moves the palm of the hand toward the ceiling to the limit of internal rotation (Fig. 3-49), that is, when scapular movement first occurs.

• End Feel. Firm.

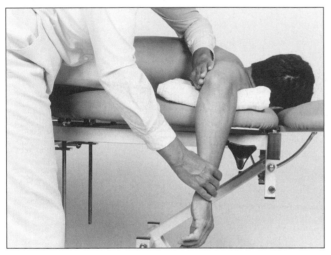

Figure 3-48.   Start position for shoulder internal rotation.

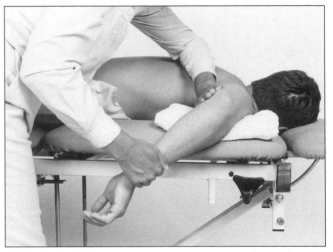

Figure 3-49.   Firm end feel at limit of shoulder internal rotation.

Measurement: Universal Goniometer

- **Start Position.** The patient is prone. The shoulder is in 90° of abduction, the elbow is flexed to 90°, and the forearm is in midposition (Fig. 3-50). A towel is placed under the humerus to achieve the abducted position. This start position is contraindicated if the patient has a history of posterior dislocation of the glenohumeral joint.

- **Goniometer Axis.** The axis is placed on the olecranon process of the ulna (Fig. 3-51).

- **Stationary Arm.** Perpendicular to the floor.

- **Movable Arm.** Parallel to the longitudinal axis of the ulna, pointing toward the ulnar styloid process.

- **End Position.** The palm of the hand is moved toward the ceiling to the limit of internal rotation (70°) (Fig. 3-52).

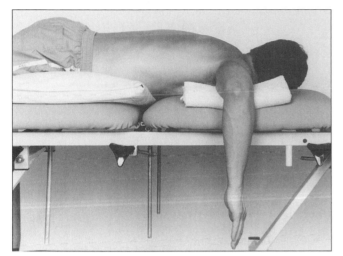

Figure 3-50.   Start position for shoulder internal rotation.

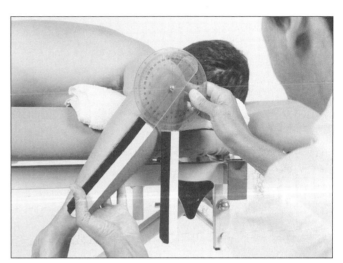

Figure 3-52.   Shoulder internal rotation.

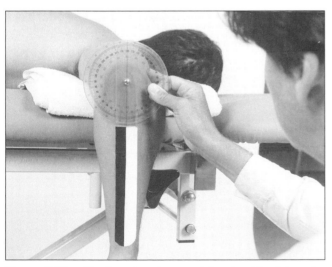

Figure 3-51.   Goniometer placement for shoulder internal rotation.

SHOULDER EXTERNAL ROTATION

AROM Assessment

• **Substitution/Trick Movement.** In supine position with the shoulder in 90° abduction: elbow extension, scapular depression, and shoulder adduction. In sitting with the arm at the side: scapular depression, shoulder adduction and trunk rotation.

PROM Assessment

• **Start Position.** The patient is supine. The shoulder is in 90° of abduction, the elbow is flexed to 90°, and the forearm is in midposition (Fig. 3-53). A towel is placed under the humerus to achieve the abducted position. This start position is contraindicated if the patient has a history of anterior dislocation of the glenohumeral joint.

• **Stabilization.** The weight of the trunk. The therapist stabilizes the scapula.

• **Therapist's Distal Hand Placement.** The therapist grasps the distal radius and ulna.

• **End Position.** The therapist moves the dorsum of the hand toward the floor to the limit of external rotation (Fig. 3-54), that is, when scapular movement first occurs.

• **End Feel.** Firm.

Measurement: Universal Goniometer

The measurement process is similar to that for internal rotation with the following exceptions:

• **Start Position.** The patient is supine (Fig. 3-55). This start position is contraindicated if the patient has a history of anterior dislocation of the glenohumeral joint.

• **End Position.** The dorsum of the hand moves toward the floor to the limit of motion in external rotation (90°) (Fig. 3-56).

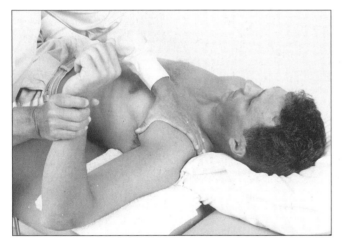

Figure 3-53.   Start position for shoulder external rotation.

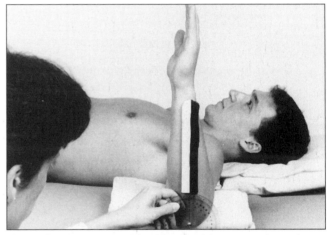

Figure 3-55.   Start position for shoulder external rotation.

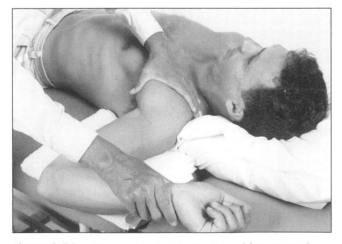

Figure 3-54.   Firm end feel at limit of shoulder external rotation.

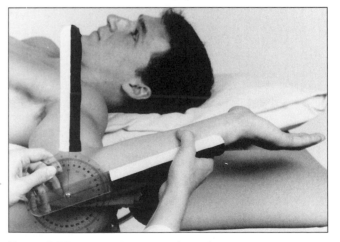

Figure 3-56.   Shoulder external rotation.

Alternate Assessment and Measurement: Internal/External Rotation. If the patient cannot achieve 90° of shoulder abduction, the end feel can be assessed (not shown) and the measurement can be taken while the patient is sitting. The starting position should be documented.

• **Start Position.** The patient is sitting. To measure shoulder internal rotation the shoulder is abducted to about 15°, the elbow is flexed to 90°, and the forearm is in midposition (Fig. 3-57). To measure external rotation (not shown) the arm is at the side in adduction, the elbow is flexed to 90°, and the forearm is in midposition.

• **Goniometer Axis.** The axis is placed under the olecranon process.

• **Stationary Arm.** Perpendicular to the trunk.

• **Movable Arm.** Parallel to the longitudinal axis of the ulna.

• **End Position.** The palm of the hand is moved toward the abdomen to the limit of shoulder internal rotation (Fig. 3-58). The therapist moves the hand away from the abdomen to the limit of external rotation.

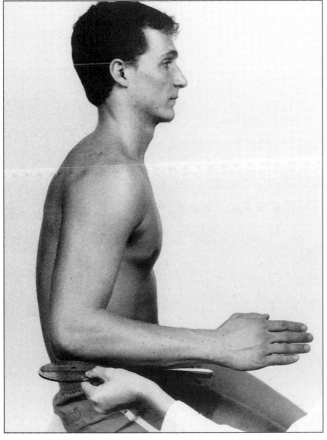

Figure 3-57.   Alternate start position for shoulder internal rotation.

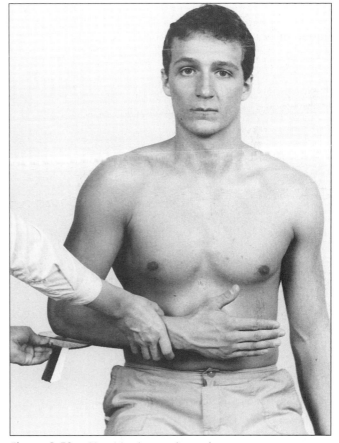

Figure 3-58.   Shoulder internal rotation.

ASSESSMENT OF MUSCLE LENGTH: PECTORALIS MAJOR

This muscle length assessment technique is contraindicated if the patient has a history of anterior dislocation of the glenohumeral joint.

• **Start Position.** The patient is supine with the shoulder in external rotation and 90° elevation through a plane midway between forward flexion and abduction. The elbow is in 90° flexion (Fig. 3-59).

• **Stabilization.** The therapist stabilizes the trunk.

• **End Position.** The shoulder is moved into horizontal abduction to the limit of motion, to put pectoralis major on full stretch (Figs. 3-60 and 3-61). With shortness of the pectoralis major muscle, shoulder horizontal abduction will be restricted.

• **End Feel.** Pectoralis major on stretch-firm.

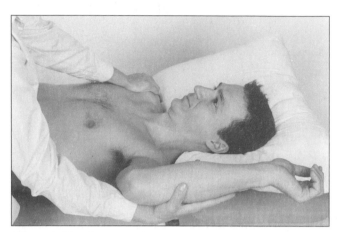

Figure 3-59.   Start position: length of pectoralis major.

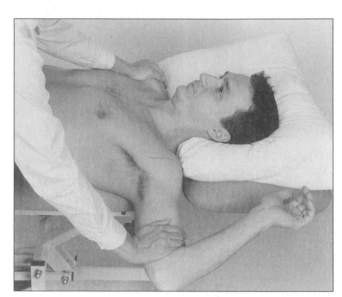

Figure 3-60.   Pectoralis major on stretch.

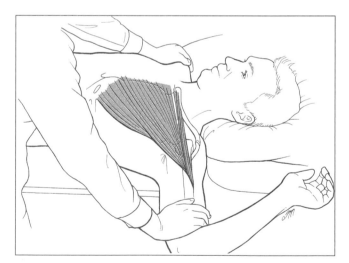

Figure 3-61.   Pectoralis major.

ASSESSMENT OF MUSCLE LENGTH: PECTORALIS MINOR[11]

This muscle length assessment technique is contraindicated if the patient has a history of posterior dislocation of the glenohumeral joint.

• **Start Position.** The patient is supine with the scapula over the side of the plinth, with the shoulder in external rotation and about 80° flexion. The elbow is flexed (Fig. 3-62).

• **Stabilization.** The weight of the trunk.

• **End Position.** The therapist moves the shoulder girdle cranially and dorsally along the shaft of the humerus to put pectoralis minor on full stretch (Figs. 3-63 and 3-64). The therapist observes decreased scapular retraction ROM in the presence of a shortened length of pectoralis minor.

• **End Feel.** Pectoralis minor on stretch-firm.

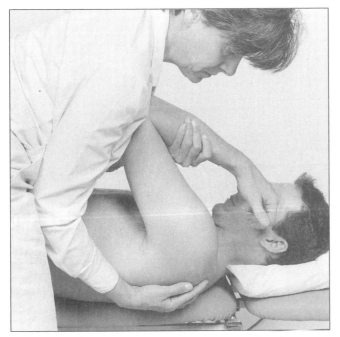

Figure 3-62. Start position: length of pectoralis minor.

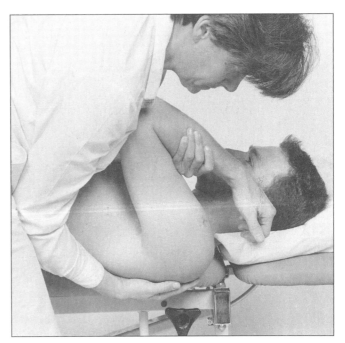

Figure 3-63. Pectoralis minor on stretch.

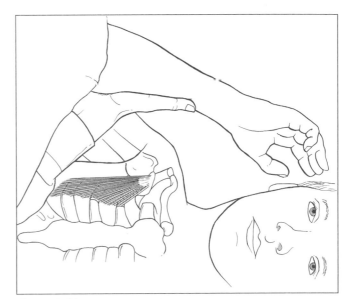

Figure 3-64. Pectoralis minor.

▼ MUSCLE STRENGTH ASSESSMENT (TABLE 3-4)

TABLE 3-4 ▼ MUSCLE ACTIONS, ATTACHMENTS, AND NERVE SUPPLY: THE SHOULDER GIRDLE[2]

Muscle	Primary Muscle Action	Muscle Origin	Muscle Insertion	Peripheral Nerve	Nerve Root
Serratus anterior	Scapular abduction; Scapular lateral rotation	Outer surfaces and superior borders of the upper 8, 9, or 10 ribs; fascia covering corresponding intercostal muscles	Costal surface of the medial border of the scapula including the superior angle and the inferior angle	Long thoracic	C567
Levator scapulae	Scapular elevation; Scapular medial rotation	Transverse processes of the upper 4 cervical vertebrae	Medial border of the scapula between the superior angle and the root of the spine	Third and fourth cervical; dorsal scapular	C345
Trapezius a. Upper fibers	Scapular elevation	Medial one third of the superior nuchal line of the occipital bone; external occipital protuberance; ligamentum nuchae	Posterior border of the lateral one-third of the clavicle	Spinal accessory	C34
b. Middle fibers	Scapular adduction	Spinous processes of T1 to T5 and the corresponding supraspinous ligament	Medial border of the acromion process and the superior border of the rest of the spine of the scapula	Spinal accessory	C34
c. Lower fibers	Scapular depression; Scapular adduction	Spinous processes of T6 to T12 and the corresponding supraspinous ligament	Tubercle at the apex of the triangular surface at the medial end of the spine of the scapula	Spinal accessory	C34

TABLE
3-4

▼ MUSCLE ACTIONS, ATTACHMENTS, AND NERVE SUPPLY: THE SHOULDER GIRDLE[2] Continued

Muscle	Primary Muscle Action	Muscle Origin	Muscle Insertion	Peripheral Nerve	Nerve Root
Rhomboid minor	Scapular adduction Scapular medial rotation	Inferior portion of the ligamentum nuchae; spinous processes of C7 and T1 and the corresponding supraspinous ligament	Base of the smooth triangular region at the root of the spine of the scapula	Dorsal scapular	C45
Rhomboid major	Scapular adduction Scapular medial rotation	Spinous processes of T2 to T5 and the corresponding supraspinous ligament	Medial border of the scapula between the root of the spine and inferior angle	Dorsal scapular	C45
Deltoid a. Anterior fibers	Shoulder flexion Shoulder internal rotation	Anterior border of the lateral one-third of the clavicle	Deltoid tuberosity on the lateral aspect of the humeral shaft	Axillary	C56
b. Middle fibers	Shoulder abduction	Lateral border and superior surface of the acromion process	Deltoid tuberosity on the lateral aspect of the humeral shaft	Axillary	C56
c. Posterior fibers	Shoulder extension Shoulder external rotation	Inferior lip of the crest of the spine of the scapula	Deltoid tuberosity on the lateral aspect of the humeral shaft	Axillary	C56
Supraspinatus	Shoulder abduction	Medial two thirds of the supraspinous fossa	Superior facet of the greater tuberosity of the humerus	Supra scapular	C56
Coracobrachialis	Shoulder flexion and adduction	Tip of the coracoid process	Middle of the medial aspect of the shaft of the humerus	Musculocutaneous	C567
Pectoralis major	Shoulder horizontal adduction Shoulder internal rotation	a. Clavicular head: anterior border of the medial third of the clavicle	Lateral lip of the intertubercular groove of the humerus	Medial and lateral pectoral	C56

Muscle	Primary Muscle Action	Muscle Origin	Muscle Insertion	Peripheral Nerve	Nerve Root
		b. Sternal head: medial half of the anterior surface of the sternum; cartilage of the first 6 or 7 ribs; aponeurosis of the external abdominal oblique		Medial and lateral pectoral	C678T1
Pectoralis minor	Scapular protraction / Scapular medial rotation	Outer surfaces of ribs 2 to 4 or 3 to 5 near the costal cartilages; fascia over corresponding external intercostals	Medial border and upper surface of the coracoid process of the scapula	Medial and lateral pectoral	C5678T1
Subscapularis	Shoulder internal rotation	Medial two thirds of the subscapular fossa of the scapula	Lesser tuberosity of the humerus; anterior aspect shoulder joint capsule	Upper and lower subscapular	C56
Infraspinatus	Shoulder external rotation	Medial two thirds of the infraspinous fossa	Middle facet of the greater tuberosity of the humerus	Suprascapular	C56
Teres minor	Shoulder external rotation	Upper two thirds of the lateral aspect of the dorsal surface of the scapula, adjacent to the lateral border of the scapula	Inferior facet of the greater tuberosity of the humerus	Axillary	C56
Teres major	Shoulder extension / Shoulder internal rotation	Posterior surface of the inferior angle of the scapula	Medial lip of the intertubercular groove of the humerus	Lower subscapular	C567

TABLE
3-4

▼ **MUSCLE ACTIONS, ATTACHMENTS, AND NERVE SUPPLY: THE SHOULDER GIRDLE²** *Continued*

Muscle	Primary Muscle Action	Muscle Origin	Muscle Insertion	Peripheral Nerve	Nerve Root
Latissius dorsi	Shoulder extension Shoulder adduction Shoulder internal rotation	Posterior layer of the thoracolumbar fascia that takes attachment from the lumbar and sacral spinous processes, the corresponding supraspinous ligament, and the posterior aspect of the crest of the ilium; spines of the lower 6 thoracic vertebrae anterior to the attachment of trapezius; lower 3 or 4 ribs; inferior angle of the scapula	Floor of the intertubercular groove of the humerus	Thoracodorsal	C678

SCAPULAR ABDUCTION AND LATERAL ROTATION

Against Gravity: Serratus Anterior

Accessory muscles: trapezius (lateral rotation) and pectoralis minor (abduction).

• **Start Position.** The patient is supine. The shoulder is flexed to 90° with slight horizontal abduction, and the elbow is extended (Fig. 3-65).

• **Stabilization.** The weight of the trunk.

• **Movement.** The patient abducts (protracts) the scapula through full ROM (Fig. 3-66).

• **Palpation.** Midaxillary line over the thorax.

• **Substitution/Trick Movement.** Pectoralis major, pectoralis minor.

• **Resistance Location.** Applied on the distal end of the humerus (Figs. 3-67 and 3-68). The isometric test is preferred because it is difficult to maintain resistance throughout range and the arc of movement is small.

• **Resistance Direction.** Scapular adduction.

• **Alternate Test (not shown).** The serratus anterior muscle can also be tested in the gravity eliminated position of sitting (see Fig. 3-69). The patient is able to hold the upper extremity in the test position and abduct the scapula by reaching upward and forward, without scapular winging, for a grade 3. For grades greater than a 3, the therapist applies resistance on the distal end of the humerus in the direction of shoulder extension and scapular adduction.

Caution: If the shoulder joint is unstable, the start positions may still be assumed; however, the therapist must support the upper extremity, and resistance is not applied. It is then only possible to assess a grade of 3 with the patient in supine or sitting.

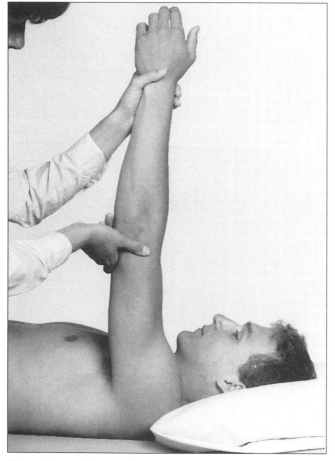

Figure 3-65. Start position: serratus anterior.

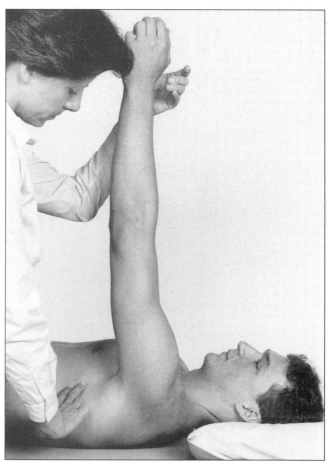

Figure 3-66. Screen position: serratus anterior.

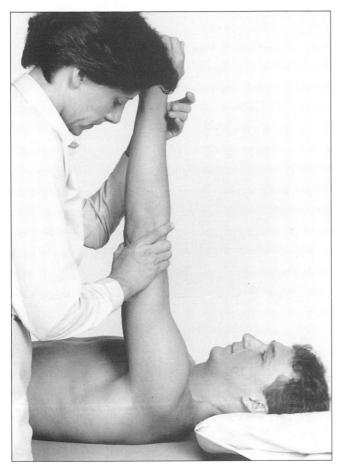

Figure 3-67. Resistance: serratus anterior.

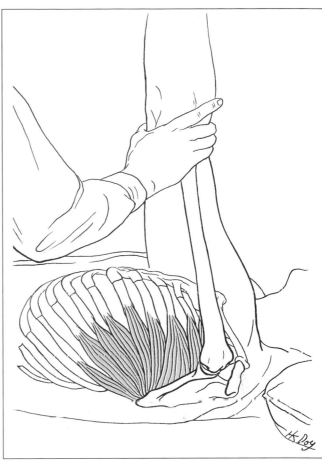

Figure 3-68. Serratus anterior.

Gravity Eliminated: Serratus Anterior

- **Start Position.** The patient is sitting. The shoulder is flexed to 90° with slight horizontal abduction, and the elbow is extended (Fig. 3-69). The therapist supports the weight of the upper extremity.

- **Stabilization.** The patient is instructed to avoid trunk rotation.

- **End Position.** The patient abducts the scapula through full ROM (Fig. 3-70).

- **Substitution/Trick Movement.** Pectoralis major and minor, upper and lower fibers of trapezius, and contralateral trunk rotation.

- **Alternate Test.** If the patient is unable to assume a sitting position, the serratus anterior muscle can be tested in the against gravity position of supine. The therapist positions and holds the scapula in abduction. The therapist palpates for quality of muscle contraction as the patient attempts to hold this position.

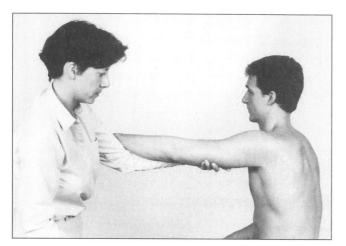

Figure 3-69. Start position: serratus anterior.

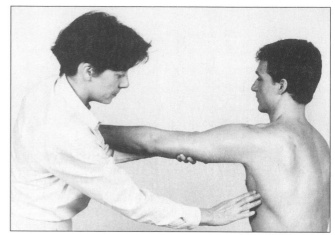

Figure 3-70. End position: serratus anterior.

Clinical Test: Serratus Anterior. This test is a quick clinical test used to assess whether the serratus anterior muscle is strong or weak. A specific grade cannot be assigned.

• **Start Position.** The patient is standing and facing a wall. The hands are placed on the wall at shoulder level, the shoulders are in slight horizontal abduction, and the elbows are extended (Fig. 3-71). The thorax is allowed to sag toward the wall so that the scapulae are adducted.

• **Movement.** The patient pushes the thorax away from the wall so that the scapulae abduct (Fig. 3-72).

• **Observation.** Weakness is demonstrated by "winging"[12] of the scapula. The medial border and inferior angle of the scapula become more prominent, and the scapula remains in an adducted and medially rotated position.

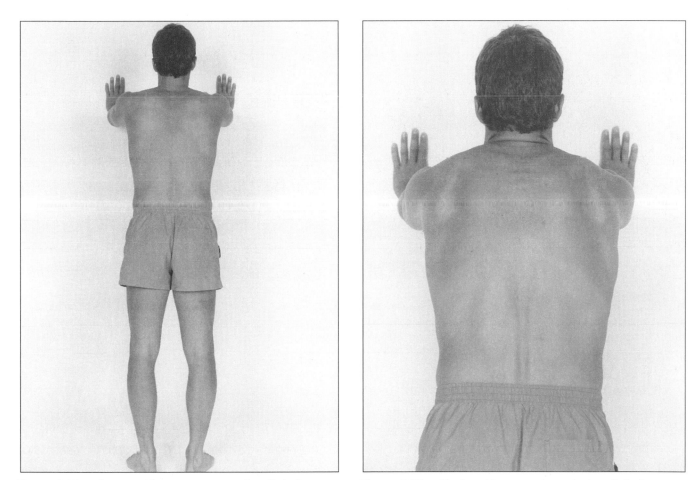

Figure 3-71.   Start position: serratus anterior clinical test.

Figure 3-72.   End position: serratus anterior clinical test.

SCAPULAR ELEVATION

Against Gravity: Upper Fibers of Trapezius and Levator Scapulae

• **Start Position.** The patient is sitting. The shoulders are slightly abducted, and the elbows are flexed to 90° (Fig. 3-73).

• **Movement.** The patient elevates the shoulder girdle(s) to bring the acromion process closer to the ear (Fig. 3-74). For the unilateral test, the therapist places the hand against the lateral aspect of the patient's head on the test side, maintaining the head in a neutral position to stabilize the origins of the muscles (Fig. 3-75).

• **Palpation.** Upper fibers of trapezius: on a point of a line midway between the inion and the acromion process. Levator scapulae: too deep to palpate.

• **Substitution/Trick Movement.** Unilateral test: lowering ear to shoulder and contralateral trunk side flexion.

• **Resistance Location.** Applied over the top of the shoulder(s) (Figs. 3-76, 3-77, and 3-78). The isometric test is preferred.

• **Resistance Direction.** Scapular depression.

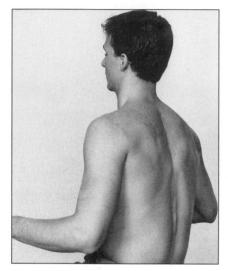

Figure 3-73. Start position: upper fibers of trapezius and levator scapulae.

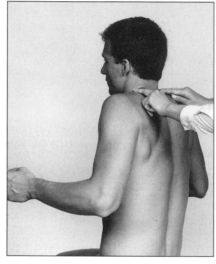

Figure 3-74. Screen position: bilateral test for upper fibers of trapezius and levator scapulae.

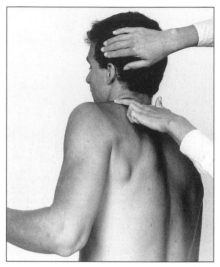

Figure 3-75. Screen position: unilateral test for upper fibers of trapezius and levator scapulae.

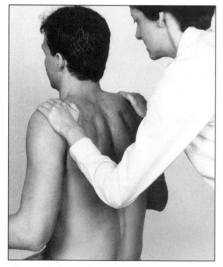

Figure 3-76. Resistance: upper fibers of trapezius and levator scapulae.

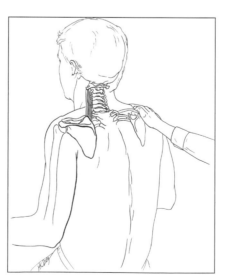

Figure 3-77. Levator scapulae.

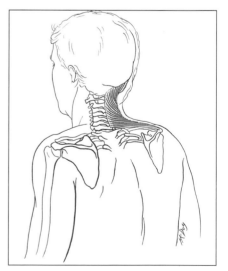

Figure 3-78. Upper fibers of trapezius.

Gravity Eliminated: Upper Fibers of Trapezius and Levator Scapulae

• **Start Position.** The patient is prone. The arm is at the side, and the shoulder is in neutral rotation (Fig. 3-79). The therapist supports the weight of the upper extremity to reduce the resistance of friction between the plinth and the upper extremity.

• **Stabilization.** The weight of the head.

• **End Position.** The patient elevates the scapula through full ROM (Fig. 3-80).

• **Substitution/Trick Movement.** Contralateral trunk side flexion.

• **Alternate Test.** If the patient is unable to assume a prone position, these muscles can be tested in the against gravity position of sitting. The therapist positions the shoulder girdle in elevation and palpates for the quality of muscle contraction while the patient attempts to hold the position.

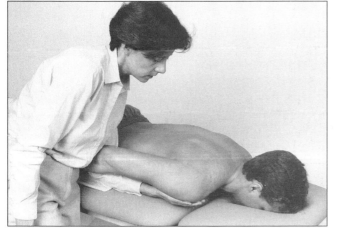

Figure 3-79. Start position: upper fibers of trapezius and levator scapulae.

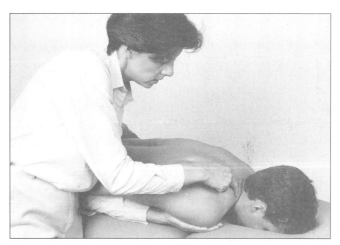

Figure 3-80. End position: upper fibers of trapezius and levator scapulae.

SCAPULAR ADDUCTION

Against Gravity: Middle Fibers of Trapezius

Accessory muscle: trapezius (upper and lower fibers).

• **Start Position.** The patient is prone. The shoulder is flexed to 90° and in neutral rotation. The arm is hanging vertically over the edge of the plinth (Fig. 3-81).

• **Stabilization.** The weight of the trunk.

• **Movement.** The patient adducts the scapula toward the midline (Fig. 3-82).

• **Palpation.** Between the medial (vertebral) border of the scapula and the vertebrae, above the spine of the scapula.

• **Substitution/Trick Movement.** Rhomboid major, rhomboid minor, and ipsilateral trunk rotation.

• **Resistance Location.** Applied over the scapula (Figs. 3-83 and 3-84). Ensure that no resistance is applied over the humerus. The isometric test is preferred.

• **Resistance Direction.** Scapular abduction.

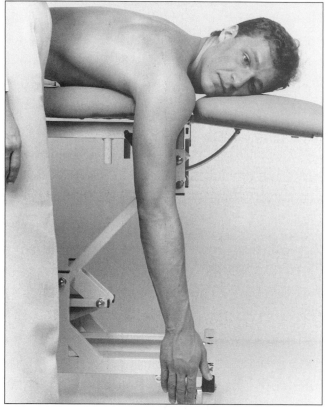

Figure 3-81.   Start position: middle fibers of trapezius.

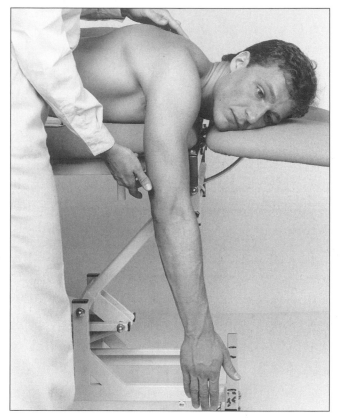

Figure 3-82.   Screen position: middle fibers of trapezius.

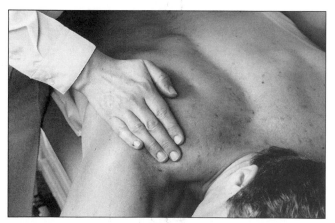

Figure 3-83.   Resistance: middle fibers of trapezius.

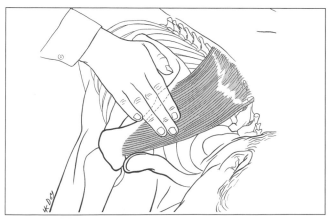

Figure 3-84.   Middle fibers of trapezius.

Gravity Eliminated: Middle Fibers of Trapezius

• **Start Position.** The patient is sitting. The shoulder is in a few degrees of horizontal abduction and internal rotation (Fig. 3-85). The arm is supported by the therapist.

• **Stabilization.** The therapist instructs the patient to avoid trunk rotation.

• **End Position.** The patient adducts the scapula through full ROM (Fig. 3-86).

• **Substitution/Trick Movement.** Shoulder horizontal abduction, and ipsilateral trunk rotation.

• **Alternate Test.** If the patient cannot assume a sitting posture, this muscle can be tested in the against gravity position of prone-lying. The shoulder is abducted to 90°, and the elbow is flexed to 90° and hanging vertically over the edge of the plinth. This position allows the therapist to position the scapula in the adducted position while palpating for the quality of muscle contraction as the patient attempts to hold the position. During positioning of the scapula, the therapist supports the glenohumeral joint and humerus anteriorly to control the movement of the scapula and avoid shoulder horizontal abduction.

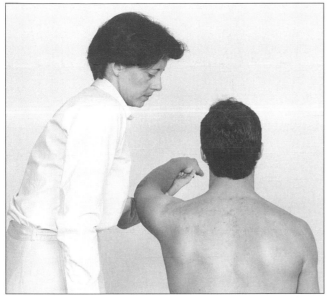

Figure 3-85.   Start position: middle fibers of trapezius.

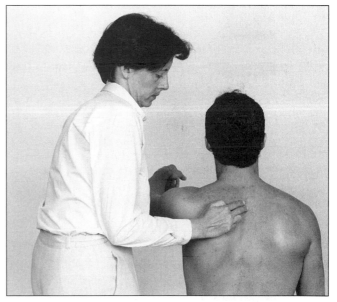

Figure 3-86.   End position: middle fibers of trapezius.

SCAPULAR ADDUCTION AND MEDIAL ROTATION

Against Gravity: Rhomboid Major and Rhomboid Minor

Accessory muscle: middle fibers of trapezius.

- **Start Position.** The patient is prone. The dorsum of the hand is placed over the buttock of the nontest side, and the shoulders remain relaxed (Fig. 3-87).

- **Stabilization.** The weight of the trunk.

- **Movement.** The patient raises the arm away from the back. The weight of the raised upper extremity provides resistance to the scapular test motion.

Note: Inability to lift the hand off the buttock may be due to shoulder muscle weakness, notably subscapu-laris, not rhomboid muscle weakness. Ensure that the hand is maintained over the nontest side buttock and that the patient adducts and medially rotates the scapula during the test (Fig. 3-88).

- **Palpation.** On a point of an oblique line between the vertebral border of the scapula and C7 to T5. Rhomboid major can be palpated medial to the vertebral border of the scapula lateral to the lower fibers of trapezius, near the inferior angle of the scapula.

- **Substitution/Trick Movement.** Tipping the scapula forward through pectoralis minor.[12]

- **Resistance Location.** Applied over the scapula (Figs. 3-89 and 3-90). Ensure that resistance is not applied over the humerus. The isometric test is preferred.

- **Resistance Direction.** Scapular abduction and lateral rotation.

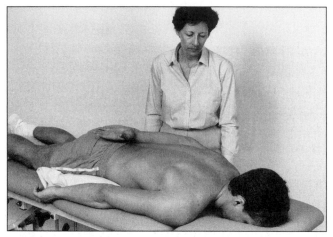

Figure 3-87.   Start position: rhomboids.

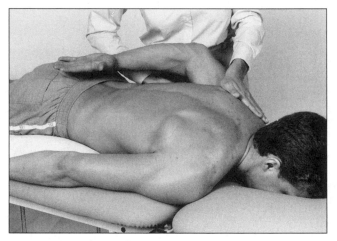

Figure 3-89.   Resistance: rhomboids.

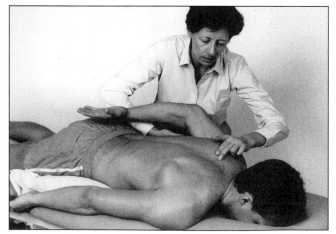

Figure 3-88.   Screen position: rhomboids.

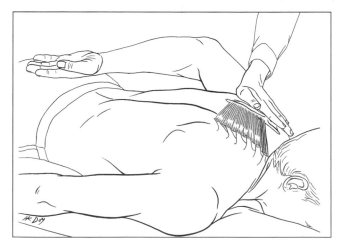

Figure 3-90.   Rhomboids.

Gravity Eliminated: Rhomboid Major and Rhomboid Minor

• **Start Position.** The patient is sitting. The dorsum of the hand is placed over the nontest side buttock, and the shoulders remain relaxed (Fig. 3-91).

• **Stabilization.** The therapist instructs the patient to avoid trunk forward flexion and/or ipsilateral trunk rotation.

• **End Position.** The patient adducts and medially rotates the scapula by moving the arm away from the back while maintaining the hand over the buttock (Fig. 3-92).

• **Substitution/Trick Movement.** Ipsilateral trunk rotation and/or trunk forward flexion, and tipping the scapula forward.

• **Alternate Test.** If a sitting posture cannot be assumed, the rhomboids can be tested in the against gravity position of prone-lying. The therapist positions the upper extremity up toward the ceiling while the therapist's hand supports the glenohumeral joint anteriorly and brings the scapula into a position of retraction and medial rotation. The therapist palpates for the quality of contraction of rhomboids while the patient attempts to hold the position.

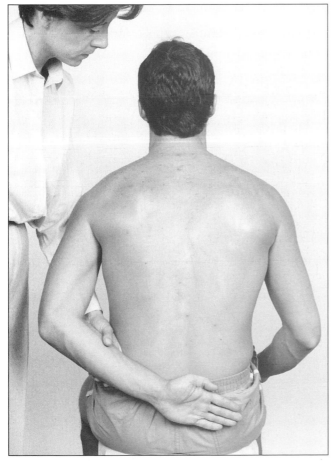

Figure 3-91.   Start position: rhomboids.

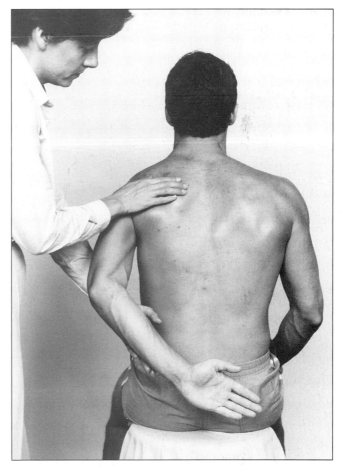

Figure 3-92.   End position: rhomboids.

SCAPULAR DEPRESSION AND ADDUCTION

Against Gravity: Lower Fibers of Trapezius

Accessory muscle: middle fibers of trapezius.

• **Start Position.** The patient is prone. The head is rotated to the opposite side, and the shoulder is abducted to about 130° (Fig. 3-93). Although the prone position is a gravity eliminated position for the movement of scapular depression, the lower fibers of trapezius, through the position of the arm, work against resistance of the weight of the arm.

• **Stabilization.** The weight of the trunk.

• **Movement.** The patient raises the arm to produce depression and adduction of the scapula (Fig. 3-94).

• **Palpation.** Medial to the inferior angle of the scapula along a line between the root of the spine of the scapula and the T12 spinous process.

• **Substitution/Trick Movement.** Trunk extension, middle fibers of trapezius.

• **Alternate Test (not shown).** If the patient is unable to position the arm in abduction, the arms can remain by the side. The isometric test is preferred for against gravity grading. The therapist positions the scapula into depression and adduction while the patient attempts to hold this position. Resistance can be added over the scapula.

• **Resistance Location.** The isometric test is preferred, and the resistance is applied over the scapula (Figs. 3-95 and 3-96).

• **Resistance Direction.** Scapular elevation and abduction.

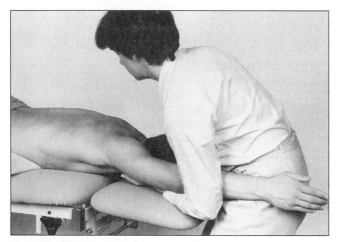

Figure 3-93.   Start position: lower fibers of trapezius.

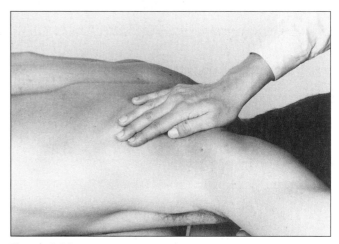

Figure 3-95.   Resistance: lower fibers of trapezius.

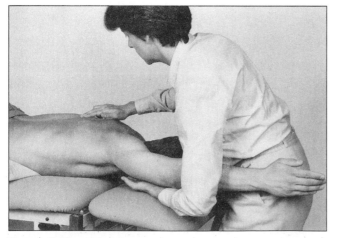

Figure 3-94.   Screen position: lower fibers of trapezius.

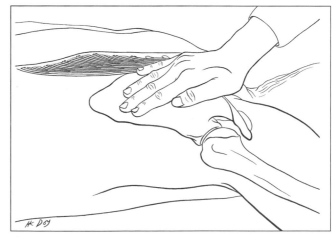

Figure 3-96.   Lower fibers of trapezius.

Gravity Eliminated: Lower Fibers of Trapezius

• **Start Position.** The patient is prone with the arms by the sides (Fig. 3-97). The therapist supports the arm through range, to reduce the resistance of friction between the plinth and the upper extremity.

• **Stabilization.** The weight of the trunk.

• **End Position.** The patient depresses and adducts the scapula through full ROM (Fig. 3-98).

• **Substitution/Trick Movement.** Ipsilateral trunk side flexion and middle fibers of trapezius.

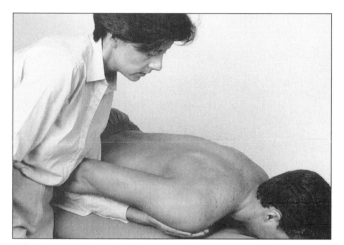

Figure 3-97. Start position: lower fibers of trapezius.

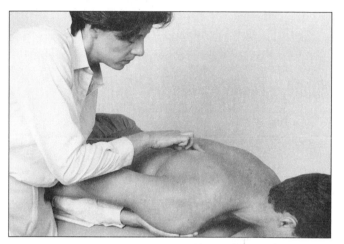

Figure 3-98. End position: lower fibers of trapezius.

SHOULDER FLEXION TO 90°

Against Gravity: Anterior Fibers of Deltoid

Accessory muscles: coracobrachialis, middle fibers of deltoid, clavicular fibers of pectoralis major, biceps brachii, upper and lower fibers of trapezius, and serratus anterior.

• **Start Position.** The patient is sitting. The arm is at the side, with the shoulder in slight abduction and the palm facing medially (Fig. 3-99).

• **Stabilization.** The therapist stabilizes the scapula and clavicle.

• **Movement.** The patient flexes the shoulder to 90°, simultaneously slightly adducting and internally rotating the shoulder joint (Fig. 3-100).

• **Palpation.** Anterior aspect of the shoulder joint just distal to the lateral one third of the clavicle.

• **Resistance Location.** Applied on the anteromedial aspect of the arm just proximal to the elbow joint (Figs. 3-101 and 3-102).

• **Resistance Direction.** Shoulder extension, slight abduction and external rotation.

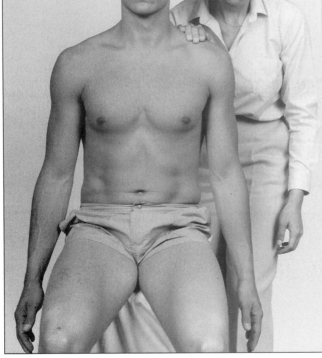

Figure 3-99. Start position: anterior fibers of deltoid.

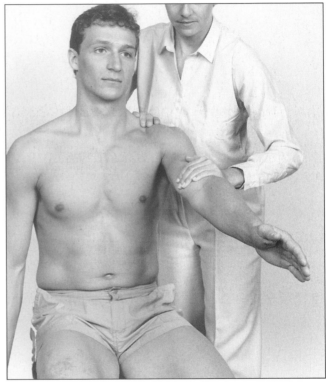

Figure 3-101. Resistance: anterior fibers of deltoid.

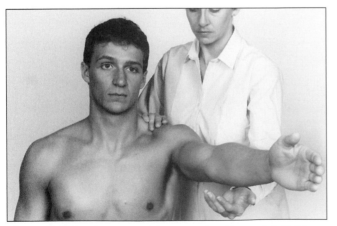

Figure 3-100. Screen position: anterior fibers of deltoid.

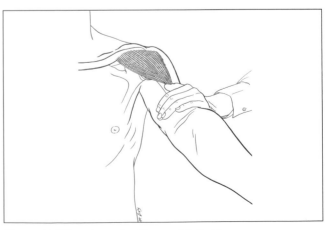

Figure 3-102. Anterior fibers of deltoid.

Gravity Eliminated: Anterior Fibers of Deltoid

• **Start Position.** The patient is in a side-lying position on the nontest side. The arm is at the side, with the shoulder in slight abduction and neutral rotation (Fig. 3-103). The therapist supports the weight of the limb.

• **Stabilization.** The therapist stabilizes the scapula and clavicle.

• **End Position.** The patient flexes the shoulder to 90°, simultaneously slightly adducting and internally rotating the shoulder joint (Fig. 3-104).

• **Substitution/Trick Movement.** Scapular elevation and trunk extension.

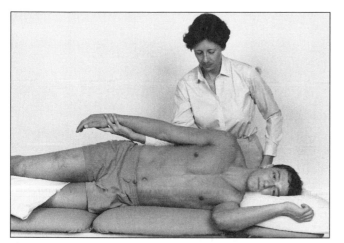

Figure 3-103.   Start position: anterior fibers of deltoid.

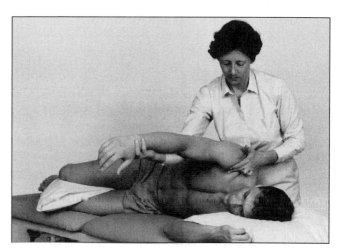

Figure 3-104.   End position: anterior fibers of deltoid.

SHOULDER FLEXION AND ADDUCTION

Against Gravity: Coracobrachialis

Accessory muscles: anterior fibers of deltoid, clavicular fibers of pectoralis major, and the short head of biceps brachii.

- **Start Position.** The patient is supine. The shoulder is in slight abduction and external rotation; the elbow is flexed with the forearm in supination (Fig. 3-105).

- **Stabilization.** The weight of the trunk.

- **Movement.** The patient flexes and adducts the shoulder while maintaining the shoulder in external rotation (Fig. 3-106).

- **Palpation.** Proximal one third of the anteromedial aspect of the arm, just anterior to the brachial pulse (Fig. 3-107).

- **Substitution/Trick Movement.** Scapular elevation.

- **Resistance Location.** Applied on the anteromedial aspect of the distal humerus (Figs. 3-108 and 3-109).

- **Resistance Direction.** Shoulder abduction and extension.

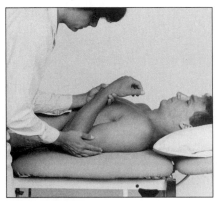

Figure 3-105.   Start position: coracobrachialis.

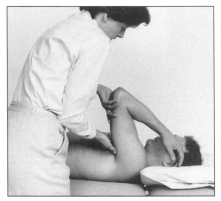

Figure 3-106.   Screen position: coracobrachialis.

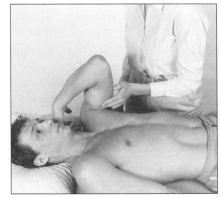

Figure 3-107.   Palpation: coracobrachialis.

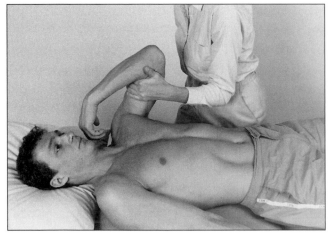

Figure 3-108.   Resistance: coracobrachialis.

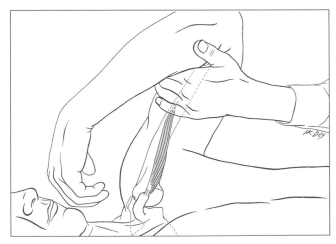

Figure 3-109.   Coracobrachialis.

Gravity Eliminated: Coracobrachialis

- **Start Position.** The patient is in a side-lying position on the nontest side. The arm is at the side, with the shoulder in slight abduction and external rotation and the elbow fully flexed with the forearm supinated (Fig. 3-110). The therapist supports the weight of the arm.

- **Stabilization.** The therapist stabilizes the scapula.

- **End Position.** The patient flexes and adducts the shoulder through full ROM (Fig. 3-111).

- **Substitution/Trick Movement.** Scapular elevation.

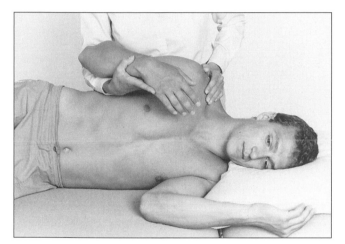

Figure 3-110.   Start position: coracobrachialis.

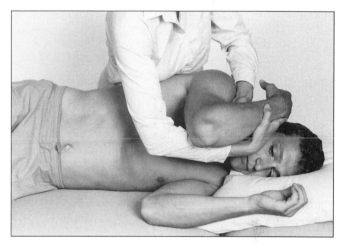

Figure 3-111.   End position: coracobrachialis.

SHOULDER EXTENSION

Against Gravity: Latissimus Dorsi and Teres Major

Accessory muscles: posterior fibers of deltoid, triceps, and teres minor.

- **Start Position.** The patient is in a prone-lying position at the edge of the plinth. The arm is at the side, with the shoulder in internal rotation. The palm faces the ceiling (Fig. 3-112).

- **Stabilization.** The weight of the trunk.

- **Movement.** The patient extends the shoulder through full ROM while maintaining slight shoulder adduction (Fig. 3-113A). The posterior fibers of deltoid are essential for full shoulder extension.[13] In the event of deltoid paralysis this test motion may be restricted to approximately one third of the full shoulder extension ROM.

- **Palpation.** Latissimus dorsi: lateral to the inferior angle of the scapula or at the posterior wall of the axilla (Fig. 3-113B) (inferior and lateral to palpation for teres major). Teres major: posterior wall of the axilla lateral to the axillary border of the scapula.

- **Substitution/Trick Movement.** Pectoralis minor.

- **Resistance Location.** Applied proximal to the elbow joint on the posteromedial aspect of the arm (Figs. 3-114 and 3-115).

- **Resistance Direction.** Shoulder flexion and slight abduction.

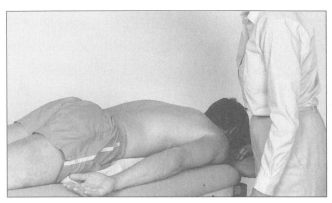

Figure 3-112. Start position: latissimus dorsi and teres major.

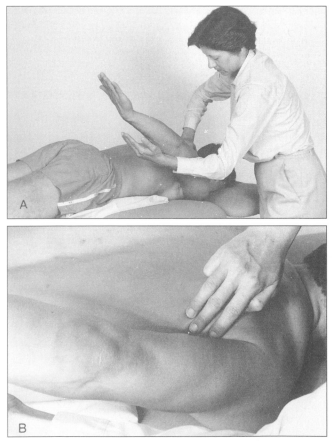

Figure 3-113. (*A*) Screen position: latissimus dorsi and teres major. (*B*) Palpation: latissimus dorsi.

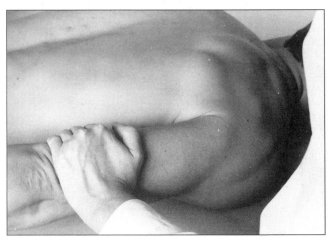

Figure 3-114. Resistance: latissimus dorsi and teres major.

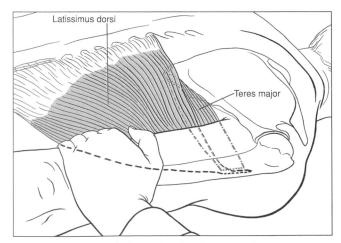

Figure 3-115. Latissimus dorsi and teres major.

Gravity Eliminated: Latissimus Dorsi and Teres Major

• **Start Position.** The patient is in a side-lying position on the nontest side, with the arm at the side and the shoulder in internal rotation. The hips and knees are flexed (Fig. 3-116). The therapist supports the weight of the arm.

• **Stabilization.** None.

• **End Position.** The patient extends the shoulder while maintaining shoulder adduction (Fig. 3-117).

• **Substitution/Trick Movement.** Pectoralis minor.

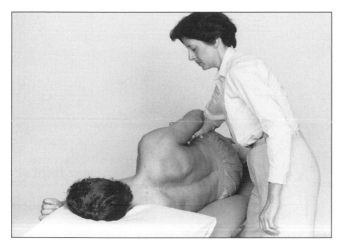

Figure 3-116.   Start position: latissimus dorsi and teres major.

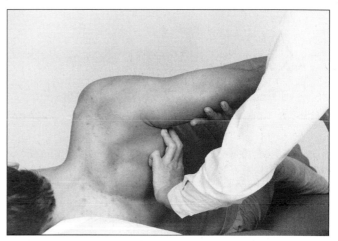

Figure 3-117.   End position: latissimus dorsi and teres major.

SHOULDER ABDUCTION TO 90°

Against Gravity: Middle Fibers of Deltoid and Supraspinatus

Accessory muscles: none.

• **Start Position.** The patient is sitting. The test arm is at the side in neutral rotation, and the elbow is extended (Fig. 3-118).

• **Stabilization.** The therapist stabilizes the scapula.

• **Movement.** The patient abducts the arm to 90° (Fig. 3-119).

• **Palpation.** Middle fibers of deltoid: inferior to the tip of the acromion process. Supraspinatus: too deep to palpate.

• **Substitution/Trick Movement.** Upper fibers of trapezius (shoulder elevation), long head of biceps (shoulder external rotation), and contralateral or ipsilateral trunk side flexion.

• **Resistance Location.** Applied proximal to the elbow joint on the lateral aspect of the arm (Figs. 3-120, 3-121, and 3-122).

• **Resistance Direction.** Shoulder adduction.

• **Alternate Test (not shown).** This test may also be performed abducting the arm in the plane of the scapula (Fig. 3-123). The scapular plane lies 30° to 45° anterior to the frontal plane.[14] Although there appears to be no difference in the strength of the shoulder abductors when tested in the frontal or scapular planes of motion,[15] assessment in the plane of the scapula may be preferred. Movement performed in the scapular plane is a more functional plane of motion and produces less stress on the capsuloligamentous structures of the glenohumeral joint. The plane of motion used should be recorded.

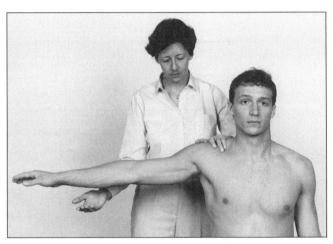

Figure 3-119. Screen position: middle fibers of deltoid and supraspinatus.

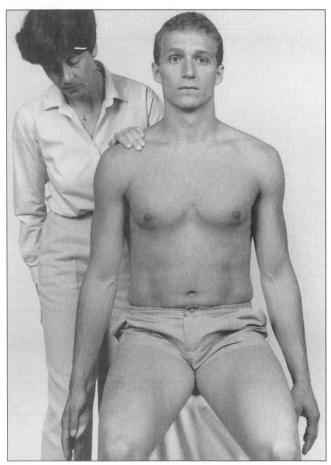

Figure 3-118. Start position: middle fibers of deltoid and supraspinatus.

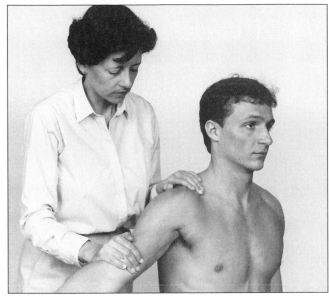

Figure 3-120. Resistance: middle fibers of deltoid and supraspinatus.

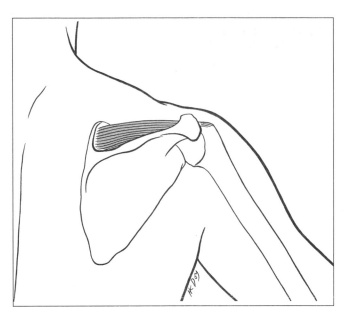

Figure 3-122. Supraspinatus.

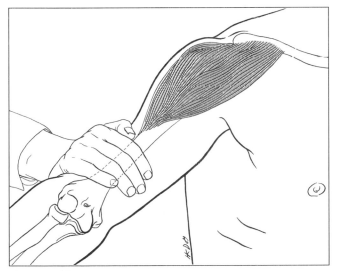

Figure 3-121. Middle fibers of deltoid.

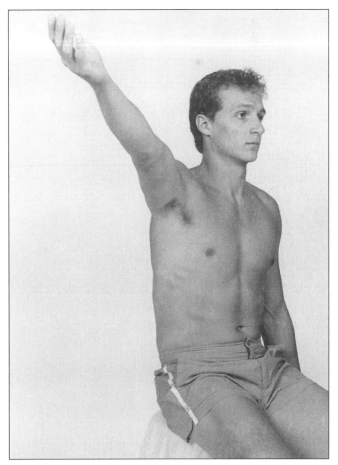

Figure 3-123. Shoulder abduction in the scapular plane.

Gravity Eliminated: Middle Fibers of Deltoid and Supraspinatus

• **Start Position.** The patient is supine. The test arm is at the side in neutral rotation with the elbow extended (Fig. 3-124). The therapist supports the weight of the arm.

• **Stabilization.** The therapist stabilizes the scapula.

• **End Position.** The patient abducts the shoulder to 90° (Fig. 3-125).

• **Substitution/Trick Movement.** Upper fibers of trapezius (shoulder elevation), long head of biceps (shoulder external rotation), and contralateral trunk side flexion.

SHOULDER ADDUCTION

The primary muscles involved in this movement are tested in the following movements:

Pectoralis major: shoulder horizontal adduction

Latissimus dorsi: shoulder extension

Teres major: shoulder extension

The shoulder adductors can be tested as a group with the patient in a supine position. The resisted gravity eliminated method is used for grades 3 to 5 and the conventional method for grades 0 to 2.

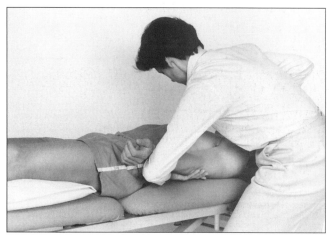

Figure 3-124.   Start position: middle fibers of deltoid and supraspinatus.

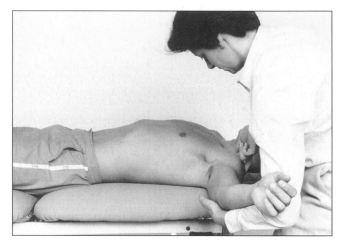

Figure 3-125.   End position: middle fibers of deltoid and supraspinatus.

SHOULDER HORIZONTAL ADDUCTION

Against Gravity: Pectoralis Major (Sternal and Clavicular Heads)

Accessory muscle: anterior fibers of deltoid.

• **Start Position.** The patient is supine. The shoulder is abducted to 90°, and the elbow is flexed to 90° (Fig. 3-126).

• **Stabilization.** The weight of the trunk.

• **Movement.** The patient horizontally adducts the shoulder through full ROM (Fig. 3-127).

• **Palpation.** Pectoralis major sternal head: anterior border of the axilla. Pectoralis major clavicular head: inferior to the middle of the anterior border of the clavicle.

• **Substitution/Trick Movement.** Trunk rotation.

• **Resistance Location.** Applied on the anterior aspect of the arm proximal to the elbow joint (Figs. 3-128 and 3-129).

• **Resistance Direction.** Shoulder horizontal abduction.

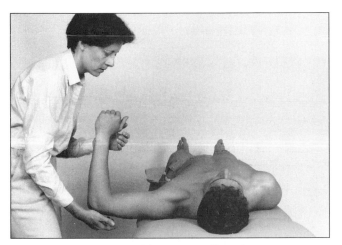

Figure 3-126.   Start position: pectoralis major.

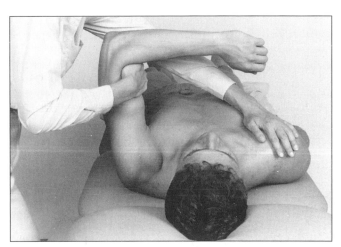

Figure 3-128.   Resistance: pectoralis major.

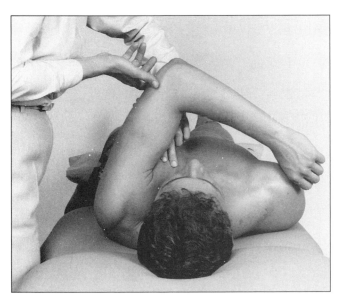

Figure 3-127.   Screen position: pectoralis major.

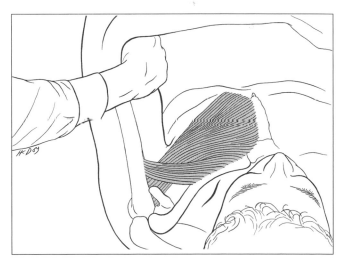

Figure 3-129.   Pectoralis major.

Gravity Eliminated: Pectoralis Major (Sternal and Clavicular Heads)

• **Start Position.** The patient is sitting. The shoulder is abducted to 90°, the elbow is flexed to 90°, and the arm is supported by the therapist (Fig. 3-130).

• **Stabilization.** The therapist stabilizes the scapula and trunk by placing the hand on top of the shoulder.

• **End Position.** The patient horizontally adducts the shoulder through full ROM (Fig. 3-131).

• **Substitution/Trick Movement.** Contralateral trunk rotation.

Against Gravity: Clavicular Head of Pectoralis Major and Sternal Head of Pectoralis Major.
If there is weakness noted during testing of both heads of the pectoralis major, specific testing (not shown) of the sternal and clavicular heads should be performed because each head has a separate innervation. The patient is positioned so that the humerus is aligned with the direct line of pull of each segment of the muscle. The patient is in the against gravity position of supine-lying. The assisted against gravity methodology is used for grading of 0 to 2 muscle strengths.

Clavicular Head

• **Start Position.** Shoulder abducted to about 70° to 75°.

• **Movement.** Adduction, forward flexion, and internal rotation of the shoulder (the hand reaches to a point above the contralateral shoulder).

• **Resistance Location.** Applied on the anteromedial aspect of the arm, proximal to the elbow joint.

• **Resistance Direction.** Abduction, extension, and slight external rotation of the shoulder.

• **Substitution/Trick Movement.** Contralateral trunk rotation, coracobrachialis, and short head of biceps brachii.

Sternal Head

• **Start Position.** Shoulder abducted to about 135°.

• **Movement.** Adduction, extension, and internal rotation of the shoulder (the hand reaches toward the contralateral hip).

• **Resistance Location.** Applied on the anteromedial aspect of the arm, proximal to the elbow joint.

• **Resistance Direction.** Abduction, flexion, and slight external rotation of the shoulder.

• **Substitution/Trick Movement.** Latissimus dorsi, teres major, and contralateral trunk rotation.

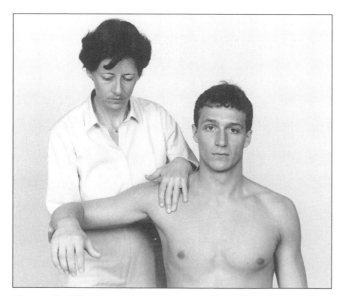

Figure 3-130.   Start position: pectoralis major.

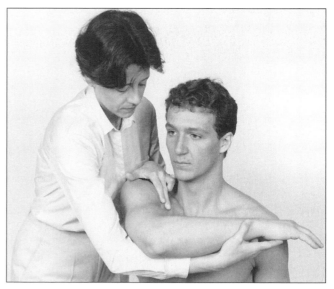

Figure 3-131.   End position: pectoralis major.

SHOULDER HORIZONTAL ABDUCTION

Against Gravity: Posterior Fibers of Deltoid

Accessory muscles: infraspinatus and teres minor.

• **Start Position.** The patient is prone. The shoulder is abducted to about 75°, the elbow is flexed to 90°, and the forearm is hanging vertically over the edge of the plinth (Fig. 3-132).

• **Stabilization.** The therapist stabilizes the scapula.

• **Movement.** The patient horizontally abducts and slightly externally rotates the shoulder (Fig. 3-133).

• **Palpation.** Inferior to the lateral aspect of the spine of the scapula.

• **Substitution/Trick Movement.** Rhomboids, middle fibers of trapezius, and ipsilateral trunk rotation.

• **Resistance Location.** Applied on the posterolateral aspect of the arm proximal to the elbow joint (Figs. 3-134 and 3-135).

• **Resistance Direction.** Shoulder horizontal adduction and slight internal rotation.

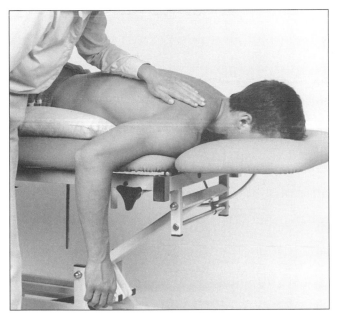

Figure 3-132.   Start position: posterior fibers of deltoid.

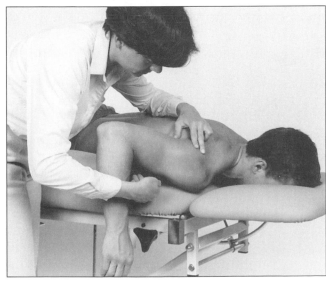

Figure 3-133.   Screen position: posterior fibers of deltoid.

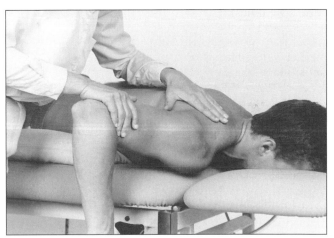

Figure 3-134.   Resistance: posterior fibers of deltoid.

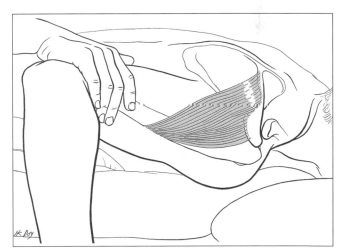

Figure 3-135.   Posterior fibers of deltoid.

Gravity Eliminated: Posterior Fibers of Deltoid

• **Start Position.** The patient is sitting. The shoulder is abducted to about 75° (Fig. 3-136). The upper extremity is supported by the therapist.

• **Stabilization.** The therapist stabilizes the scapula.

• **End Position.** The patient horizontally abducts and slightly externally rotates the shoulder (Fig. 3-137).

• **Substitution/Trick Movement.** Rhomboids, middle fibers of trapezius, and ipsilateral trunk rotation.

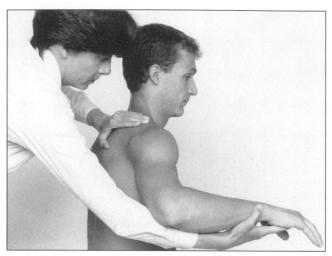

Figure 3-136. Start position: posterior fibers of deltoid.

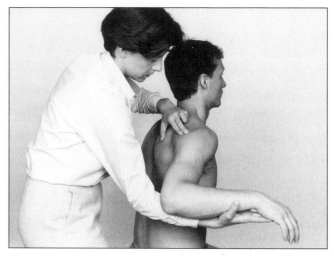

Figure 3-137. End position: posterior fibers of deltoid.

SHOULDER INTERNAL ROTATION

Against Gravity: Subscapularis

Accessory muscles: teres major, pectoralis major, latissimus dorsi, and anterior fibers of deltoid.

• **Start Position.** The patient is prone. The shoulder is abducted to 90°, the elbow is flexed to 90°, the arm proximal to the elbow is resting on the plinth (Fig. 3-138).

• **Stabilization.** The therapist stabilizes the humerus to prevent shoulder adduction.

• **Movement.** The patient internally rotates the shoulder by moving the palm of the hand toward the ceiling (Fig. 3-139).

• **Palpation.** Subscapularis is too deep to palpate.

• **Substitution/Trick Movement.** Triceps (elbow extension) and pectoralis minor (scapular protraction).

• **Alternate Test.** If the patient has a history of posterior dislocation of the glenohumeral joint and/or is unable to assume the prone position or achieve 90° of shoulder abduction, the gravity eliminated position of sitting is assumed (Fig. 3-141), and the resisted gravity eliminated methodology is used.

• **Resistance Location.** Applied proximal to the wrist joint (Figs. 3-140, 3-141, and 3-142). Application of resistance stresses the shoulder and elbow joints, and caution should be exercised.

• **Resistance Direction.** Shoulder external rotation.

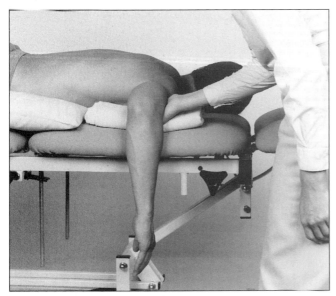

Figure 3-138. Start position: subscapularis.

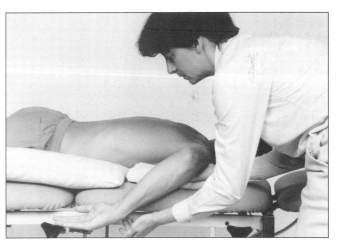

Figure 3-139. Screen position: subscapularis.

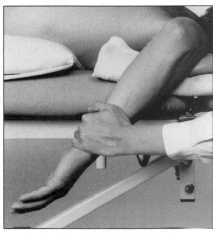

Figure 3-140. Resistance: subscapularis.

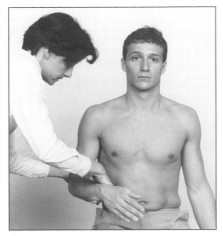

Figure 3-141. Alternate position: subscapularis.

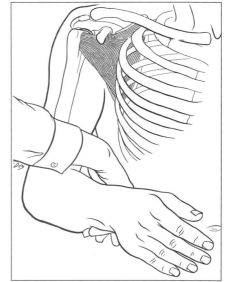

Figure 3-142. Subscapularis.

Gravity Eliminated: Subscapularis

- **Start Position.** The patient is sitting. The shoulder is slightly abducted in neutral rotation and the elbow is flexed to 90° with the forearm in midposition (Fig. 3-143).

- **Stabilization.** The therapist stabilizes the humerus to prevent shoulder abduction.

- **End Position.** The patient internally rotates the shoulder by bringing the palm of the hand toward the abdomen (Fig. 3-144).

- **Substitution/Trick Movement.** Triceps (elbow extension), shoulder abduction, and pronation of the forearm.

Subscapularis Alternate Test. The patient must have full shoulder internal rotation ROM to assume this test position. This test maximizes the activity of subscapularis and minimizes the activity of the accessory muscles: latissimus dorsi, pectoralis major[16,17] and teres major.[16]

- **Start Position.** The patient is sitting. The shoulder is internally rotated and the dorsum of the hand is placed over the midlumbar spine (Fig. 3-145).

- **Stabilization.** The therapist instructs the patient to avoid trunk forward flexion and/or ipsilateral trunk rotation.

- **End Position (not shown).** The patient moves the hand away from the back.

- **Palpation.** Subscapularis is too deep to palpate.

- **Substitution/Trick Movement.** Ipsilateral trunk rotation and/or trunk forward flexion, and scapular anterior tilt, retraction, medial rotation and elevation.

- **Resistance Location (not shown).** Applied proximal to the wrist joint. Application of resistance stresses the shoulder and elbow joints, and caution should be exercised.

- **Resistance Direction.** Shoulder external rotation. The resisted gravity eliminated method is used to assess for grades greater than 2 and the conventional gravity eliminated method is used to assess for grades less than 2.

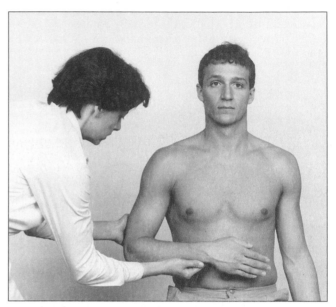

Figure 3-144. End position: subscapularis.

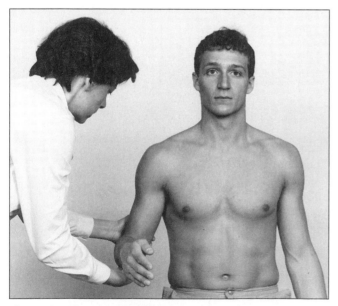

Figure 3-143. Start position: subscapularis.

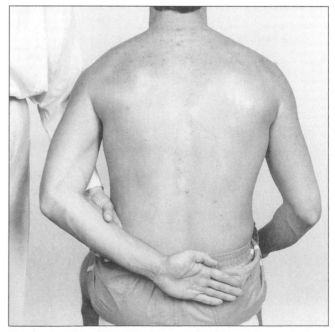

Figure 3-145. Alternate test start position: subscapularis.

SHOULDER EXTERNAL ROTATION

Against Gravity: Infraspinatus and Teres Minor

Accessory muscle: posterior fibers of deltoid.

- **Start Position.** The patient is prone. The shoulder is abducted to 90°, the elbow is flexed to 90°, and the arm proximal to the elbow is resting on the plinth (Fig. 3-146).

- **Stabilization.** The therapist stabilizes the humerus to prevent shoulder adduction.

- **Movement.** The patient externally rotates the shoulder by moving the dorsum of the hand toward the ceiling (Fig. 3-147).

- **Palpation.** Infraspinatus: over the body of the scapula just inferior to the spine of the scapula. Teres minor: not palpable.

- **Substitution/Trick Movement.** Triceps (elbow extension) and lower fibers of trapezius (scapular depression).

- **Alternate Test.** If the patient has a history of anterior dislocation of the glenohumeral joint and/or is unable to assume the prone position or achieve 90° of shoulder abduction, the gravity eliminated position of sitting is assumed and the resisted gravity eliminated methodology is used.

- **Resistance Location.** Applied proximal to the wrist joint on the posterior aspect of the forearm (Figs. 3-148, 3-149, and 3-150). Application of resistance stresses the elbow and shoulder joints, and caution should be exercised.

- **Resistance Direction.** Shoulder internal rotation.

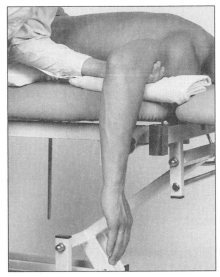

Figure 3-146. Start position: infraspinatus and teres minor.

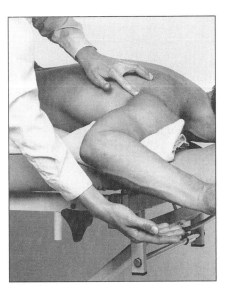

Figure 3-147. Screen position: infraspinatus and teres minor.

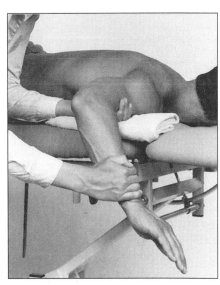

Figure 3-148. Resistance: infraspinatus and teres minor.

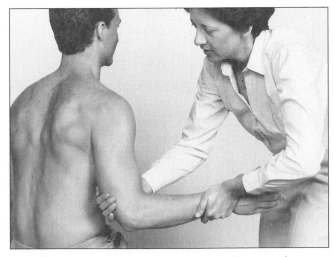

Figure 3-149. Alternate position: infraspinatus and teres minor.

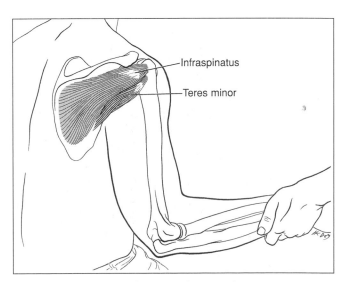

Figure 3-150. Infraspinatus and teres minor.

Gravity Eliminated: Infraspinatus and Teres Minor

• **Start Position.** The patient is sitting. The arm is at the side, with the shoulder adducted in neutral rotation, and the elbow is flexed to 90° with the forearm in midposition (Fig. 3-151).

• **Stabilization.** The therapist stabilizes the humerus.

• **End Position.** The patient externally rotates the shoulder by taking the hand away from the body (Fig. 3-152).

• **Substitution/Trick Movement.** Triceps (elbow extension), lower fibers of trapezius (scapular depression), and forearm supination.

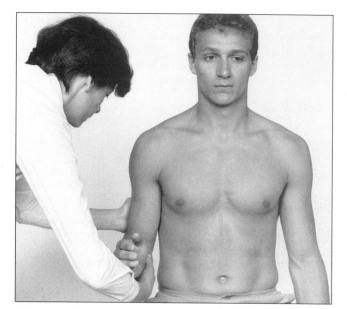

Figure 3-151.   Start position: infraspinatus and teres minor.

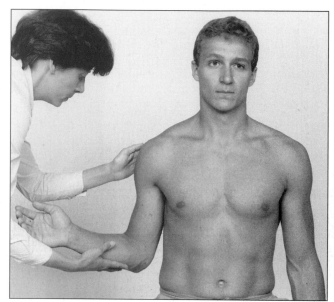

Figure 3-152.   End position: infraspinatus and teres minor.

▼ FUNCTIONAL APPLICATION: SHOULDER COMPLEX

JOINT FUNCTION

The function of the shoulder complex is to position or move the arm in space for the purpose of hand function. The shoulder complex is the most mobile joint complex in the body, providing ROM that exceeds that of any other joint. Because of this mobility, stability is sacrificed.[5,18–22]

FUNCTIONAL RANGE OF MOTION

The glenohumeral joint may by abducted and adducted, flexed and extended, and internally and externally rotated. In the performance of functional activities, the glenohumeral movements are accompanied at varying points in the ROM by scapular, clavicular, and trunk motion. These motions extend the functional range capabilities of the shoulder joint, and without their contribution, movement of the upper limbs would be severely restricted.[19,21,22] The functional movements of the shoulder complex are described, with the purpose of explaining the interdependence of the components of the shoulder complex and trunk throughout movement.

Elevation of the Arm Over the Head

This functional motion of elevation to 170° to 180° may be achieved through forward flexion in the sagittal plane or abduction in the frontal plane. Due to the position of the scapula, which lies 30° to 45° anterior to the frontal plane,[14] many daily functional activities are performed in the plane of the scapula. The plane of the scapula is the plane of reference for diagonal movements of shoulder elevation (Fig. 3-153). The plane used by an individual depends on the motion requirements of the activity and the position of the hand required for the task (Table 3-5).

To attain the full 180° of elevation through flexion or abduction, movement of the glenohumeral joint is accompanied by movement at the sternoclavicular, acromioclavicular, and scapulothoracic joints. The final degrees of motion can only be achieved through contribution of the spinal movement of trunk extension and/or contralateral side flexion.[1,14,18] The total shoulder complex functions in a coordinated way to provide smooth movement and to gain a large excursion of movement for the upper extremity. The coordinated movement pattern achieved through scapulothoracic and glenohumeral movement is described as a scapulohumeral rhythm.[5,14,18,20]

There are individual variations as to the contribution of all joints to the movement. Variation depends on the plane of elevation, the arc of elevation, the amount of load on the arm, and individual anatomical differ-

ences.[22] Recognizing these variations, it is generally felt that the range of glenohumeral to scapular motion throughout elevation is in the ratio of 2 : 1; that is, 2° of glenohumeral motion to every degree of scapular motion.[5,20,21,24] The scapulohumeral rhythm is described for elevation through flexion and for elevation through abduction. An understanding of the rhythm is essential in understanding the significance of limitations in joint ROM at the shoulder complex.

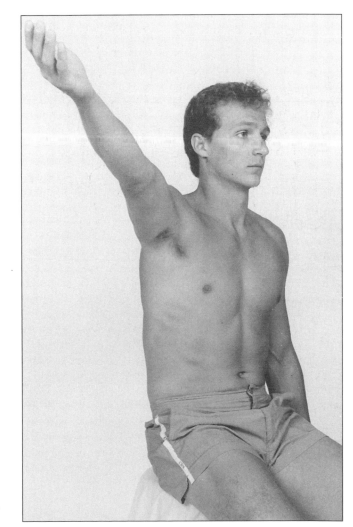

Figure 3-153. Elevation: plane of the scapula.

TABLE
3-5

▼ SHOULDER HORIZONTAL ADDUCTION/ABDUCTION AND OTHER SHOULDER ROM* REQUIRED FOR SELECTED FUNCTIONAL ACTIVITIES†

Activity	Horizontal Adduction ROM (degrees)‡	Other Shoulder ROM (degrees)	
Washing axilla	104 ± 12	flexion	52 ± 14
Eating	87 ± 29	flexion	52 ± 8
Combing hair	54 ± 27	abduction	112 ± 10
	Horizontal Abduction Rom (degrees)‡		
Reaching maximally up back	69 ± 11	extension	56 ± 13
Reaching perineum	86 ± 13	extension	38 ± 10

*Values are mean ± SD for eight normal subjects.
†This table was adapted from Matsen FA, Lippitt SB, Sidles JA, Harryman DT. *Practical Evaluation and Management of the Shoulder.* Philadelphia: WB Saunders; 1994:22, 23.[23]
‡The 0° start position for establishing the degrees of horizontal adduction and horizontal abduction is 90° shoulder abduction (see Fig. 3-41).

Scapulohumeral Rhythm

During the initial 60° of shoulder flexion in the sagittal plane or the initial 30° of abduction in the frontal plane, there is an inconsistent scapulohumeral rhythm. It is during this phase that the scapula is seeking stability in relationship to the humerus.[5,24-26] The scapula is in a setting phase where it may remain stationary, or it may slightly medially or laterally rotate[24] (Fig. 3-154). The glenohumeral joint is the main contributor to movement in this phase. Feeding activities that are performed within this phase of shoulder elevation include eating using a spoon or a fork and drinking from a cup. These activities are carried out within the ranges of 5° to 45° shoulder flexion and 5° to 30° shoulder abduction.[27]

Following the setting phase, there is a predictable scapulohumeral rhythm throughout the remaining arc of movement to 170° (Fig. 3-155). For every 15° of movement between 30° abduction or 60° flexion and 170° of abduction/flexion, 10° occurs at the glenohumeral joint and 5° occurs at the scapulothoracic joint. Movement of the scapula following the setting phase consists of the primary scapular movement of lateral rotation, accompanied by secondary rotations of posterior tilting (sagittal plane) and a posterior rotation (transverse plane) as the humeral angle is increased with elevation of the arm in the scapular plane.[28]

Range to 170° through abduction depends on a normal scapulohumeral rhythm and the ability to externally rotate the humerus fully through elevation. When the abducted arm reaches a position of 90°, movement through full range of elevation cannot continue as a result of the greater tuberosity of the humerus contacting the superior margin of the glenoid fossa and the coracoacromial arch.[1,26,29] External rotation of the humerus places the greater tuberosity posteriorly, allowing the humerus to move freely under the coracoacromial arch. Full shoulder elevation through flexion depends on scapulohumeral rhythm and the ability to rotate the humerus internally through range.[30]

The final degrees of elevation are achieved through contralateral trunk side flexion (Fig. 3-156) and/or trunk extension. From the discussion of scapulohumeral rhythm, it becomes apparent that restriction in movement at any of the joints of the shoulder complex will limit the ability to position the hand for function.

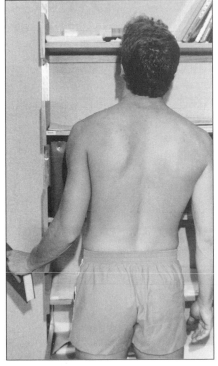

Figure 3-154. Setting phase of the scapula during elevation of the arm through abduction. The scapula remains stationary.

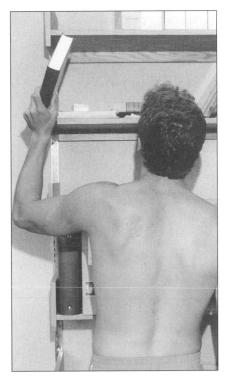

Figure 3-155. Scapulohumeral rhythm: during elevation beyond 60° of flexion or 30° of abduction, the scapula abducts and laterally rotates.

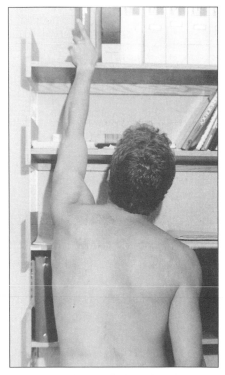

Figure 3-156. Full elevation through abduction: full range is achieved through contralateral trunk side flexion.

Shoulder Extension

The range of 60° of shoulder extension is primarily obtained through the glenohumeral joint.[29] A consistent scapulohumeral rhythm is not present in this movement. In the performance of functional activities, extension is often accompanied by adduction and medial rotation of the scapula.

Forty-three to 69° of shoulder extension is required to reach maximally up the back,[23] for example, when doing up a bra, (see Fig. 3-157), and 28° to 48° shoulder extension is necessary to reach the perineum[23] when performing toilet hygiene.

Horizontal Adduction and Abduction

The movements of horizontal adduction and abduction allow the arm to be moved around the body at shoulder level for such activities as washing the axilla or the back (see Fig. 3-160) and sliding windows open or closed. Although, by definition, horizontal adduction and abduction movements take place in the transverse plane, many activities of daily living (ADL) require similar motions in planes located above or below shoulder level. These movements may also be referred to as horizontal adduction and abduction, until these movements approach the frontal plane and are then referred to as either adduction or abduction. Table 3-5 provides examples of the ROM required for selected ADL, to bring the arm in front of body (horizontal adduction) or behind the body (horizontal abduction) and position the arm for other shoulder movements needed to perform these activities.

Internal and External Rotation

The range of movement varies with the position of the arm. Both ranges average 68° when the arm is at the side, whereas when the arm is abducted to 90°, 70° of internal and 90° of external rotation can be achieved.[9] Full external rotation is required to place the hand behind the neck when performing self-care activities such as combing the hair and manipulating the clasp of a necklace.

Mallon and colleagues[31] analyzed joint motions occurring at the shoulder complex and elbow in placing the arm behind the back. The analysis revealed the presence of a coordinated pattern of motion occurring between scapular and glenohumeral joint motion. At the beginning of the ROM, internal rotation occurs almost exclusively at the glenohumeral joint as the hand is brought across in front of the body and to a position alongside the ipsilateral hip. As the movement continues and the hand is brought behind the low back, motion at the scapulothoracic joint augments glenohumeral joint internal rotation. The elbow is then flexed to reach up the spine to the level of the thorax.

Internal shoulder rotation is needed to do up the buttons on a shirt. Five to 25° of shoulder internal rotation is required to eat using a spoon or fork and to drink from a cup.[27] Full glenohumeral joint internal rotation, augmented by scapulothoracic and elbow joint motion, positions the hand behind the back to reach into a back pocket, perform toilet hygiene, and do up a bra (Fig. 3-157).

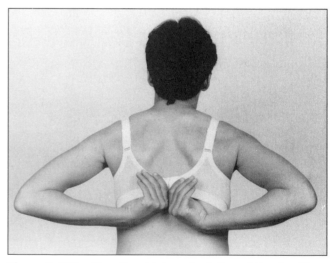

Figure 3-157. Functional internal rotation of the shoulders.

MUSCLE FUNCTION

Shoulder Elevation

The ability to perform activities involving elevation of the arm depends on joint integrity for freedom of movement and on the strength and function of the muscles of the shoulder girdle that produce and control movement.[5] The muscles responsible for the smooth, coordinated action involved in elevation can be divided into four functional groups:

1. Scapular stabilizers and motivators
2. Humeral stabilizers
3. Humeral flexors or abductors
4. Humeral rotators

The scapular stabilizers and motivators include the trapezius, rhomboids, serratus anterior, and levator scapulae. During the setting phase of the scapula there is minimal activity in these muscles. The specific contribution of scapular muscles depends on individual variation and whether the scapula, in its stabilizing role, is stationary, or slightly medially or laterally rotated.[24] Following the setting phase, a scapulohumeral rhythm exists with movements of the scapula and humerus occurring simultaneously. The setting phase and simultaneous movement can be visualized by observing the position of the scapula in Figures 3-154 and 3-155. As the arm is elevated there is a gradual increase in the activity of the scapular muscles to full range[24] as these muscles primarily rotate the scapula laterally or upward. The purpose of scapular rotation is to place the glenoid fossa and other lateral parts of the scapula in positions where the humerus can be raised without limitation imposed by bony and ligamentous structures.[32] The upper and lower fibers of trapezius and the serratus anterior are the prime movers responsible for the lateral rotation of the scapula.[14,28,33] The serratus anterior appears to play a more prominent role in elevation through flexion, drawing the scapula more anteriorly around the chest wall, while the trapezius appears to be more important in abduction.[5]

The second group of muscles stabilizes the humeral head in the glenoid fossa. Because the glenohumeral joint is not a static fulcrum, this stabilization is referred to as dynamic stability.[34] The functional significance of the movement or stabilizing contribution of these muscles becomes apparent through the following descriptions of specific muscle contribution throughout elevation. Throughout the full range of movement, the head of the humerus is stabilized in the glenoid fossa by the action of subscapularis, supraspinatus, infraspinatus, the upper half of teres minor[34,35] and the long head of biceps.[36] Through electromyographic studies, Saha[34] found that in abduction, the subscapularis and infraspinatus stabilize in the range of 0° to 150° and the infraspinatus is the primary stabilizer throughout the remainder of range. Supraspinatus provides stabilization in the pendant arm position.[20,35]

The third group of muscles acts to move the humerus in the sagittal or frontal plane. These muscles are active throughout a range of movement of 0° to 180°. These muscles proximally attach on the scapula and distally attach on the humerus and include the shoulder abductors and shoulder flexors. The middle fibers of the deltoid and supraspinatus elevate the humerus through abduction; the anterior fibers of deltoid and the clavicular portion of pectoralis major and coracobrachialis elevate the humerus through flexion.

As the shoulder muscles contract to flex or abduct the arm, the rotator cuff muscles stabilize or dynamically "fix" the head of the humerus in the glenoid fossa, thus creating a fulcrum or "fixed point" around which the humerus moves in abduction or flexion. This stabilization checks or prevents the occurrence of other, unwanted, movements of the humerus that would be created by the contraction forces of the shoulder abductor or flexor muscles during elevation.

The purpose of the fourth group is to rotate the humerus externally or internally. Elevation through abduction is accompanied by external rotation of the humerus.[1,18,26,29] The anterior fibers of deltoid also function to rotate the humerus internally,[37] as flexion is accompanied by internal rotation.[30]

The function of elevation of the shoulder is to position and move the arm in space for the purpose of hand function. Hand activity places additional demands on the muscles of the shoulder girdle responsible for elevation. Sporrong and coworkers[38] evaluated activity in four muscles of the shoulder girdle, a scapular stabilizer and motivator (trapezius), the humeral stabilizers (supraspinatus, infraspinatus), and a humeral motivator (deltoid), with a small load, similar in weight to an industrial handtool, held in the hand in elevated arm positions while sitting. When increased hand-grip forces were applied to the load, muscle activity increased in the shoulder girdle muscles, most notably in the humeral stabilizers.

Shoulder Adduction and Extension

From elevation of the arm through flexion or abduction the arm is brought down to the side of the body through extension or adduction. When quick movement or force is required for an activity such as closing a window, climbing a ladder, or serving the ball in tennis (Fig. 3-158), the latissimus dorsi and teres major adduct and extend the humerus. Although latissimus dorsi functions with or without resistance as a factor, teres major is only active in activities where resistance is a factor.[35] In this instance, teres major is accompanied by the action of rhomboids, functioning to rotate the scapula medially.[1,35] When the arm is taken posteriorly from the side, in a sagittal plane, the latissimus dorsi and teres major are assisted by the posterior fibers of deltoid.

The functional significance of the latissimus dorsi, through its attachment on the crest of the ilium, is apparent in activities that require weight bearing with the hands.[18] In activities, such as crutch walking or rising from a sitting position (Fig. 3-159), the latissimus dorsi depresses the shoulder girdle to raise the trunk and pelvis. The sternal fibers of pectoralis major assist latissimus dorsi to elevate the trunk on the fixed humerus as in performing a weight relief raise[39] or during depression transfers[40] for patients with low-level paraplegia.

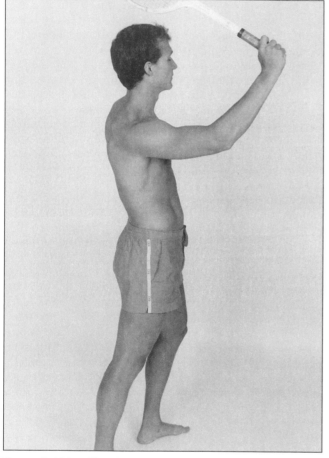

Figure 3-158. Shoulder extension.

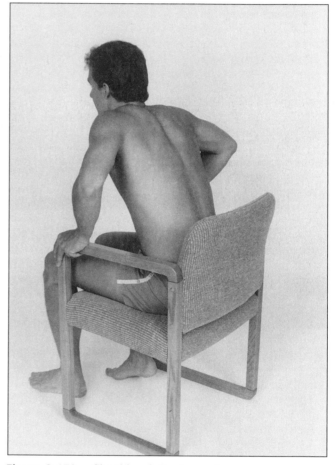

Figure 3-159. Shoulder girdle depression.

Flexion and Adduction

Pectoralis major is a flexor and adductor of the arm. The functional significance of its integrity is illustrated in self-care activities where the arm is flexed and adducted. This pattern of movement is evident in many self-care activities, including dressing, bathing (Fig. 3-160), and hygiene tasks.

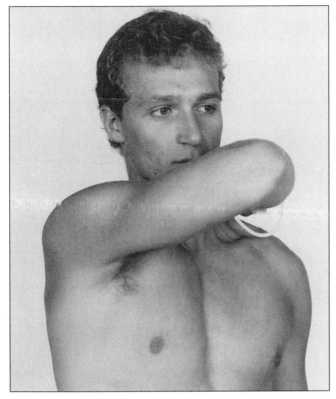

Figure 3-160. Flexion and adduction.

Internal Rotation

The subscapularis is the only pure internal rotator of the shoulder.[41] The teres major, latissimus dorsi, pectoralis major, and the anterior deltoid combine internal rotation with other movements previously described. Subscapularis internally rotates the humerus when the arm is positioned in front of or behind the body. The muscle plays a major role in lifting the hand away from the region of the midlumbar spine,[16] for example, as one positions a pillow behind the back when sitting.

Internal rotation has a functional link with pronation of the forearm, as both actions occur simultaneously with performance of many activities[18] and pronation can be amplified by internal rotation of the shoulder (Fig. 3-161).

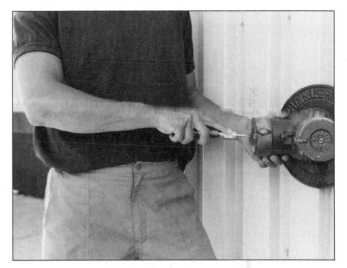

Figure 3-161. Functional association: should internal rotation and forearm pronation.

External Rotation

This movement is achieved through the action of infraspinatus, teres minor, and posterior deltoid. External rotation has a functional link with the supinators of the forearm when the elbow is extended.[18] Both muscle groups are concerned with turning the palm to face the ceiling. Examples of activities that illustrate this combined action are inserting a light bulb into a ceiling socket, releasing a bowling ball from the extended arm, and manipulating the foot into a shoe (Fig. 3-162).

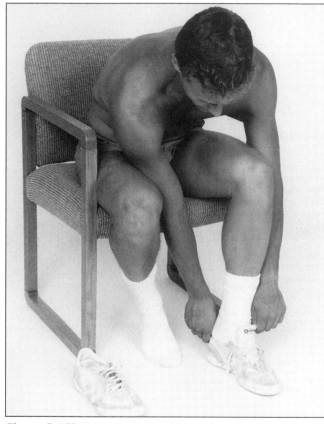

Figure 3-162. Functional association: shoulder external rotation and forearm supination.

REFERENCES

1. Kapandji IA. *The Physiology of the Joints*. Vol 1. 5th ed. New York: Churchill Livingstone; 1982.
2. Soames RW, ed. Skeletal system. Salmons S, ed. Muscle. *Gray's Anatomy*. 38th ed. New York: Churchill Livingstone; 1995.
3. Norkin CC, White DJ. *Measurement of Joint Motion: A Guide to Goniometry*. 2nd ed. Philadelphia: FA Davis; 1995.
4. Daniels L, Worthingham C. *Muscle Testing: Techniques of Manual Examination*. 5th ed. Philadelphia: WB Saunders; 1986.
5. Norkin CC, Levangie PK. *Joint Structure & Function: A Comprehensive Analysis*. 2nd ed. Philadelphia: FA Davis; 1992.
6. Woodburne RT. *Essentials of Human Anatomy*. 5th ed. London: Oxford University Press; 1973.
7. Cyriax J. *Textbook of Orthopaedic Medicine, vol. 1. Diagnosis of Soft Tissue Lesions*. 8th ed. London: Bailliere Tindall; 1982.
8. Magee DJ. *Orthopedic Physical Assessment*. 3rd ed. Philadelphia: WB Saunders; 1997.
9. American Academy of Orthopaedic Surgeons. *Joint Motion: Method of Measuring and Recording*. Chicago: Author; 1965.
10. Gajdosik RL, Hallett JP, Slaughter LL. Passive insufficiency of two-joint shoulder muscles. *Clin Biomech*. 1994;9:377–378.
11. Evjenth O, Hamberg J. *Muscle Stretching in Manual Therapy A Clinical Manual: The Extremities*, Vol. 1. Alfta, Sweden: Alfta Rehab Forlag; 1984.
12. Brunnstrom MA. Muscle testing around the shoulder girdle. *J Bone Joint Surg [Am]*. 1941;23:263–272.
13. Nishijima N, Yamamuro T, Fujio K, Ohba M. The swallowtail sign: a test of deltoid function. *J Bone Joint Surg [Br]*. 1994;77B:152–153.
14. Soderberg GL. *Kinesiology: Application to Pathological Motion*. 2nd ed. Baltimore: Williams & Wilkins; 1997.
15. Whitcomb LJ, Kelley MJ, Leiper CI. A comparison of torque production during dynamic strength testing of shoulder abduction in the coronal plane and the plane of the scapula. *J Orthop Sports Phys Ther*. 1995;21:227–232.
16. Greis PE, Kuhn JE, Schultheis J, Hintermeister R, Hawkins R. Validation of the lift-off test and analysis of subscapularis activity during maximal internal rotation. *Am J Sports Med*. 1996;24:589–593.
17. Kelly BT, Kadrmas WR, Speer KP. The manual muscle examination for rotator cuff strength. *Am J Sports Med*. 1996;24:581–588.
18. Smith LK, Weiss EL, Lehmkuhl LD. *Brunnstrom's Clinical Kinesiology*. 5th ed. Philadelphia: FA Davis; 1996.
19. MacConaill MA, Basmajian JV. *Muscles and Movements*. 2nd ed. New York: RE Kreiger; 1977.
20. Cailliet R. *Shoulder Pain*. 3rd ed. Philadelphia: FA Davis; 1991.
21. Rosse C. The shoulder region and the brachial plexus. In: Rosse C, Clawson DK, eds. *The Musculoskeletal System in Health and Disease*. New York: Harper & Row; 1980.
22. Zuckerman JD, Matsen FA. Biomechanics of the shoulder. In: Nordin M, Frankel VM. *Basic Biomechanics of the Musculoskeletal System*. 2nd ed. Philadelphia: Lea & Febiger; 1989.
23. Matsen FA, Lippitt SB, Sidles JA, Harryman DT. *Practical Evaluation and Management of the Shoulder*. Philadelphia: WB Saunders; 1994.

24. Inman VT, Saunders M, Abbot LC. Observations on the function of the shoulder joint. *J Bone Joint Surg.* 1944; 26:1–30.
25. Dvir Z, Berme N. The shoulder complex in elevation of the arm: a mechanism approach. *J Biomech.* 1978;11: 219–225.
26. Kent BE. Functional anatomy of the shoulder complex: a review. *Phys Ther* 1971;51:867–888.
27. Safaee-Rad R, Shwedyk E, Quanbury AO, Cooper JE. Normal functional range of motion of upper limb joints during performance of three feeding activities. *Arch Phys Med Rehabil.* 1990;71:505–509.
28. Ludewig PM, Cook TM, Nawoczenski DA. Three-dimensional scapular orientation and muscle activity at selected positions of humeral elevation. *J Orthop Sports Phys Ther.* 1996;24:57–65.
29. Peat M. The shoulder complex: a review of some aspects of functional anatomy. *Physiother Can.* 1977;29: 241–246.
30. Blakey RL, Palmer ML. Analysis of rotation accompanying shoulder flexion. *Phys Ther.* 1984;64:1214–1216.
31. Mallon WJ, Herring CL, Sallay PI, Moorman CT III, Crim JR. Use of vertebral levels to measure presumed internal rotation at the shoulder: A radiologic analysis. *J Shoulder Elbow Surg.* 1996;5:299–306.
32. Duvall EN. Critical analysis of divergent views of movement of the shoulder joint. *Arch Phys Med Rehabil.* 1955;36:149–153.
33. Johnson G, Bogduk N, Nowitzke A, House D. Anatomy and actions of the trapezius muscle. *Clinical Biomechanics.* 1994;9:44–50.
34. Saha AK. Dynamic stability of the glenohumeral joint. *Acta Orthop Scand.* 1971;42:491–505.
35. Basmajian JV, DeLuca CJ. *Muscles Alive: Their Functions Revealed by Electromyography.* 5th ed. Baltimore: Williams & Wilkins; 1985.
36. Pagnani MJ, Deng X-H, Warren RF, Torzilli PA, O'Brien SJ. Role of the long head of the biceps brachii in glenohumeral stability: A biomechanical study in cadavers. *J Shoulder Elbow Surg.* 1996;5:255–262.
37. Moore KL. *Clinically Oriented Anatomy.* Baltimore: Williams & Wilkins; 1980.
38. Sporrong H, Palmerud G, Herberts P. Hand grip increases shoulder muscle activity: an EMG analysis with static hand contractions in 9 subjects. *Acta Orthop Scand.* 1996;67:485–490.
39. Reyes ML, Gronley JK, Newsam CJ, Mulroy SJ, Perry J. Electromyographic analysis of shoulder muscles of men with low-level paraplegia during a weight relief raise. *Arch Phys Med Rehabil.* 1995;76:433–439.
40. Perry J, Gronley JK, Newsam CJ, Reyes ML, Mulroy SJ. Electromyographic analysis of shoulder muscles during depression transfers in subjects with low-level paraplegia. *Arch Phys Med Rehabil.* 1996;77:350–355.
41. Lehmkuhl LD, Smith LK. *Brunnstrom's Clinical Kinesiology.* 4th ed. Philadelphia: FA Davis; 1983.

ELBOW
AND FOREARM

▼ **SURFACE ANATOMY** (Figs. 4-1 and 4-2)

Structure	Location
1. Acromion process	Lateral aspect of the spine of the scapula at the tip of the shoulder.
2. Medial epicondyle of the humerus	Medial projection at the distal end of the humerus.
3. Lateral epicondyle of the humerus	Lateral projection at the distal end of the humerus.
4. Olecranon process	Posterior aspect of the elbow; proximal end of the shaft of the ulna.
5. Head of the radius	Distal to the lateral epicondyle of the humerus.
6. Styloid process of the radius	Bony prominence on the lateral aspect of the forearm at the distal end of the radius.
7. Head of the third metacarpal	Bony prominence at the base of the third digit.
8. Head of the ulna	Round bony prominence on the posteromedial aspect of the forearm at the distal end of the ulna.

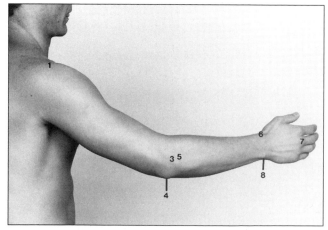

Figure 4-1.   Posterolateral aspect of the arm.

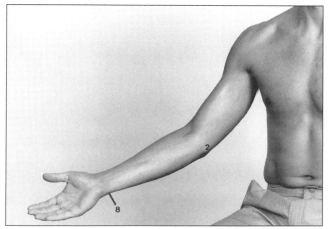

Figure 4-2.   Anteromedial aspect of the arm.

ASSESSMENT PROCESS: THE ELBOW AND FOREARM

1. The therapist observes:
   a. Function
   b. Posture, body symmetry, atrophy, and skin condition
   c. Active range of movement (AROM) at the elbow, the forearm, the shoulder, and the wrist
2. The therapist assesses passive range of motion (PROM) by:
   a. Estimating joint PROM
   b. Determining the end feels at the joint
   c. Establishing the presence or absence of pain
   d. Determining the presence of a capsular or noncapsular pattern
3. The therapist measures PROM through goniometry.
4. The therapist assesses muscle strength through manual muscle testing.

TABLE
4-1

▼ JOINT STRUCTURE: ELBOW AND FOREARM MOVEMENTS

	Flexion	Extension	Supination	Pronation
Articulation[1,2]	Humeroulnar, humeroradial	Humeroulnar, humeroradial	Humeroradial, superior radioulnar, inferior radioulnar, interosseous membrane	Humeroradial, superior radioulnar, inferior radioulnar, interosseous membrane
Plane	Sagittal	Sagittal	Horizontal	Horizontal
Axis	Frontal	Frontal	Longitudinal	Longitudinal
Normal limiting factors[1,3–5]	Soft tissue apposition of the anterior forearm and upper arm; coronoid process contacting the coronoid fossa and the radial head contacting the radial fossa; tension in the posterior capsule and triceps	Olecranon process contacting the olecranon fossa; tension in the elbow flexors and anterior joint capsule	Tension in the pronator muscles, quadrate ligament, palmar radioulnar ligament of the inferior radioulnar joint, oblique cord, and interosseous membrane	Contact of the radius on the ulna; tension in the quadrate ligament, the dorsal radioulnar ligament of the inferior radioulnar joint, interosseous membrane; supinator, and biceps brachii muscles with elbow in extension
Normal end feel[3,6,7]	Soft/hard/firm	Hard/firm	Firm	Hard/firm
Normal active range of motion[8]	0–150°	150–0°	0–80–90°	0–80–90°
Capsular pattern[6,7]	Elbow joint: flexion, extension, and rotation full and painless			
	Superior radioulnar joint: equal limitation of supination and pronation			
	Inferior radioulnar joint: full rotation with pain at extremes of rotation			

RANGE OF MOTION ASSESSMENT AND MEASUREMENT

The articulations and joint axes of the elbow and fore-arm are illustrated in Figures 4-3 and 4-4 and the joint structure is described in Table 4-1.

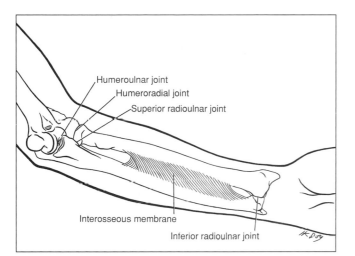

Figure 4-3.   Elbow and forearm articulations.

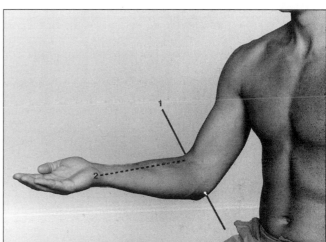

Figure 4-4.   Elbow joint and forearm axes: (*1*) flexion-extension and (*2*) supination-pronation.

ELBOW FLEXION-EXTENSION/HYPEREXTENSION

AROM Assessment

• **Substitution/Trick Movement.** Flexion—shoulder flexion. Extension—shoulder extension.

PROM Assessment

• **Start Position.** The patient is supine or sitting. The arm is in the anatomical position with the elbow in extension (Fig. 4-5). A towel is placed under the distal end of the humerus to accommodate the ROM. Due to biceps muscle tension, unusually muscular men may not be able to achieve 0°. Up to 15° of hyperextension is not uncommon in women[8-10] or children because the olecranon is smaller.[10]

• **Stabilization.** The therapist stabilizes the humerus.

• **Therapist's Distal Hand Placement.** The therapist grasps the distal radius and ulna.

• **End Positions.** The therapist applies slight traction to and moves the forearm in an anterior direction, applying slight overpressure at the limit of elbow flexion (Fig. 4-6).

The therapist applies slight traction to and moves the forearm in a posterior direction, applying slight overpressure at the limit of elbow extension/hyperextension (Fig. 4-7).

• **End Feels.** Flexion—soft/hard/firm; extension/hyperextension—hard/firm.

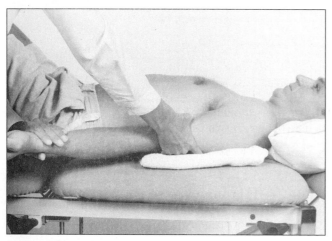

Figure 4-5. Start position for elbow flexion and extension/hyperextension.

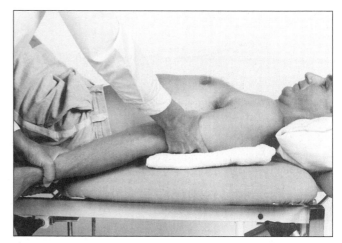

Figure 4-7. Hard or soft end feel at limit of elbow hyperextension.

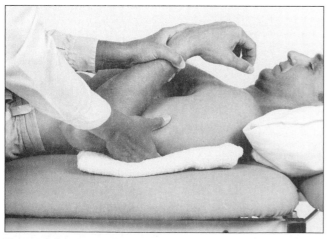

Figure 4-6. Soft or hard end feel at limit of elbow flexion.

Measurement: Universal Goniometer

• **Start Position.** The patient is supine or sitting. The arm is in the anatomical position with the elbow in extension (0°) (Fig. 4-8). A towel is placed under the distal end of the humerus to accommodate the ROM. Due to biceps muscle tension, unusually muscular men may not be able to achieve 0°.

• **Stabilization.** The therapist stabilizes the humerus.

• **Goniometer Axis.** The axis is placed over the lateral epicondyle of the humerus.

• **Stationary Arm.** Parallel to the longitudinal axis of the humerus, pointing toward the tip of the acromion process.

• **Movable Arm.** Parallel to the longitudinal axis of the radius, pointing toward the styloid process of the radius.

• **End Position.** From the start position of elbow extension, the forearm is moved in an anterior direction so that the hand approximates the shoulder to the limit of elbow flexion (150°) (Fig. 4-9).

• **Hyperextension.** The forearm is moved in a posterior direction beyond 0° of extension (Fig. 4-10). Up to 15° of hyperextension is not uncommon in women[8-10] or children because the olecranon is smaller.[10]

Alternate Measurement. The patient is sitting (Figs. 4-11 and 4-12).

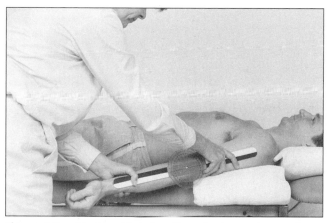

Figure 4-8. Start position for elbow flexion and extension.

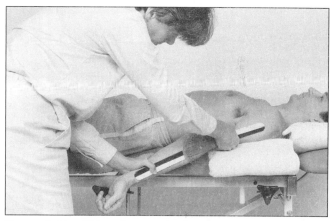

Figure 4-10. Elbow hyperextension.

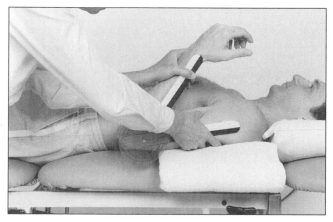

Figure 4-9. Elbow flexion.

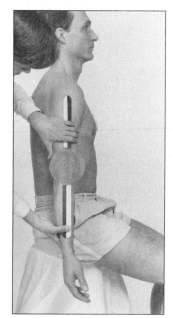

Figure 4-11. Elbow extension 0°.

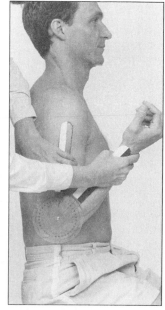

Figure 4-12. Elbow flexion.

SUPINATION—PRONATION

AROM Assessment

• **Substitution/Trick Movement.** Supination—adduction and external rotation of the shoulder, and ipsilateral trunk side flexion. Pronation—abduction and internal rotation of the shoulder, and contralateral trunk side flexion.

PROM Assessment

• **Start Position.** The patient is sitting. The arm is at the side, and the elbow is flexed to 90° with the forearm in midposition (see Fig. 4-13A).

• **Stabilization.** The therapist stabilizes the humerus.

• **Therapist's Distal Hand Placement.** The therapist grasps the distal radius and ulna (Fig. 4-13 A and B).

• **End Positions.** The forearm is rotated externally from midposition so that the palm faces upward and toward the ceiling to the limit of forearm supination (Fig. 4-14 A and B).

The forearm is rotated internally so that the palm faces downward and toward the floor to the limit of forearm pronation (Fig. 4-15 A and B).

• **End Feels.** Supination—firm; pronation—hard/firm.

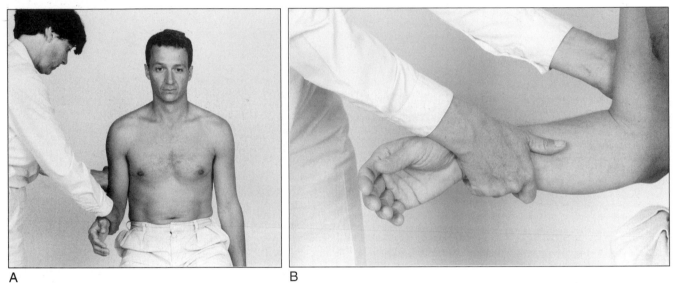

A   B

Figure 4-13.   A. Start position for supination and pronation. B. Therapist's hand position.

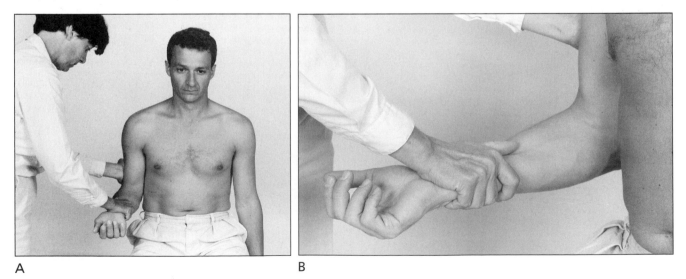

A   B

Figure 4-14.   A. Firm end feel at limit of supination. B. Therapist's hand position.

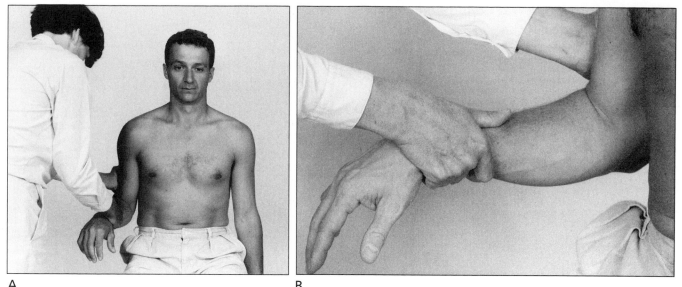

A   B

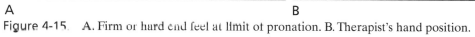

Figure 4-15.   A. Firm or hard end feel at limit of pronation. B. Therapist's hand position.

ELBOW AND FOREARM

Measurement: Universal Goniometer

- **Start Position.** The patient is sitting. The arm is at the side, and the elbow is flexed to 90° with the forearm in midposition. A pencil is held in the tightly closed fist with the pencil protruding from the radial aspect of the hand[9] (Fig. 4-16).

- **Stabilization.** The patient stabilizes the humerus using the nontest hand.

- **Goniometer Axis.** The axis is placed over the head of the third metacarpal.

- **Stationary Arm.** Perpendicular to the floor.

- **Movable Arm.** Parallel to the pencil.

- **End Position.** The forearm is rotated externally from midposition so that the palm faces upward and toward the ceiling (80–90° from midposition) (Fig. 4-17).

- **Substitution/Trick Movement.** Altered grasp of the pencil, wrist extension and/or radial deviation.

- **End Position.** The forearm is rotated internally so that the palm faces downward and toward the floor (80–90° from midposition) (Fig. 4-18).

- **Substitution/Trick Movement.** Altered grasp of the pencil, wrist flexion and/or ulnar deviation.

Alternate Measurement. This measurement is indicated if the patient is unable to grasp a pencil.

- **Start Position.** The arm is at the side, and the elbow is flexed to 90° with the forearm in midposition. The wrist is in neutral, and the fingers are extended (Fig. 4-19).

- **Stabilization.** The patient stabilizes the humerus using the nontest hand.

- **Goniometer Axis.** The axis is placed at the tip of the middle digit.

- **Stationary Arm.** Perpendicular to the floor.

- **Movable Arm.** Parallel to the tips of the four extended fingers.

- **End Position.** The forearm is rotated externally so that the palm faces upward and toward the ceiling (80–90° from midposition) (Fig. 4-20).

- **Substitution/Trick Movement.** Finger hyperextension, wrist extension, wrist deviations.

- **End Position.** The forearm is rotated internally so that the palm faces downward and toward the floor (80–90° from midposition) (Fig. 4-21).

- **Substitution/Trick Movement.** Finger flexion, wrist flexion, wrist deviations.

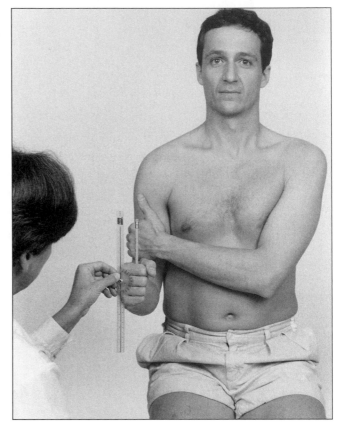

Figure 4-16.   Start position for supination and pronation.

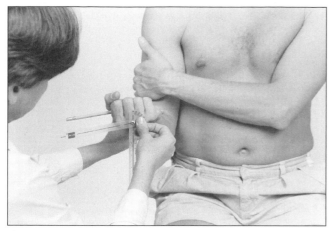

Figure 4-17.   Supination.

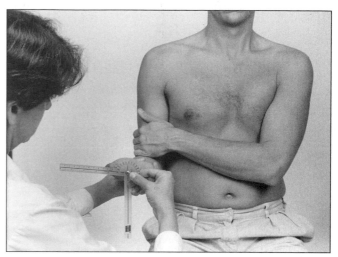

Figure 4-20.   Supination.

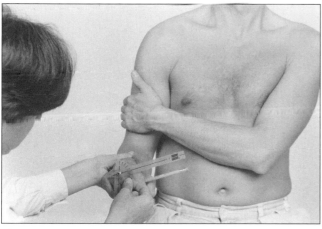

Figure 4-18.   Pronation.

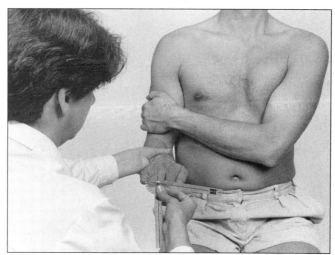

Figure 4-21.   Pronation.

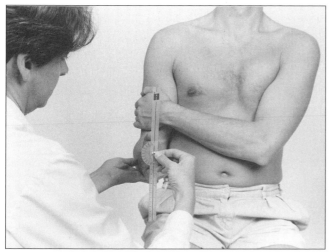

Figure 4-19.   Start position for supination and pronation.

MEASUREMENT OF MUSCLE LENGTH: BICEPS BRACHII

• **Start Position.** The patient is supine with the shoulder in extension over the edge of the plinth, the elbow is flexed, and the forearm is pronated (Fig. 4-22).

• **Stabilization.** The therapist stabilizes the humerus.

• **End Position.** The elbow is extended to the limit of motion so that biceps brachii is put on full stretch (Figs. 4-23 and 4-24).

• **Goniometer Placement.** The goniometer is placed the same as for elbow flexion-extension.

• **End Feel.** Biceps brachii on stretch-firm.

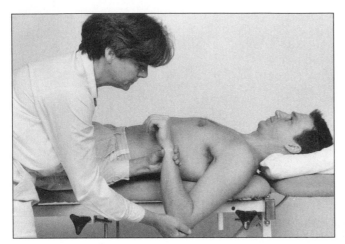

Figure 4-22.   Start position: length of biceps brachii.

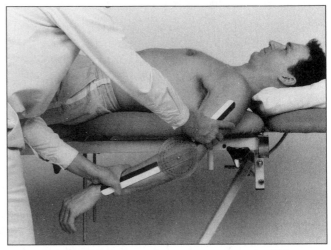

Figure 4-23.   Goniometer measurement: length of biceps brachii.

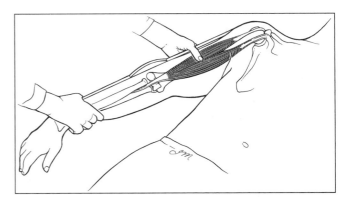

Figure 4-24.   Biceps brachii on stretch.

MEASUREMENT OF MUSCLE LENGTH: TRICEPS

- **Start Position.** The patient is sitting with the shoulder in full elevation through forward flexion and external rotation. The elbow is in extension (Fig. 4-25).

- **Stabilization.** The therapist stabilizes the humerus.

- **End Position.** The elbow is flexed to the limit of motion so that triceps is put on full stretch (Figs. 4-26 and 4-27).

- **Goniometer Placement.** The goniometer is placed the same as for elbow flexion-extension.

- **End Feel.** Triceps on stretch-firm.

Alternate Position. If the patient has decreased shoulder flexion ROM.

- **Start Position.** The patient is supine with the shoulder in 90° flexion and the elbow in extension (Fig. 4-28).

- **Stabilization.** The therapist stabilizes the humerus.

- **End Position.** The elbow is flexed to the limit of motion to put triceps on stretch (Fig. 4-29).

- **Goniometer Placement.** The goniometer is placed the same as for elbow flexion-extension.

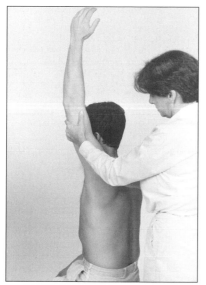

Figure 4-25. Start position: length of triceps.

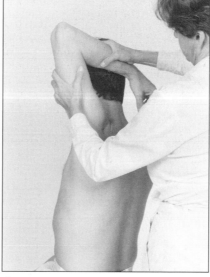

Figure 4-26. End position: triceps on stretch.

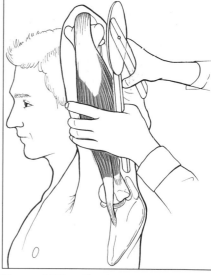

Figure 4-27. Goniometer measurement: length of triceps.

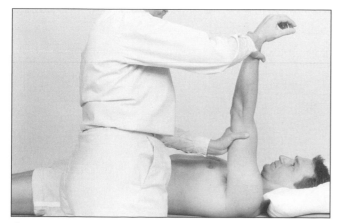

Figure 4-28. Alternate start position: triceps length.

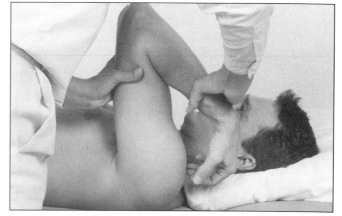

Figure 4-29. End position: triceps on stretch.

TABLE 4-6 ▼ MUSCLE ACTIONS, ATTACHMENTS, AND NERVE SUPPLY: THE ELBOW AND FOREARM[2]

Muscle	Primary Muscle Action	Muscle Origin	Muscle Insertion	Peripheral Nerve	Nerve Root
Biceps brachii	Elbow flexion Forearm supination	a. Short head: apex of the coracoid process of the scapula b. Long head: supraglenoid tubercle of the scapula	a. Posterior aspect of the radial tuberosity b. Bicipital aponeurosis: deep fascia covering origins of the flexor muscles of the forearm	Musculocutaneous	C56
Brachialis	Elbow flexion	Distal one half of the anterior aspect of the humerus; medial and lateral intermuscular septa	Tuberosity of the ulna; rough impression on the anterior surface of the coronoid process	Musculocutaneous, Radial	C56(7)
Brachioradialis	Elbow flexion	Proximal two thirds of the lateral supracondylar ridge of the humerus; lateral intermuscular septum	Lateral side of the distal end of the radius, just proximal to the styloid process	Radial	C56
Triceps	Elbow extension	a. Long head: infraglenoid tubercle of the scapula b. Lateral head: posterolateral surface of the humerus between the radial groove and the insertion of teres minor; lateral intermuscular septum c. Medial head: posterior surface of the humerus below the radial groove between the trochlea of the humerus and the insertion of teres major; medial and lateral intermuscular septa	Posteriorly, on the proximal surface of the olecranon; some fibers continue distally to blend with the antebrachial fascia	Radial	C678

TABLE
4-2

▼ **MUSCLE ACTIONS, ATTACHMENTS, AND NERVE SUPPLY: THE ELBOW AND FOREARM**[2] *Continued*

Muscle	Primary Muscle Action	Muscle Origin	Muscle Insertion	Peripheral Nerve	Nerve Root
Supinator	Forearm supination	Lateral epicondyle of the humerus; radial collateral ligament of the elbow joint; annular ligament of the superior radioulnar joint; from the supinator crest of the ulna and the posterior part of the depression anterior to it	Anterolateral and posterolateral surfaces of the proximal one third of the radius	Posterior interosseous branch of radial	C67
Pronator teres	Forearm pronation	a. Humeral head: just proximal to the medial epicondyle; common forearm flexor muscle tendon b. Ulnar head: medial side of the coronoid process of the ulna	Midway along the lateral surface of the radial shaft	Median	C67
Pronator quadratus	Forearm pronation	Distal one fourth of the anterior surface of the shaft of the ulna	Distal one fourth of the anterior border and surface of the shaft of the radius; triangular area proximal to the ulnar notch of the radius	Anterior interosseous branch of median	C78

ELBOW AND FOREARM

ELBOW FLEXION

Against Gravity: Biceps Brachii

Accessory muscles: brachialis, brachioradialis, pronator teres,[2] and extensor carpi radialis longus and brevis.[11]

• **Start Position.** The patient is supine or sitting. The arm is at the side, the elbow is extended, and the forearm is supinated (Fig. 4-30).

• **Stabilization.** The therapist stabilizes the humerus.

• **Movement.** The patient flexes the elbow through full ROM (Fig. 4-31).

• **Palpation.** Anterior aspect of the antecubital fossa.

• **Substitution/Trick Movement.** Brachialis may substitute for biceps brachii, because it is an elbow flexor, irrespective of forearm positioning.[12]

• **Resistance Location.** Applied proximal to the wrist joint on the anterior aspect of the forearm (Figs. 4-32 and 4-33).

• **Resistance Direction.** Forearm pronation and elbow extension.

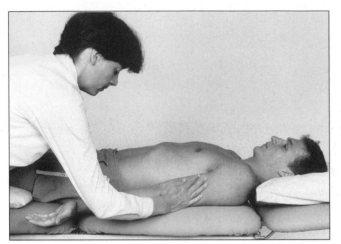

Figure 4-30.   Start position: biceps brachii.

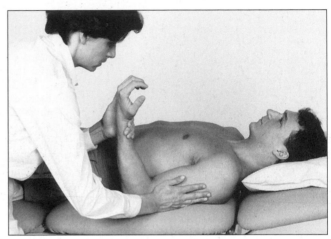

Figure 4-32.   Resistance: biceps brachii.

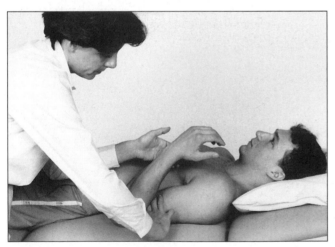

Figure 4-31.   Screen position: biceps brachii.

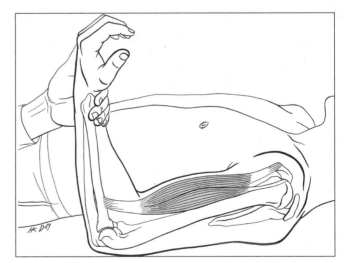

Figure 4-33.   Biceps brachii.

Gravity Eliminated: Biceps Brachii

• **Start Position.** The patient is sitting with the arm supported on a powder board. The shoulder is abducted to 90°, the elbow is extended, and the forearm is supinated (Fig. 4-34).

• **Alternate Start Position.** The patient is in a side-lying position. The therapist supports the weight of the upper extremity (Fig. 4-35).

• **Stabilization.** The therapist stabilizes the humerus.

• **End Position.** The patient flexes the elbow through full ROM (Fig. 4-36).

• **Substitution/Trick Movement.** Brachialis.

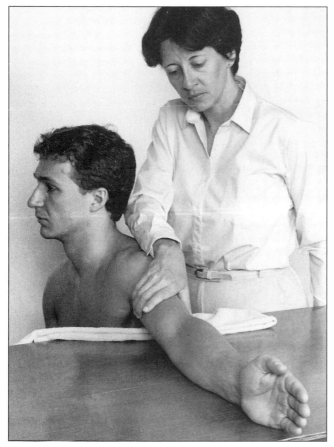

Figure 4-34.   Start position: biceps brachii.

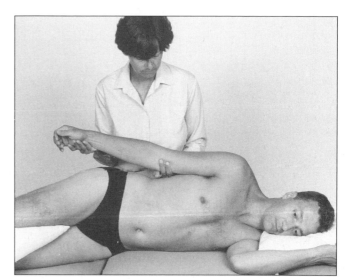

Figure 4-35.   Alternate start position.

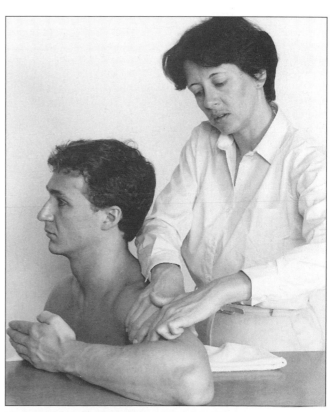

Figure 4-36.   End position: biceps brachii.

Against Gravity: Brachialis and Brachioradialis

Accessory muscles: biceps brachii, pronator teres,[2] and extensor carpi radialis longus and brevis.[11]

- **Start Position.** The patient is supine or sitting. The arm is at the side, the elbow is extended, and the forearm is in pronation (Fig. 4-37).

- **Stabilization.** The therapist stabilizes the humerus.

- **Movement.** The patient flexes the elbow through full ROM (Fig. 4-38).

- **Palpation.** Brachialis: medial to biceps brachii tendon. Brachioradialis: anterolateral aspect of the forearm, just distal to the elbow crease. Because both muscles are active when the forearm is pronated,[12] muscle contraction must be confirmed by palpation and/or observation.

- **Resistance Location.** Applied proximal to the wrist joint on the posterior aspect of the forearm (Figs. 4-39, 4-40, and 4-41).

- **Resistance Direction.** Elbow extension.

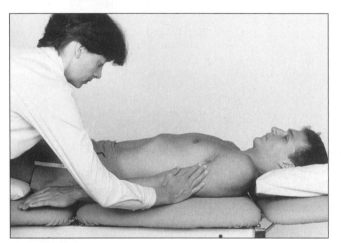

Figure 4-37. Start position: brachialis and brachioradialis.

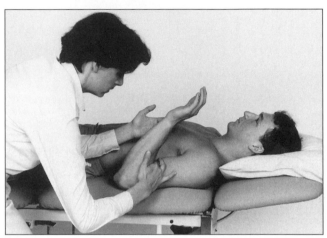

Figure 4-38. Screen position: brachialis and brachioradialis.

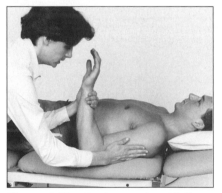

Figure 4-39. Resistance: brachialis and brachioradialis.

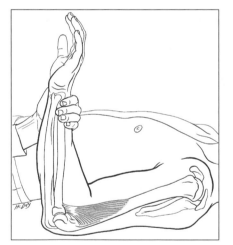

Figure 4-40. Brachialis.

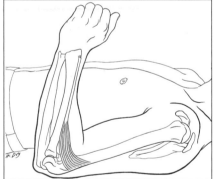

Figure 4-41. Brachioradialis.

Gravity Eliminated: Brachialis and Brachioradialis

• **Start Position.** The patient is sitting with the arm supported on a powder board. The shoulder is abducted to 90°, the elbow is extended, and the forearm is pronated (Fig. 4-42). An alternate position is side-lying (not shown).

• **Stabilization.** The therapist stabilizes the humerus.

• **End Position.** The patient flexes the elbow through full ROM (Fig. 4-43).

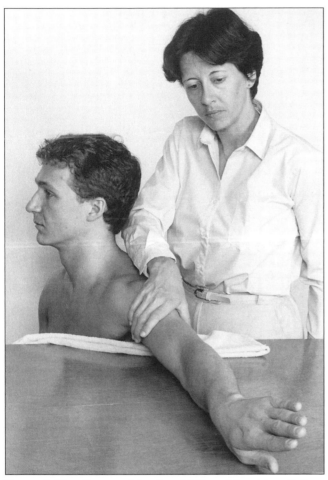

Figure 4-42. Start position: brachialis and brachioradialis.

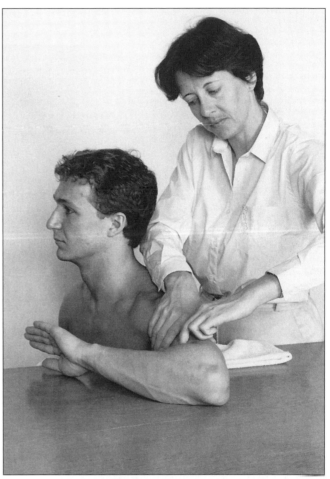

Figure 4-43. End position: brachialis and brachioradialis.

ELBOW AND FOREARM

ELBOW EXTENSION

Against Gravity: Triceps

Accessory muscle: anconeus.

- **Start Position.** The patient is supine. The shoulder is internally rotated and flexed to 90°, the elbow is flexed, and the forearm is supinated (Fig. 4-44).

- **Stabilization.** The therapist stabilizes the humerus.

- **Movement.** The patient extends the elbow through full ROM (Fig. 4-45). Ensure that the patient does not lock the elbow in full extension (close-packed position).

- **Palpation.** Just proximal to the olecranon process.

- **Resistance Location.** Applied proximal to the wrist joint on the posterior aspect of the forearm (Figs. 4-46 and 4-47).

- **Resistance Direction.** Elbow flexion.

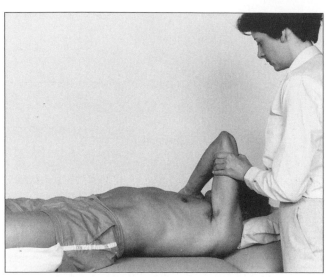

Figure 4-44.   Start position: triceps.

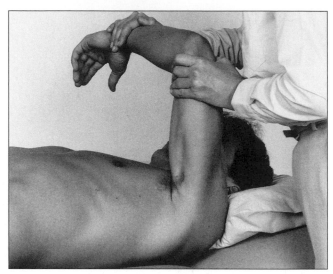

Figure 4-46.   Resistance: triceps.

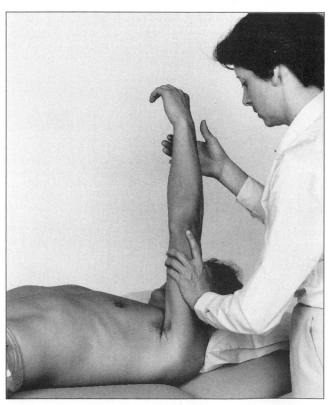

Figure 4-45.   Screen position: triceps.

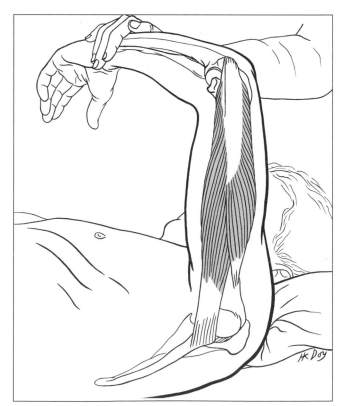

Figure 4-47.   Triceps.

Gravity Eliminated: Triceps

• **Start Position.** The patient is sitting with the arm supported on a powder board. The shoulder is abducted to 90°, the elbow is flexed, and the forearm is supinated (Fig. 4-48).

• **Alternate Start Position.** The patient is in a side-lying position. The therapist supports the weight of the upper extremity (Fig. 4-49).

• **Stabilization.** The therapist stabilizes the humerus.

• **End Position.** The patient extends the elbow through full ROM, avoiding the close-packed position (Fig. 4-50).

• **Substitution/Trick Movement.** Scapular depression and shoulder external rotation, permitting gravity to complete the ROM.

Alternate Against Gravity Assessment: Triceps. This test is indicated if the patient has shoulder muscle weakness.

The patient is prone. A towel is placed under the humerus for patient comfort during application of stabilization and resistance. The shoulder is abducted, and the elbow is flexed with the forearm and hand hanging vertically over the edge of the plinth (Fig. 4-51). The patient extends the elbow through the full ROM, avoiding the close-packed position (Fig. 4-52). Resistance is applied proximal to the wrist joint on the posterior aspect of the forearm (Fig. 4-53).

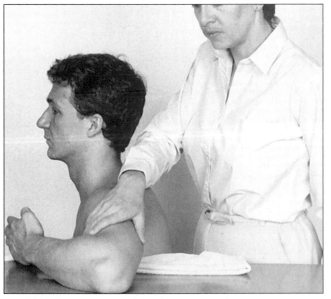

Figure 4-48.   Start position: triceps.

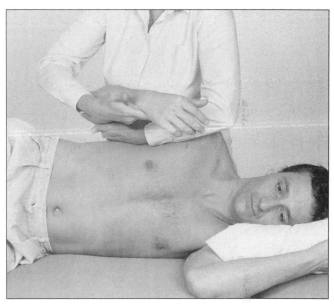

Figure 4-49.   Alternate start position.

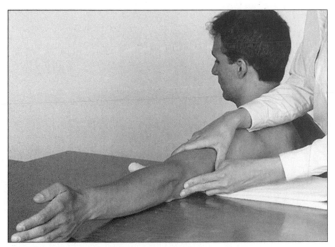

Figure 4-50.   End position: triceps.

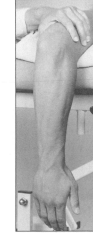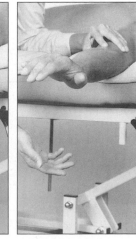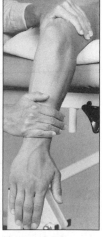

Figure 4-51.
Start position:
triceps.

Figure 4-52.   Screen
position: triceps.

Figure 4-53.
Resistance:
triceps.

SUPINATION

Against Gravity: Supinator and Biceps Brachii

• Start Position. The patient is sitting. The arm is at the side, the elbow is flexed to 90°, and the forearm is pronated (Fig. 4-54).

• Stabilization. The therapist stabilizes the humerus.

• Movement. The patient supinates the forearm through full ROM (Fig. 4-55). Because gravity assists supination beyond midposition, slight resistance, equal to the weight of the forearm, may be applied by the therapist.

• Palpation. Biceps brachii: anterior aspect of the antecubital fossa. Supinator: posterior aspect of the forearm, distal to the head of the radius.

• Substitution/Trick Movement. Shoulder external rotation, shoulder adduction, and ipsilateral trunk side flexion.

• Resistance Location. Applied on the posterior surface of the distal end of the radius with counterpressure on the anterior aspect of the ulna (Figs. 4-56 and 4-57).

• Resistance Direction. Forearm pronation.

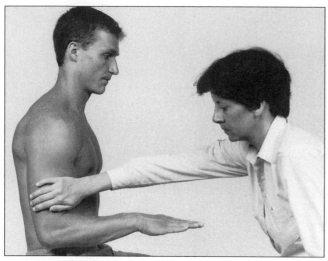

Figure 4-54.   Start position: supinator and biceps brachii.

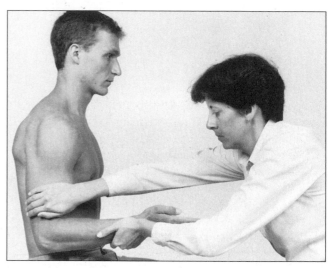

Figure 4-56.   Resistance: supinator and biceps brachii.

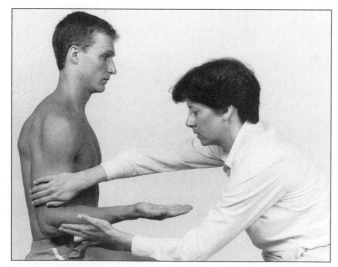

Figure 4-55.   Screen position: supinator and biceps brachii.

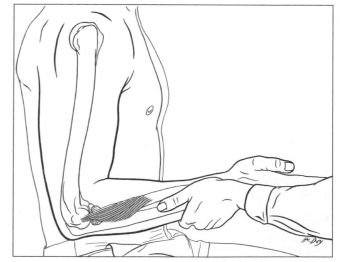

Figure 4-57.   Supinator.

Gravity Eliminated: Supinator and Biceps Brachii

• **Start Position.** The patient is supine with the arm at the side, the elbow flexed to 90°, and the forearm pronated (Fig. 4-58).

• **Alternate Start Position (not shown).** The patient is sitting, the shoulder and elbow are flexed to 90°, and the forearm is pronated.

• **Stabilization.** The therapist stabilizes the humerus.

• **End Position.** The patient supinates the forearm through full ROM (Fig. 4-59).

• **Substitution/Trick Movement.** Shoulder adduction and external rotation.

Isolation of Supinator. The biceps brachii does not supinate the forearm when the elbow is in extension and the movement is performed slowly and without resistance.[5,12]

• **Start Position.** The patient is sitting, the arm is at the side, the elbow extended, and the forearm is pronated.

• **Stabilization.** The therapist stabilizes the humerus.

• **Movement.** The patient supinates the forearm through full ROM. The therapist palpates supinator during the movement (Fig. 4-60).

• **Alternate Start Position (not shown).** Using this test position the biceps brachii is placed in a maximally shortened position, that is, a position of active insufficiency. In this position the biceps is put on slack and no longer has the ability to develop effective tension, thus isolating supinator.

• **Start Position.** The patient is supine, the shoulder is flexed 90°, the elbow is fully flexed and the forearm pronated.

• **Stabilization.** The therapist stabilizes the humerus.

• **Movement.** The patient slowly supinates the forearm. The therapist palpates supinator during the movement.

In the presence of supinator muscle weakness the patient will be unable to maintain the forearm in the fully supinated position using biceps alone.[13]

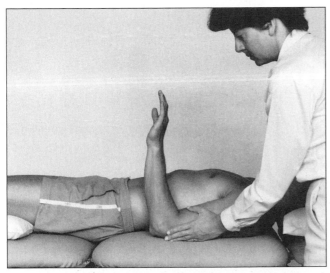

Figure 4-58.   Start position: supinator and biceps brachii.

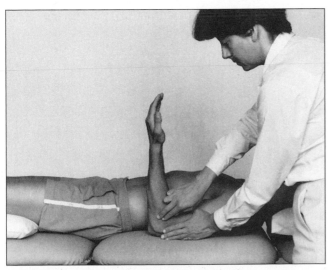

Figure 4-59.   End position: supinator and biceps brachii.

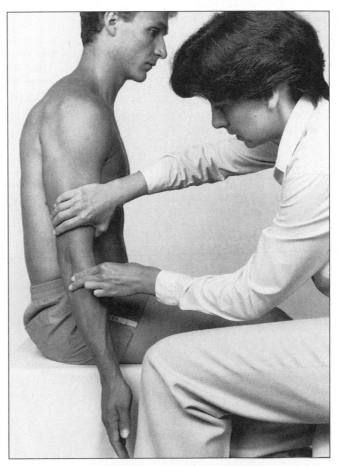

Figure 4-60.   Clinical test for isolation of supinator.

PRONATION

Against Gravity: Pronator Teres and Pronator Quadratus

• Start Position. The patient is sitting. The arm is at the side, the elbow is flexed to 90°, and the forearm is supinated (Fig. 4-61).

• Stabilization. The therapist stabilizes the humerus.

• Movement. The patient pronates the forearm through full ROM (Fig. 4-62). Because gravity assists pronation beyond midposition, slight resistance, equal to the weight of the forearm, may be applied by the therapist.

• Palpation. Pronator teres: proximal one-third of the anterior surface of the forearm on a diagonal line from the medial epicondyle of the humerus to the middle of the lateral border of the radius. Pronator quadratus: too deep to palpate.

• Substitution/Trick Movement. Shoulder abduction and internal rotation, and contralateral trunk side flexion.

• Resistance Location. Applied on the anterior surface of the distal end of the radius with counterpressure on the posterior aspect of the ulna (Figs. 4-63, 4-64, and 4-65).

• Resistance Direction. Forearm supination.

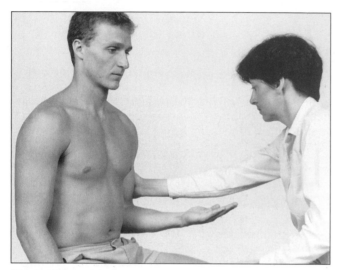

Figure 4-61. Start position: pronator teres and pronator quadratus.

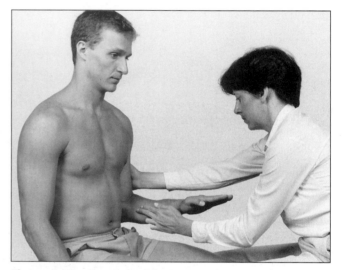

Figure 4-62. Screen position: pronator teres and pronator quadratus.

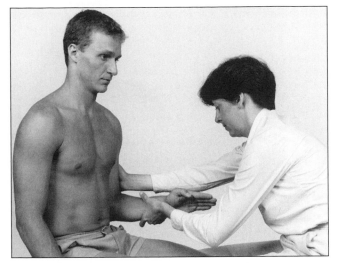

Figure 4-63. Resistance: pronator teres and pronator quadratus.

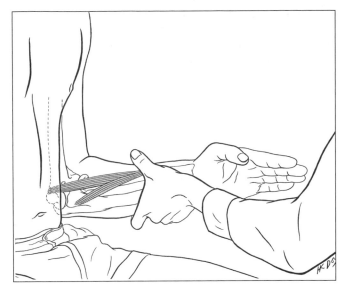

Figure 4-64. Pronator teres.

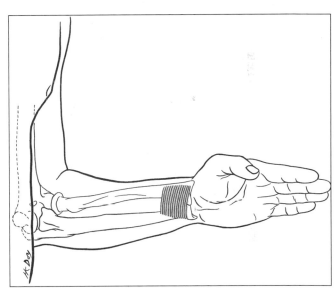

Figure 4-65. Pronator quadratus.

Gravity Eliminated: Pronator Teres and Pronator Quadratus

• **Start Position.** The patient is supine with the arm at the side, the elbow flexed to 90°, and the forearm supinated (Fig. 4-66).

• **Alternate Start Position (not shown).** The patient is sitting, the shoulder and elbow are flexed to 90°, and the forearm is supinated.

• **Stabilization.** The therapist stabilizes the humerus.

• **End Position.** The patient pronates the forearm through full ROM (Fig. 4-67).

• **Substitution/Trick Movement.** Shoulder abduction and internal rotation.

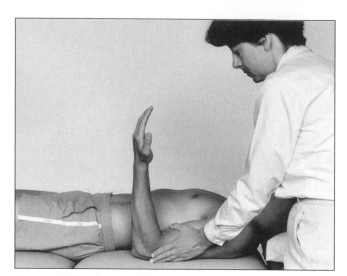

Figure 4-66. Start position: pronator teres and pronator quadratus.

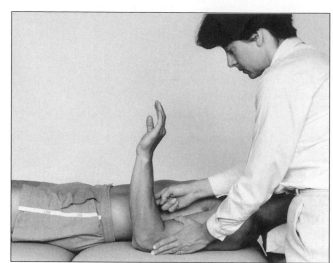

Figure 4-67. End position: pronator teres and pronator quadratus.

▼ FUNCTIONAL APPLICATION: ELBOW AND FOREARM

JOINT FUNCTION

The function of the elbow complex is to serve the hand.[1,5,14] Elbow extension moves the hand away from the body; elbow flexion moves the hand toward the body. Hand orientation in space and hand mobility are enhanced through supination and pronation of the forearm. The elbow complex, including the forearm, contributes to many skilled and forceful hand movements involved in daily self-care, leisure, and work functions. The elbow complex also provides the power necessary to perform lifting activities[15] and activities involving raising and lowering of the body using the hands.[14]

FUNCTIONAL RANGE OF MOTION

The normal AROM at the elbow is from 0° of extension to 150° of flexion, 80° to 90° of forearm pronation, and 80° to 90° of forearm supination. However, many daily functions are performed with less than these ranges. The ROM requirements for the activities of daily living are influenced by furniture design, the placement of utensils, and the patient's posture. Many self-care activities can be accomplished within the arc of movement from 30° to 130° of flexion and from 50° of pronation to 50° of supination.[15] Writing, pouring from a pitcher, reading a newspaper, and performing perineal hygiene are examples of activities performed within these ROMs. Feeding activities such as drinking from a cup (Fig. 4-68), eating using a fork or spoon (see Fig. 4-74), and cutting with a knife (Fig. 4-69) may be performed within an arc of movement from about 45° to 136° of flexion and from about 59° supination to 47° pronation.[15–18]

Daily functions that may involve extreme ranges of elbow motion include combing or washing the hair (flexion, pronation, and supination), reaching a back zipper at the neck level (flexion, pronation), using the telephone (135–140° flexion[15,17]), tying a shoe (16° flexion),[15] throwing a ball (extension), walking with crutches (extension) (Fig. 4-70), using the arms to elevate the body when getting up from a chair (15° flexion)[17] (see Fig. 4-73), and playing tennis (extension).

Less elbow ROM is required to perform most upper extremity activities when elbow flexion and extension ROM is restricted and compensatory motions are allowed at normal adjacent joints. In this case, functional elbow ROM is from 75° to 120° flexion.[19] These compensatory motions occur at the thoracic and lumbar spines, shoulder (primarily scapulothoracic and clavicular joints), and the wrist.[20]

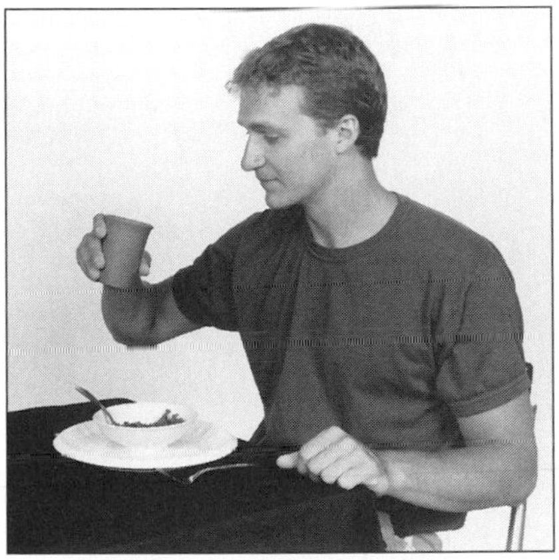

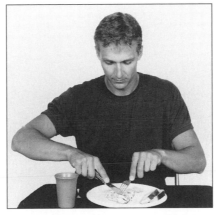

Figure 4-68. Elbow range within the arc of movement from 45° to 136° of flexion and from 47° of pronation to 59° of supination.

Figure 4-69. Elbow range within the arc of movement from 45° to 136° of flexion and from 47° of pronation to 59° of supination.

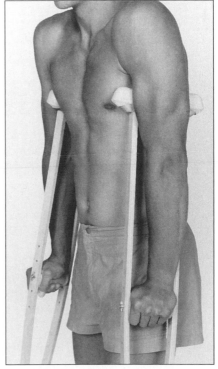

Figure 4-70. Elbow extension required to walk with crutches.

Chapter 4 Elbow and Forearm   191

ELBOW AND FOREARM

MUSCLE FUNCTION

Elbow Flexion

Biceps brachii, brachialis, and brachioradialis are the flexors of the elbow. The role of the three flexors in functional activities is partially determined by the position of the elbow joint, the position of the forearm, the magnitude of the applied load, and the speed of motion.[5] Of clinical and functional significance is the electromyographic data that indicate a fine interplay between the action of the flexors during activity and a wide range of muscle response between individuals.[12] The movement combinations required for a specific task are an important consideration in specifying the contribution of each muscle to function and in analyzing movement compensation due to paralysis.

Biceps Brachii

The biceps brachii acts as an elbow flexor and forearm supinator. This action is well illustrated in activities involving both movements, such as using a corkscrew, feeding utensil, or screwdriver (Fig. 4-71). Biceps functions most efficiently at 90° of elbow flexion.[1,11] The muscle does not contribute to supination when the elbow is extended, unless supination is strongly resisted,

and does not function as an elbow flexor when the forearm is pronated.[12] Thus, the weakest elbow flexion strength is associated with forearm pronation.[21] The greatest elbow flexion strength occurs with the forearm in midposition.[11,21] Because the biceps brachii acts on three joints (ie, the shoulder, elbow and radioulnar), its efficiency is affected by the position of the shoulder.[11,14] The biceps brachii is more efficient when the shoulder is extended than when flexed. This efficiency can be illustrated in pulling activities such as rowing, playing tug-of-war games, pulling the beater of a loom, and sweeping the floor. These activities require shoulder extension and elbow flexion.

Brachialis

The brachialis has been labelled the servile muscle among the elbow flexors,[22] because it is active in all positions of the forearm, with and without resistance.[12] Because the attachments of the brachialis are at the proximal end of the ulna, and the distal end of the humerus, this muscle is unaffected by changes in the position of the forearm resulting from rotation of the radius and the position of the shoulder.[5] Although all flexors are recruited for a task such as hammering (Fig. 4-72), the brachialis is the ideal selection because its sole function is elbow flexion.

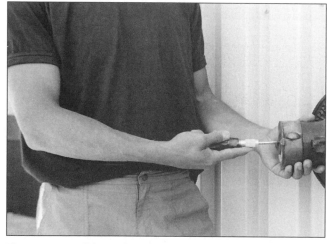

Figure 4-71. Biceps function.

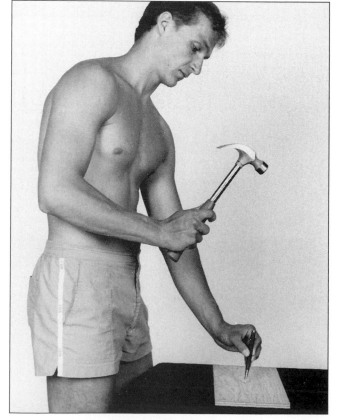

Figure 4-72. Brachialis function.

Brachioradialis

This elbow flexor functions as a reserve flexor muscle, contributing to elbow flexion when speed of movement and force are required in the semipronated or pronated forearm position.[12] Its action can be illustrated in activities such as drinking from a cup (see Fig. 4-68), typing, or playing a keyboard instrument.

Elbow Extension: Triceps

The triceps is the extensor muscle at the elbow. The role of the anconeus is controversial. The anconeus has been described as a muscle that is active in slow movements,[12] has a stabilizing function during supination and pronation,[12] assists in elbow extension,[5] and has negligible action in extension.[22]

Because the long head of triceps crosses two joints, the effectiveness of this muscle is affected by the position of the shoulder. The long head becomes stretched with the elbow and shoulder joints in flexion. Therefore, the triceps is more effective in elbow extension when the shoulder is flexed.[14] This is illustrated in such activities as pushing a broom or vacuum cleaner or sawing wood.

The medial head of triceps can be identified as the servile portion of the muscle because it is always active during elbow extension. The lateral and long heads are recruited when force is required.[12] The function of the triceps is illustrated in activities that involve elevation of the body, such as getting up from a chair (Fig. 4-73), walking with axillary crutches (see Fig. 4-70), or performing push-ups.

Forearm Supination: Supinator and Biceps Brachii

The supinator, acting alone, produces supination in all positions of the elbow.[12,22] The biceps is recruited in elbow flexion when force and speed are demanded. Most daily activities demand varying amounts of force and the combined movements of elbow flexion and forearm supination. This combination functions to maintain or move the hand closer to the body and to rotate the hand so that the palm faces the ceiling (Fig. 4-74). The supinators and external rotators of the shoulder are functionally linked when the elbow is extended,[14] because supination and shoulder external rotation occur simultaneously during activity.

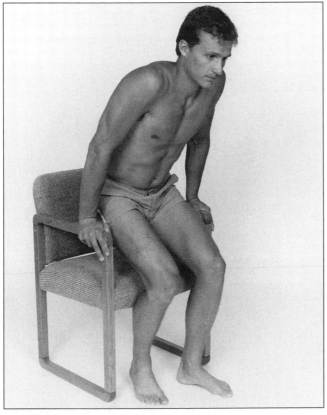

Figure 4-73.   Triceps function.

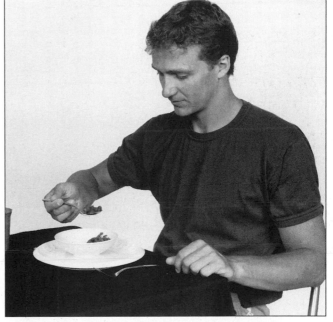

Figure 4-74.   Supinator and biceps brachii function.

Forearm Pronation: Pronator Teres and Pronator Quadratus

Both muscles are active in pronation of the forearm. The pronator quadratus has been described as the most consistent muscle of the two, with the pronator teres being recruited for activities demanding fast or powerful movement,[12,22] such as pitching a ball or playing racket sports. The pronators are recruited for many self-maintenance activities, including writing, washing one's body (Fig. 4-75), dressing, and hygiene tasks. The pronators are functionally linked to the internal rotators of the shoulder,[14] because pronation and internal rotation of the shoulder occur simultaneously in many activities.

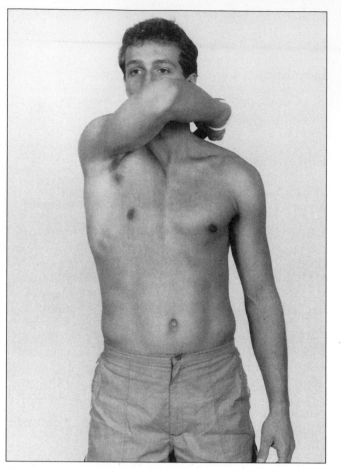

Figure 4-75.   Pronator teres and pronator quadratus function.

REFERENCES

1. Kapandji IA. *The Physiology of the Joints.* Vol. 1. 5th ed. New York: Churchill Livingstone; 1982.
2. Soames RW, ed. Skeletal System. Salmons S, ed. Muscle. *Gray's Anatomy.* 38th ed. New York: Churchill Livingstone; 1995.
3. Norkin CC, White DJ. *Measurement of Joint Motion: A Guide to Goniometry.* 2nd ed. Philadelphia: FA Davis; 1995.
4. Daniels L, Worthingham C. *Muscle Testing: Techniques of Manual Examination.* 5th ed. Philadelphia: WB Saunders; 1986.
5. Norkin CC, Levangie PK. *Joint Structure & Function: A Comprehensive Analysis.* 2nd ed. Philadelphia: FA Davis; 1992.
6. Cyriax J. *Textbook of Orthopaedic Medicine. Vol 1. Diagnosis of Soft Tissue Lesions.* 8th ed. London: Bailliere Tindall; 1982.
7. Magee DJ. *Orthopedic Physical Assessment.* 3rd ed. Philadelphia: WB Saunders; 1997.
8. American Academy of Orthopaedic Surgeons. *Joint Motion: Method of Measuring and Recording.* Chicago: Author; 1965.
9. Hoppenfeld S. *Physical Examination of the Spine and Extremities.* New York: Appleton-Century-Crofts; 1976.
10. Kaltenborn FM. *Mobilization of the Extremity Joints.* 3rd ed. Oslo: Olaf Norlis Bokhandel; 1985.
11. Soderberg GL. *Kinesiology: Application to Pathological Motion.* 2nd ed. Baltimore: Williams & Wilkins; 1997.
12. Basmajian JV, DeLuca CJ. *Muscles Alive: Their Function Revealed by Electromyography.* 5th ed. Baltimore: Williams & Wilkins; 1985.
13. Kendall FP, McCreary EK, Provance PG. *Muscles Testing and Function.* 4th ed. Baltimore: Williams & Wilkins; 1993.
14. Smith LK, Lawrence Weiss EL, Lehmkuhl LD. *Brunnstrom's Clinical Kinesiology.* 5th ed. Philadelphia: FA Davis; 1996.
15. Morrey BF, Askew LJ, An KN, Chao EY. A biomechanical study of normal functional elbow motion. *J Bone Joint Surg.* 1981;63A:872–876.
16. Safaee-Rad R, Shwedyk E, Quanbury AO, Cooper JE. Normal functional range of motion of upper limb joints during performance of three feeding activities. *Arch Phys Med Rehabil.* 1990;71:505–509.
17. Packer TL, Peat M, Wyss U, Sorbie C. Examining the elbow during functional activities. *The Occupational Therapy Journal of Research.* 1990;10:323–333.
18. Cooper JE, Shwedyk E, Quanbury AO, Miller J, Hildebrand D. Elbow joint restriction: effect on functional upper limb motion during performance of three feeding activities. *Arch Phys Med Rehabil.* 1993;74:805–809.
19. Vasen AP, Lacey SH, Keith MW, Shaffer JW. Functional range of motion of the elbow. *J Hand Surg.* 1995;20A: 288–292.
20. O'Neill OR, Morrey BF, Tanaka S, An K-N. Compensatory motion in the upper extremity after elbow arthrodesis. *Clin Orthop.* 1992;281:89–96.
21. Morrey BF, An KN, Chao EYS. Functional evaluation of the elbow. In: Morrey BF, ed. *The Elbow and Its Disorders.* 2nd ed. Toronto: WB Saunders; 1993.
22. Rosse C. The arm, forearm, and wrist. In: Rosse C, Clawson DK, eds. *The Musculoskeletal System in Health and Disease.* New York: Harper & Row; 1980.

ELBOW AND FOREARM

WRIST AND HAND

▼ **SURFACE ANATOMY** (Figs. 5-1 and 5-2)

Structure	Location
1. Styloid process of the ulna	Bony prominence on the posteromedial aspect of the forearm at the distal end of the ulna.
2. Styloid process of the radius	Bony prominence on the lateral aspect of the forearm at the distal end of the radius.
3. Metacarpal bones	The bases and shafts are felt through the extensor tendons on the dorsal surface of the wrist and hand. The heads are the bony prominences at the bases of the digits.
4. Capitate bone	In the small depression proximal to the base of the third metacarpal bone.
5. Pisiform bone	Medial bone of the proximal row of carpal bones; proximal to the base of the hypothenar eminence.
6. Thumb web space	The web of skin connecting the thumb to the hand.
7. Distal palmar crease	Transverse crease commencing on the medial side of the palm and extending laterally to the web between the index and middle fingers.
8. Proximal palmar crease	Transverse crease commencing on the lateral side of the palm, extending medially and fading out on the hypothenar eminence.
9. Thenar eminence	The pad on the palm of the hand at the base of the thumb; bound medially and distally by the longitudinal palmar crease.
10. Hypothenar eminence	The pad on the medial side of the base of the palm.

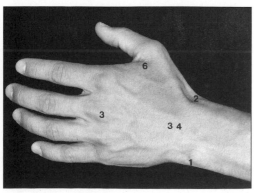

Figure 5-1. Dorsal aspect of the wrist and hand.

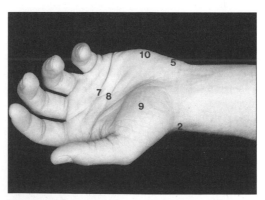

Figure 5-2. Volar aspect of the wrist and hand.

▼ ASSESSMENT PROCESS: THE WRIST AND HAND

1. The therapist observes:
   a. Function
   b. Posture, symmetry, atrophy, skin and nail condition, and color
   c. Active range of motion (AROM) at the elbow, wrist, fingers, and thumb
2. The therapist assesses passive ranges of motion (PROM) by:
   a. Estimating joint PROM
   b. Determining the end feels at the joint
   c. Establishing the presence or absence of pain
   d. Determining the presence of a capsular or noncapsular pattern
3. The therapist measures PROM through goniometry.
4. The therapist assesses muscle strength through manual muscle testing.
5. The therapist uses a dynamometer for assessing grip strength and a pinch meter to assess pinch strength. This type of measurement is beyond the scope of the manual muscle testing presented in this volume. Measurement issues and procedures and normal values are provided in the literature.[1-7]

TABLE
5-1 ▼ **JOINT STRUCTURE: WRIST MOVEMENTS**

	Flexion	Extension	Radial Deviation	Ulnar Deviation
Articulation[8,9]	Radiocarpal Midcarpal	Midcarpal Radiocarpal	Midcarpal Radiocarpal	Radiocarpal (predominant) Midcarpal
Plane	Sagittal	Sagittal	Frontal	Frontal
Axis	Frontal	Frontal	Sagittal	Sagittal
Normal limiting factors[8,10–12]	Tension in the posterior radiocarpal ligament and posterior joint capsule	Tension in the anterior radiocarpal ligament and anterior joint capsule; contact between the radius and the carpal bones	Tension in the ulnar collateral ligament, ulnocarpal ligament, and ulnar portion of the joint capsule; contact between the radial styloid process and the scaphoid bone	Tension in the radial collateral ligament and radial portion of the joint capsule
Normal end feel[10,13,14]	Firm	Firm/hard	Firm/hard	Firm
Normal active range of motion[15]	0–80°	0–70°	0–20°	0–30°

Capsular pattern[13,14]: Flexion and extension are equally restricted

▼ RANGE OF MOTION ASSESSMENT AND MEASUREMENT

The joint articulations and axes of the wrist and hand are illustrated in Figures 5-3 through 5-7 and the joint structure is described in Tables 5-1, 5-2, and 5-3.

GENERAL SCAN: WRIST AND HAND AROM

The AROM of the wrist and hand is scanned (not shown) to provide a general indication of the available ROM and/or muscle strength at the wrist and hand before proceeding with a detailed assessment of the region. The patient is first instructed to make a fist. The therapist ob-

serves the AROM of finger flexion, thumb flexion and adduction, and wrist extension. The patient is then instructed to open the hand and spread the fingers as far apart as possible. The therapist observes the AROM for finger extension and abduction, thumb extension, and wrist flexion.

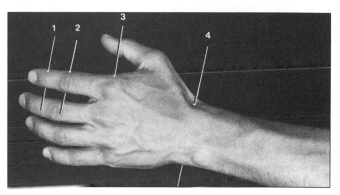

Figure 5-5. Wrist and finger axes: (*1*) distal interphalangeal flexion-extension; (*2*) proximal interphalangeal flexion-extension; (*3*) metacarpophalangeal flexion-extension; (*4*) wrist flexion-extension.

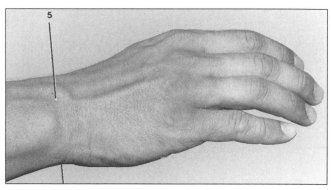

Figure 5-6. Wrist axis: (*5*) ulnar-radial deviation.

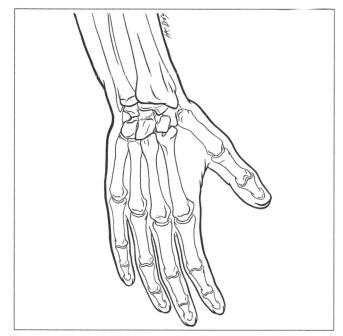

Figure 5-3. Wrist, finger, and thumb articulations.

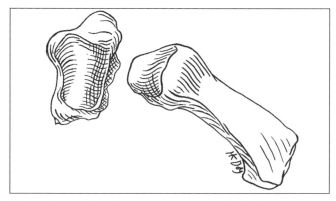

Figure 5-4. Thumb carpometacarpal articulation.

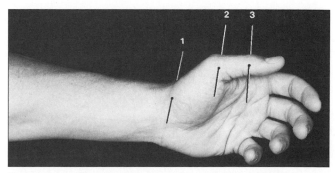

Figure 5-7. Thumb axes: (*1*) carpometacarpal flexion-extension; (*2*) metacarpophalangeal flexion-extension; (*3*) interphalangeal flexion-extension.

TABLE 5-6

▼ JOINT STRUCTURE: FINGER MOVEMENTS

	Flexion	Extension	Abduction	Adduction
Articulation[8,9]	Metacarpophalangeal (MCP)	MCP	MCP	MCP
	Proximal interphalangeal (PIP)	PIP		
	Distal interphalangeal (DIP)	DIP		
Plane	Sagittal	Sagittal	Frontal	Frontal
Axis	Frontal	Frontal	Sagittal	Sagittal
Normal limiting factors[8,10–12]	MCP: tension in the posterior joint capsule, collateral ligaments; contact between the proximal phalanx and the metacarpal PIP: contact between the middle and proximal phalanx; soft tissue apposition of the middle and proximal phalanges; tension in the posterior joint capsule, and collateral ligaments DIP: tension in the posterior joint capsule, collateral ligaments, and oblique retinacular ligament	MCP: tension in the anterior joint capsule, palmar fibrocartilagenous plate (palmar ligament) PIP: tension in the anterior joint capsule, palmar ligament DIP: tension in the anterior joint capsule, palmar ligament	Tension in the collateral ligaments, fascia, and skin of the web spaces	Contact between adjacent fingers
Normal end feel[10,13,14]	MCP: firm/hard PIP: hard/soft/firm DIP: firm	MCP: firm PIP: firm DIP: firm	Firm	
Normal active range of motion[15]	MCP: 0–90° PIP: 0–100° DIP: 0–90°	MCP: 0–45° PIP: 0° DIP: 0°		

Capsular pattern:[13,14] Metacarpophalangeal and interphalangeal joints: flexion, extension

TABLE 5-3

▼ JOINT STRUCTURE: THUMB MOVEMENTS

	Flexion	Extension	Palmar Abduction	Adduction
Articulation[8,9]	Carpometacarpal (CM) Metacarpophalangeal (MCP) Interphalangeal (IP)	CM MCP IP	CM MCP	CM MCP
Plane	CM: oblique frontal MCP: frontal IP: frontal	CM: oblique frontal MCP: frontal IP: frontal	CM: oblique sagittal	CM: oblique sagittal
Axis	CM: oblique sagittal MCP: sagittal IP: sagittal	CM: oblique sagittal MCP: sagittal IP: sagittal	CM: oblique frontal	CM: oblique frontal
Normal limiting factors[8,10,11]	CM: soft tissue apposition between the thenar eminence and the palm; tension in the posterior joint capsule, extensor pollicis brevis, and abductor pollicis brevis MCP: contact between the first metacarpal and the proximal phalanx; tension in the posterior joint capsule, collateral ligaments, and extensor pollicis brevis IP: tension in the collateral ligaments, and posterior joint capsule; contact between the distal phalanx, fibrocartilagenous plate and the proximal phalanx	CM: tension in the anterior joint capsule, flexor pollicis brevis, and first dorsal interosseous MCP: tension in the anterior joint capsule, palmar ligament, and flexor pollicis brevis IP: tension in the anterior joint capsule, palmar ligament	Tension in the fascia and skin of the first web space, first dorsal interosseous, and adductor pollicis	Soft tissue apposition between the thumb and index finger
Normal end feel[10,13,14]	CM: soft/firm MCP: hard/firm IP: hard/firm	CM: firm MCP: firm IP: firm	Firm	Soft
Normal active range of motion[15]	CM: 0–15° MCP: 0–50° IP: 0–80°	CM: 0–20° MCP: 0° IP: 0–20°	0–70°	0°

Capsular pattern:[13,14] CM joint: abduction, extension
MCP and IP joints: flexion, extension

WRIST AND HAND

WRIST FLEXION-EXTENSION

AROM Assessment

• Substitution/Trick Movement. Wrist ulnar or radial deviation.

PROM Assessment

• Start Position. The patient is sitting. The forearm is resting on a table in pronation, the wrist is in neutral position, the hand is over the end of the table, and the fingers are relaxed (Fig. 5-8).

• Stabilization. The therapist stabilizes the forearm.

• Therapist's Distal Hand Placement. The therapist grasps the metacarpals.

• End Positions. The therapist applies slight traction to and moves the hand anteriorly to the limit of motion to assess wrist flexion (Fig. 5-9). The therapist applies slight traction to and moves the hand posteriorly to the limit of motion for wrist extension (Fig. 5-10). The fingers should be relaxed when assessing the end feels.

• End Feels. Wrist flexion—firm; wrist extension—firm or hard.

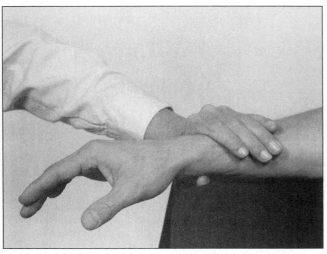

Figure 5-8.   Start position for wrist flexion and extension.

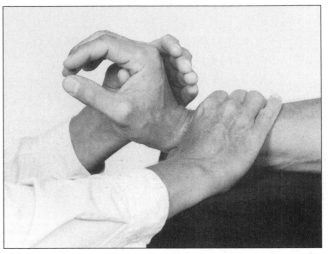

Figure 5-10.   Firm or hard end feel at limit of wrist extension.

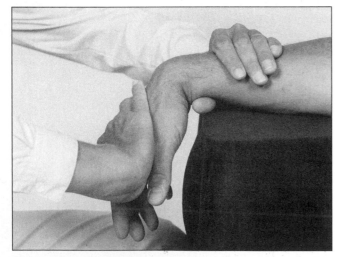

Figure 5-9.   Firm end feel at limit of wrist flexion.

Measurement: Universal Goniometer

• **Start Position.** The patient is sitting. The forearm is resting on a table in pronation, the wrist is in a neutral position, and the fingers are slightly extended for measurement of flexion and slightly flexed for measurement of extension. The hand is over the end of the table (Fig. 5-11).

• **Stabilization.** The therapist stabilizes the forearm.

• **Goniometer Axis.** The axis is placed at the level of the ulnar styloid process.

• **Stationary Arm.** Parallel to the longitudinal axis of the ulna.

• **Movable Arm.** Parallel to the longitudinal axis of the fifth metacarpal.

• **End Positions.** Wrist flexion: the wrist is moved in a volar direction (80°) (Fig. 5-12). Wrist extension: the wrist is moved in a dorsal direction to the limit of motion of 70° (Fig. 5-13). For both movements, ensure the mobile fourth and fifth metacarpals are not moved away from the start position throughout the assessment procedure and ensure that no wrist deviation occurs if full range cannot be obtained.

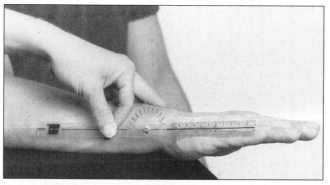

Figure 5-11.   Start position for wrist flexion and extension.

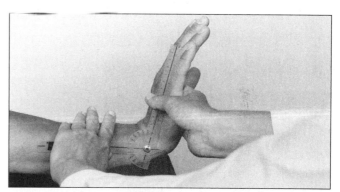

Figure 5-13.   End position for wrist extension.

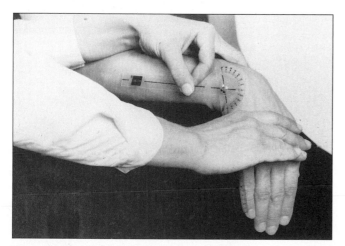

Figure 5-12.   End position for wrist flexion.

WRIST ULNAR AND RADIAL DEVIATION

AROM Assessment

• **Substitution/Trick Movement.** Ulnar or radial deviation of the fingers, wrist flexion, and wrist extension.

PROM Assessment

• **Start Position.** The patient is sitting. The forearm is resting on a table in pronation, the wrist is in neutral position, the hand is over the end of the table, and the fingers are relaxed (see Fig. 5-8).

• **Stabilization.** The therapist stabilizes the forearm.

• **Therapist's Distal Hand Placement.** The therapist grasps the metacarpals from the radial aspect of the hand to assess wrist ulnar deviation. The therapist grasps the metacarpals from the ulnar aspect of the hand to assess wrist radial deviation.

• **End Positions.** The therapist applies slight traction and moves the hand in an ulnar direction to the limit of motion to assess wrist ulnar deviation (Fig. 5-14). The therapist applies slight traction to and moves the hand in a radial direction to the limit of motion for wrist radial deviation (Fig. 5-15).

• **End Feels.** Ulnar deviation—firm; radial deviation—firm or hard.

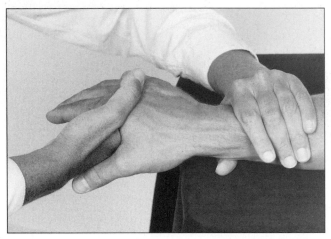

Figure 5-14.   Firm end feel at limit of wrist ulnar deviation.

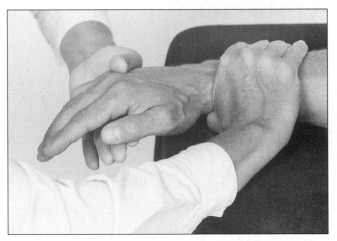

Figure 5-15.   Firm or hard end feel at limit of wrist radial deviation.

Measurement: Universal Goniometer

• **Start Position.** The patient is sitting. The forearm is pronated and the palmar surface of the hand is resting lightly on a table. The wrist remains in a neutral position and the fingers are relaxed (Fig. 5-16).

• **Stabilization.** The therapist stabilizes the forearm.

• **Goniometer Axis.** The axis is placed on the dorsal aspect of the wrist joint over the capitate bone.

• **Stationary Arm.** Along the midline of the forearm.

• **Movable Arm.** Parallel to the longitudinal axis of the shaft of the third metacarpal.

• **End Positions.** Ulnar deviation (Fig. 5-17): the wrist is adducted to the ulnar side to the limit of motion (30°). Radial deviation (Fig. 5-18): the wrist is abducted to the radial side to the limit of motion (20°). Ensure that the wrist is not moved into flexion or extension.

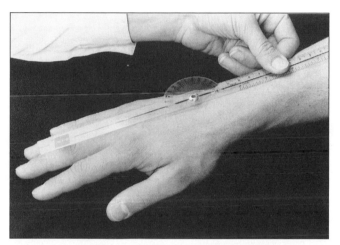

Figure 5-16. Start position for ulnar and radial deviation of the wrist.

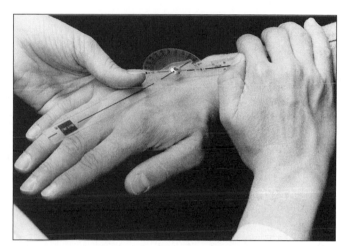

Figure 5-18. End position: radial deviation.

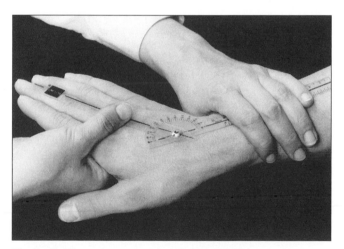

Figure 5-17. End position: ulnar deviation.

FINGER METACARPOPHALANGEAL FLEXION–EXTENSION

PROM Assessment

• **Start Position.** The patient is sitting. The forearm is resting on a table in midposition, the wrist is in neutral position, and the fingers are relaxed (Fig. 5-19).

• **Stabilization.** The therapist stabilizes the metacarpal.

• **Therapist's Distal Hand Placement.** The therapist grasps the proximal phalanx.

• **End Positions.** The therapist applies slight traction to and moves the proximal phalanx in an anterior direction to the limit of motion to assess metacarpophalangeal (MCP) joint flexion (Fig. 5-20). The therapist applies slight traction to and moves the proximal phalanx in a posterior direction to the limit of motion for MCP joint extension (Fig. 5-21).

• **End Feels.** MCP joint flexion—firm or hard; MCP joint extension—firm.

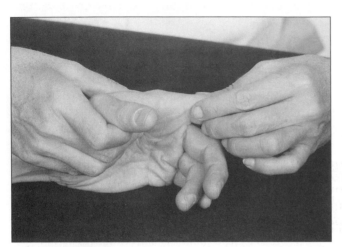

Figure 5-19.   Start position: MCP joint flexion and extension.

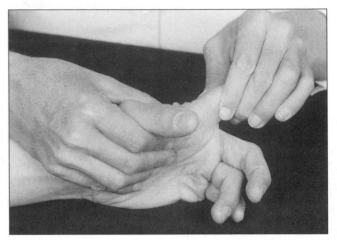

Figure 5-21.   Firm end feel at the limit of MCP extension.

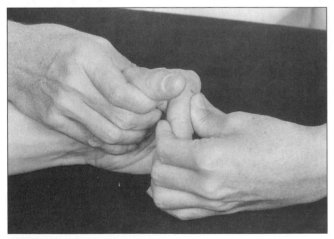

Figure 5-20.   Firm or hard end feel at the limit of MCP flexion.

FINGER METACARPOPHALANGEAL FLEXION

Measurement: Universal Goniometer

• **Start Position.** The patient is sitting. The forearm is resting on a table, the elbow is flexed, the wrist is slightly extended, and the MCP joint of the finger being measured is in 0° of extension (Fig. 5-22).

• **Stabilization.** The therapist stabilizes the metacarpal.

• **Goniometer Axis.** The axis is placed on the dorsal aspect of the MCP joint being measured.

• **Stationary Arm.** Parallel to the longitudinal axis of the shaft of the metacarpal.

• **Movable Arm.** Parallel to the longitudinal axis of the proximal phalanx.

• **End Position.** All fingers are moved toward the palm to the limit of motion of 90° (Fig. 5-23). Range increases progressively from the index to the fifth finger.[8] The interphalangeal (IP) joints are allowed to extend, so that flexion at the MCP joint is not restricted due to tension of the long finger extensor tendons.

• **Alternate Goniometer Placement.** The index and fifth MCP joints may be measured on the lateral aspect of the joint (Fig. 5-24). Should joint enlargement prevent measurement on the dorsal aspect, the index and fifth fingers may be measured and range estimated for the middle and fourth fingers.[16]

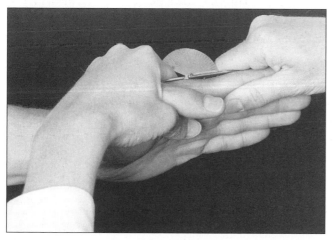

Figure 5-22.   Start position for MCP flexion.

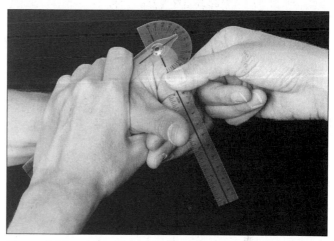

Figure 5-24.   Alternate goniometer placement for MCP flexion.

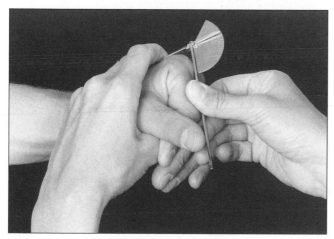

Figure 5-23.   End position: MCP flexion.

FINGER METACARPOPHALANGEAL EXTENSION

Measurement: Universal Goniometer

- **Start Position.** The patient is sitting. The forearm is resting on a table, the elbow is flexed, the wrist is slightly flexed, and the MCP joint of the finger being measured is in 0° of extension (Fig. 5-25).

- **Stabilization.** The therapist stabilizes the metacarpal.

- **Goniometer Axis.** The axis is placed on the volar surface of the MCP joint being measured.

- **Stationary Arm.** Parallel to the longitudinal axis of the shaft of the metacarpal.

- **Movable Arm.** Parallel to the longitudinal axis of the proximal phalanx.

- **End Position.** The finger is moved in a dorsal direction to the limit of motion of 45° (Fig. 5-26). The IP joints are allowed to flex, so that extension at the MCP joint is not restricted due to tension of the long finger flexor tendons.

- **Alternate Goniometer Placement.** The index and fifth MCP joints may be measured on the lateral aspect of the MCP joint (Fig. 5-27).

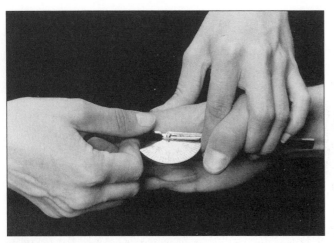

Figure 5-25.   Start position for MCP extension.

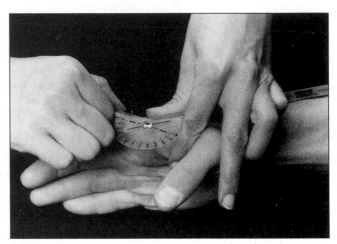

Figure 5-27.   Alternate goniometer placement for MCP extension.

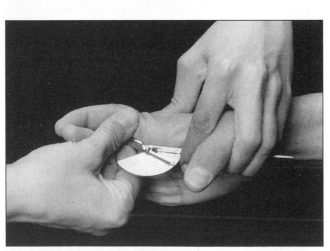

Figure 5-26.   End position: MCP extension.

FINGER METACARPOPHALANGEAL ABDUCTION–ADDUCTION

PROM Assessment. Metacarpophalangeal abduction (not shown).

• **Start Position.** The patient is sitting. The forearm is resting on a table, the wrist is in neutral position, and the fingers are in the anatomical position.

• **Stabilization.** The therapist stabilizes the metacarpal.

• **Therapist's Distal Hand Placement.** The therapist grasps the sides of the proximal phalanx.

• **End Position.** The therapist applies slight traction to and moves the proximal phalanx to the limit of motion to assess MCP joint abduction.

• **End Feel.** MCP joint abduction—firm.

Measurement: Universal Goniometer

• **Start Position.** The patient is sitting. The elbow is flexed to 90°, the forearm is pronated and resting on a table, the wrist is in neutral position, and the fingers are in the anatomical position (Fig. 5-28).

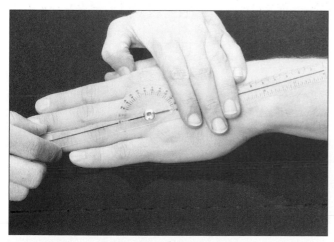

Figure 5-28.   Start position: MCP abduction and adduction.

• **Stabilization.** The therapist stabilizes the metacarpal bones.

• **Goniometer Axis.** The axis is placed on the dorsal surface of the MCP joint being measured.

• **Stationary Arm.** Parallel to the longitudinal axis of the shaft of the metacarpal.

• **Movable Arm.** Parallel to the longitudinal axis of the proximal phalanx.

• **End Positions.** The finger is moved away from the midline of the hand to the limit of motion in abduction (Fig. 5-29). The finger is moved toward the midline of the hand to the limit of motion in adduction (Fig. 5-30). The remaining fingers are moved to allow full adduction.

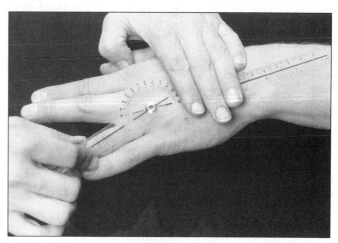

Figure 5-29.   End position: MCP abduction of the fourth finger.

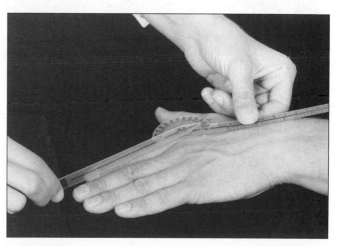

Figure 5-30.   End position: MCP adduction of the index finger.

ALTERNATE MEASUREMENT: METACARPOPHALANGEAL ABDUCTION

To gain a composite measure of finger spread and thumb web stretch, finger abduction and thumb extension can be measured in centimeters. A sheet of paper is placed under the patient's hand. The therapist stabilizes the wrist and metacarpals. The patient spreads all fingers and thumb and the therapist traces the contour of the hand (Fig. 5-31). The patient's hand is removed and a linear measure of the distances between the midpoint of the tip of each finger and the index finger and thumb is recorded in centimeters (Fig. 5-32).

FINGER INTERPHALANGEAL FLEXION-EXTENSION

PROM Assessment

• **Start Position.** The patient is sitting. The forearm is resting on a table, the wrist is in neutral position, and the fingers are relaxed.

• **Stabilization.** The therapist stabilizes the proximal phalanx for assessment of the proximal interphalangeal (PIP) joint and the middle phalanx for the distal interphalangeal (DIP) joint.

• **Therapist's Distal Hand Placement.** The therapist grasps the middle phalanx to assess the PIP joint and the distal phalanx to assess the DIP joint.

• **End Positions.** The therapist applies slight traction to and moves the middle or distal phalanx in an anterior direction to the limit of motion to assess PIP (not shown) or DIP joint flexion, respectively (Fig. 5-33). The therapist applies slight traction to and moves the middle or distal phalanx in a posterior direction to the limit of motion for PIP joint (not shown) or DIP joint extension, respectively (Fig. 5-34).

• **End Feels.** PIP joint flexion—hard, soft, or firm; DIP joint flexion—firm; PIP joint extension—firm; DIP joint extension—firm.

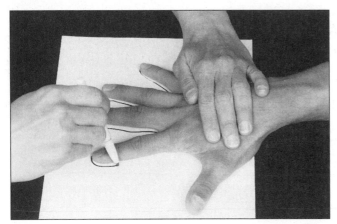

Figure 5-31. Alternate measurement: hand placement for MCP abduction.

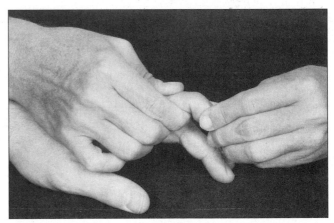

Figure 5-33. Firm end feel at limit of DIP joint flexion.

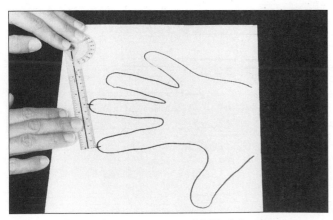

Figure 5-32. Ruler measurement: MCP abduction.

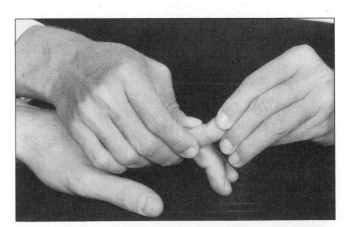

Figure 5-34. Firm end feel at limit of DIP joint extension.

Measurement: Universal Goniometer

• **Start Position.** The patient is sitting. The forearm is resting on a table in either midposition or pronation. The wrist and fingers are in the anatomical position (0° extension at the MCP and IP joints).

• **Stabilization.** The therapist stabilizes the proximal phalanx for measurement of the PIP joint and the middle phalanx for the DIP joint.

• **Goniometer Axis.** To measure IP joint flexion, the axis is placed over the dorsal surface of the PIP or DIP joint being measured (Fig. 5-35). To measure IP joint extension, the axis is placed over the palmar surface of the PIP or DIP joint being measured.

• **Stationary Arm.** PIP joint: parallel to the longitudinal axis of the proximal phalanx. DIP joint: parallel to the longitudinal axis of the middle phalanx.

• **Movable Arm.** PIP joint: parallel to the longitudinal axis of the middle phalanx. DIP joint: parallel to the longitudinal axis of the distal phalanx.

• **End Positions.** The PIP joint or DIP joint (not shown) is flexed to the limit of motion (100° or 90°, respectively) (Fig. 5-36). The PIP joint or DIP joint (not shown) is extended to the limit of motion (0°) (Fig. 5-37).

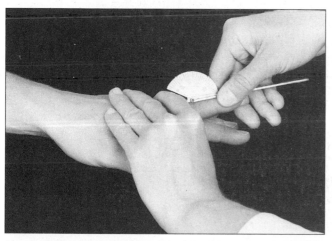

Figure 5-35.   Start Position: PIP joint flexion.

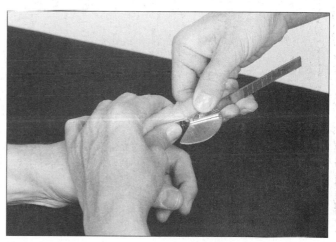

Figure 5-37.   End position: PIP joint extension.

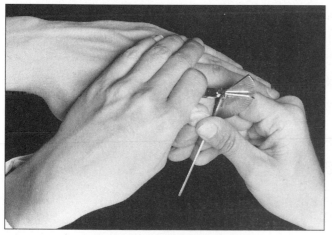

Figure 5-36.   End position: PIP joint flexion.

FINGER METACARPOPHALANGEAL AND INTERPHALANGEAL FLEXION

When evaluating impairment of hand function, a linear measurement of finger flexion should be used in conjunction with goniometry. This measure is particularly relevant in evaluating the extent of impairment[17] associated with grasp. The patient is sitting. The elbow is flexed and the forearm is resting on a table in supination. Two measurements are taken.

1. The patient flexes the IP joints while maintaining 0° of extension at the MCP joints (Fig. 5-38). A ruler measurement is taken from the pulp or tip of the middle finger to the distal palmar crease.
2. The patient flexes the MCP and IP joints (Fig. 5-39). A ruler measurement is taken from the pulp of the finger to the proximal palmar crease.

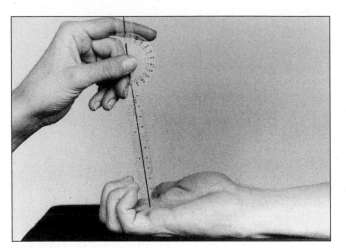

Figure 5-38.   Decreased finger IP flexion.

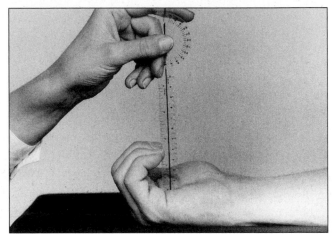

Figure 5-39.   Decreased finger MCP and IP flexion.

THUMB CARPOMETACARPAL FLEXION–EXTENSION

PROM Assessment

• **Start Position.** The patient is sitting. The elbow is flexed with the forearm in midposition and resting on a table. The wrist is in neutral position, the fingers are relaxed, and the thumb is in the anatomical position (Fig. 5-40).

• **Stabilization.** The therapist stabilizes the trapezium, forearm, and wrist (see Fig. 5-40).

• **Therapist's Distal Hand Placement.** The therapist grasps the first metacarpal (Fig. 5-41).

• **End Positions.** The therapist applies slight traction to and moves the first metacarpal in an ulnar direction to the limit of motion to assess thumb carpometacarpal (CM) joint flexion (Fig. 5-42). The therapist applies slight traction to and moves the first metacarpal in a radial direction to the limit of motion for thumb CM joint extension (Fig. 5-43).

• **End Feels.** Thumb CM joint flexion—soft or firm; thumb CM joint extension—firm.

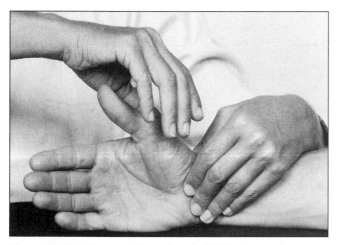

Figure 5-40. Start position: thumb CM flexion and extension. The therapist stabilizes the trapezium between the left thumb and index finger.

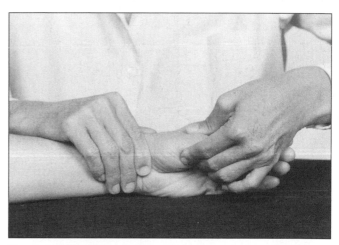

Figure 5-42. Soft or firm end feel at the limit of thumb CM flexion.

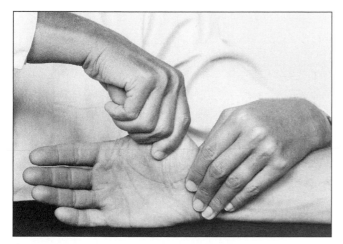

Figure 5-41. Therapist's distal hand grasps the first metacarpal.

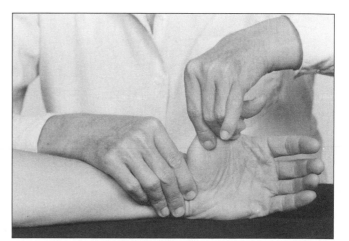

Figure 5-43. Firm end feel at the limit of thumb CM extension.

Measurement: Universal Goniometer

• **Start Position.** The patient is sitting. The elbow is flexed with the forearm in midposition and resting on a table. The wrist is in slight ulnar deviation, the fingers assume the anatomical position, and the thumb maintains contact with the metacarpal and proximal phalanx of the index finger (Fig. 5-44).

• **Stabilization.** The therapist stabilizes the forearm and wrist.

• **Goniometer Axis.** The axis is placed over the CM joint.

• **Stationary Arm.** Parallel to the longitudinal axis of the radius.

• **Movable Arm.** Parallel to the longitudinal axis of the thumb metacarpal.

Note: Although the goniometer arms are not aligned at 0° in this start position, this position is recorded as the 0° start position. The number of degrees the metacarpal is moved away from this 0° start position is recorded as the ROM for the movement. For example, if the goniometer read 10° at the start position for CM joint flexion-extension (see Fig. 5-44) and 25° at the end position for CM joint flexion (see Fig. 5-45), the CM joint flexion ROM would be 15°.

• **End Positions.** Flexion (Fig. 5-45): the thumb is flexed across the palm to the limit of motion (15°). Extension (Fig. 5-46): the thumb is extended away from the palm to the limit of motion (20°).

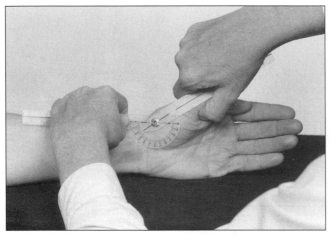

Figure 5-44. Start position: thumb CM flexion and extension.

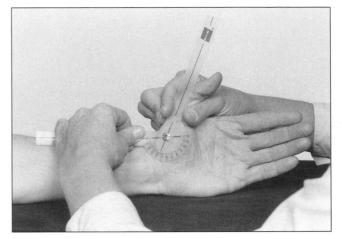

Figure 5-46. End position: thumb CM extension.

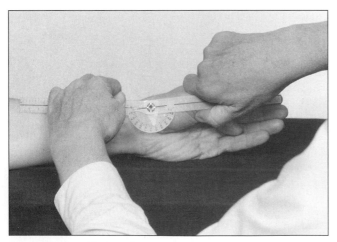

Figure 5-45. End position: thumb CM flexion.

THUMB METATCARPOPHALANGEAL AND INTERPHALANGEAL FLEXION–EXTENSION

PROM Assessment

• **Start Position.** The patient is sitting. The elbow is flexed and the forearm is resting on a table in midposition. The wrist is in the neutral position and the fingers are relaxed. The MCP and IP joints of the thumb are in extension (0°).

• **Stabilization.** First MCP joint: the therapist stabilizes the first metacarpal. IP joint: the therapist stabilizes the proximal phalanx.

• **Therapist's Distal Hand Placement.** First MCP joint: the therapist grasps the proximal phalanx. IP joint: the therapist grasps the distal phalanx.

• **End Positions.** The therapist applies slight traction to and moves the proximal phalanx across the palm to the limit of motion to assess thumb MCP flexion (Fig. 5-47), and to the limit of motion in a radial direction for thumb MCP extension (Fig. 5-48). The therapist applies slight traction to and moves the distal phalanx in an anterior (Fig. 5-49), or a posterior direction (Fig. 5-50) to the limit of motion for thumb IP flexion or extension, respectively.

• **End Feels.** Thumb MCP flexion—hard or firm; thumb IP flexion—hard or firm; thumb MCP and IP extension—firm.

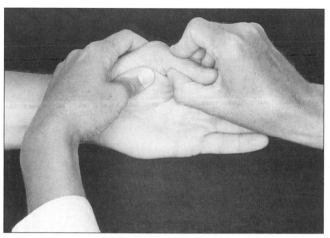

Figure 5-47.   Hard or firm end feel at the limit of thumb MCP flexion.

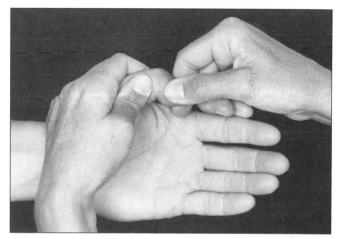

Figure 5-49.   Hard or firm end feel at the limit of thumb IP flexion.

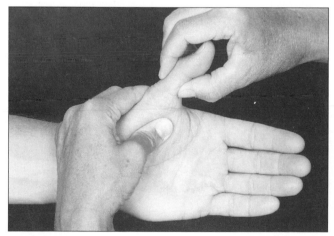

Figure 5-48.   Firm end feel at the limit of thumb MCP extension.

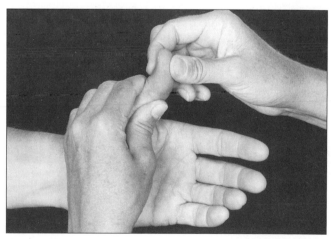

Figure 5-50.   Firm end feel at the limit of thumb IP extension.

Measurement: Universal Goniometer

• **Start Position.** The patient is sitting. The elbow is flexed and the forearm is resting on a table in midposition. The wrist and fingers are in the anatomical position. The MCP and IP joints are in extension (0°).

• **Stabilization.** MCP joint: the therapist stabilizes the first metacarpal. IP joint: the therapist stabilizes the proximal phalanx.

• **Goniometer Axis.** The axis is placed over the dorsal or lateral aspect of the MCP joint (Fig. 5-51) or IP joint (Fig. 5-52) of the thumb.

• **Stationary Arm.** MCP joint: parallel to the longitudinal axis of the shaft of the thumb metacarpal. IP joint: parallel to the longitudinal axis of the proximal phalanx.

• **Movable Arm.** MCP joint: parallel to the longitudinal axis of the proximal phalanx. IP joint: parallel to the longitudinal axis of the distal phalanx.

• **End Positions.** The MCP joint is flexed so that the thumb moves across the palm to the limit of MCP flexion (50°) (Fig. 5-53). The IP joint is flexed to the limit of motion (80°) (Fig. 5-54).

The goniometer is positioned on the lateral or volar surface of the thumb to assess MCP and IP joint extension. The MCP joint is extended to the limit of extension (0°).

• **Hyperextension.** Hyperextension of the IP joint of the thumb (see Fig. 5-50) occurs beyond 0° of extension. The IP joint can actively be hyperextended to 10° and passively to 30°.[8]

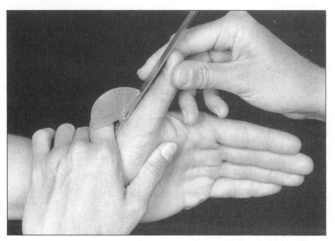

Figure 5-51. Start position: thumb MCP flexion.

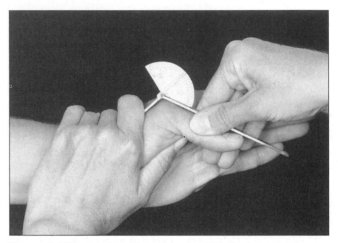

Figure 5-53. End position: thumb MCP flexion.

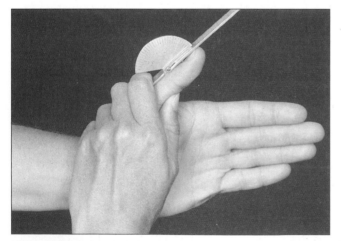

Figure 5-52. Start position: thumb IP flexion.

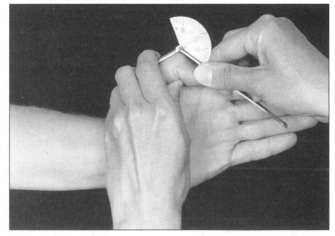

Figure 5-54. End position: thumb IP flexion.

THUMB CARPOMETACARPAL ABDUCTION

PROM Assessment (not shown)

• **Start Position.** The patient is sitting. The forearm is in midposition resting on a table, the wrist is in neutral position, and the fingers and thumb are relaxed.

• **Stabilization.** The therapist stabilizes the second metacarpal.

• **Therapist's Distal Hand Placement.** The therapist grasps the first metacarpal.

• **End Position.** The therapist applies slight traction to and moves the first metacarpal away from the second metacarpal in an anterior direction perpendicular to the plane of the palm, to the limit of motion to assess CM joint abduction.

• **End Feel.** CM joint abduction—firm.

Measurement: Universal Goniometer

• **Start Position.** The patient is sitting. The elbow is flexed and the forearm is resting on a table in midposition. The wrist and fingers are in the anatomical position. The thumb maintains contact with the metacarpal and proximal phalanx of the index finger (Fig. 5-55).

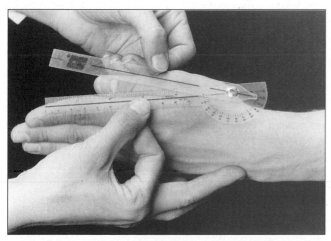

Figure 5-55.   Start position: thumb abduction.

• **Goniometer Axis.** The axis is placed at the junction of the bases of the first and second metacarpals.

• **Stationary Arm.** Parallel to the longitudinal axis of the second metacarpal.

• **Movable Arm.** Parallel to the longitudinal axis of the first metacarpal. In the start position described, the goniometer will indicate 15° to 20°. This is recorded as 0°.[16] For example, if the goniometer read 15° at the start position for CM joint abduction (see Fig. 5-55) and 60° at the end position for CM joint abduction (see Fig. 5-56), the first CM joint abduction ROM would be 45°.

• **End Position.** The thumb is abducted to the limit of motion (70°) so that the thumb column moves in the plane perpendicular to the palm (Fig. 5-56).

Measurement: Ruler. As an alternate measurement to goniometry, thumb abduction may be measured by using a ruler or tape measure. With the thumb in the abducted position, a ruler measurement is taken from the lateral aspect of the midpoint of the MCP joint of the index finger to the dorsal aspect of the midpoint of the MCP joint of the thumb (Fig. 5-57).

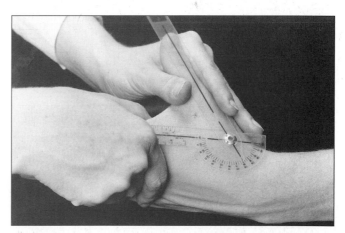

Figure 5-56.   End position: thumb abduction.

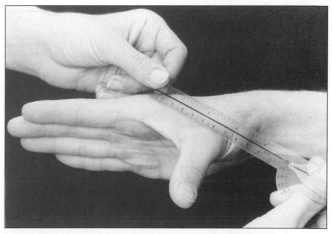

Figure 5-57.   Ruler measurement: thumb abduction.

THUMB OPPOSITION

Measurement: Ruler. On completion of full range of opposition (Fig. 5-58), between the thumb and fifth finger, it is normally possible to place the pads of the thumb and fifth finger in the same plane.[18] An evaluation of a deficit in opposition (Fig. 5-59) can be obtained by taking a linear measurement between the center of the tip of the thumb pad and the center of the tip of the fifth finger pad.

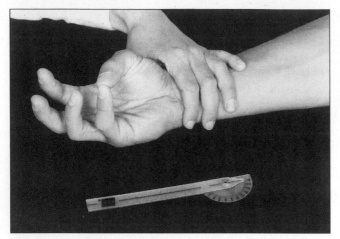

Figure 5-58.   Full opposition range of movement.

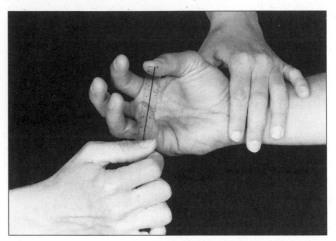

Figure 5-59.   Opposition deficit.

ASSESSMENT OF MUSCLE LENGTH: FLEXOR DIGITORUM SUPERFICIALIS, FLEXOR DIGITORUM PROFUNDUS, FLEXOR DIGITI MINIMI, AND PALMARIS LONGUS

• **Start Position.** The patient is in supine or sitting with the elbow in extension, the forearm supinated, and the fingers extended (Fig. 5-60).

• **Stabilization.** The therapist manually stabilizes the humerus. The radius and ulna are stabilized against the therapist's thigh.

• **End Position.** The therapist maintains the fingers in extension and applies slight traction to and extends the wrist to the limit of motion so that the long finger flexors are put on full stretch (Figs. 5-61 and 5-62).

• **Assessment.** If the finger flexors are shortened, wrist extension ROM will be restricted proportional to the decrease in muscle length. The therapist either observes the available PROM or uses a goniometer to measure and record the available wrist extension PROM.

• **End Feel.** Finger flexors on stretch-firm.

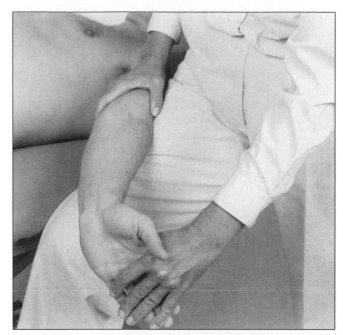

Figure 5-61. Flexor digitorum superficialis, flexor digitorum profundus, and flexor digiti minimi on stretch.

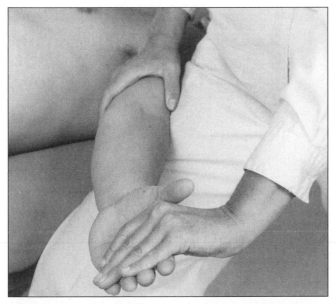

Figure 5-60. Start position: length of flexor digitorum superficialis, flexor digitorum profundus, and flexor digiti minimi.

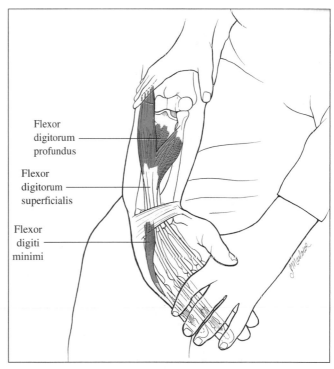

Flexor digitorum profundus

Flexor digitorum superficialis

Flexor digiti minimi

Figure 5-62. Flexor digitorum superficialis, flexor digitorum profundus, and flexor digiti minimi on stretch.

ASSESSMENT OF MUSCLE LENGTH: EXTENSOR DIGITORUM COMMUNIS, EXTENSOR INDICIS PROPRIUS, AND EXTENSOR DIGITI MINIMI

• **Start Position.** The patient is in supine or sitting position. The elbow is extended, the forearm is pronated, and the fingers are flexed (Fig. 5-63).

• **Stabilization.** The therapist stabilizes the radius and ulna.

• **End Position.** The therapist applies slight traction to and flexes the wrist to the limit of motion so that the long finger extensors are fully stretched (Figs. 5-64 and 5-65).

• **Assessment.** If the finger extensors are shortened, wrist flexion ROM will be restricted proportional to the degree of muscle shortening. The therapist either observes the available ROM or uses a goniometer to measure and record the available wrist flexion ROM.

• **End Feel.** Long finger extensors on stretch-firm.

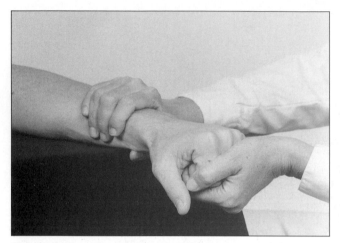

Figure 5-63. Start position: length of extensor digitorum communis, extensor indicis proprius, and extensor digiti minimi.

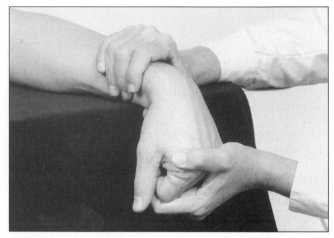

Figure 5-64. Extensor digitorum communis, extensor indicis proprius, and extensor digiti minimi on stretch.

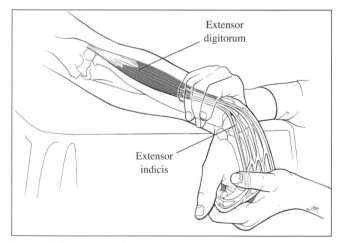

Figure 5-65. Long finger extensors on stretch.

ASSESSMENT OF MUSCLE LENGTH: LUMBRICALES

• **Start Position.** The patient is in sitting or supine position with the elbow flexed, forearm in midposition or supination, and the wrist in extension. The IP joints of the fingers are flexed (Fig. 5-66).

• **Stabilization.** The therapist stabilizes the metacarpals.

• **End Position.** The therapist simultaneously applies overpressure to flex the IP joints and extend the MCP joints of the fingers to the limit of motion so that lumbricales are put on full stretch (Figs. 5-67 and 5-68). The lumbricales may be stretched as a group or individually.

• **Assessment.** If the lumbricales are shortened, MCP joint extension ROM will be restricted proportional to the degree of muscle shortness. The therapist either observes the available PROM or uses a goniometer to measure and record the available MCP joint extension PROM.

• **End Feel.** Lumbricales on stretch-firm.

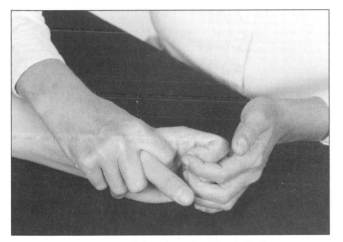

Figure 5-66. Start position: length of lumbricales.

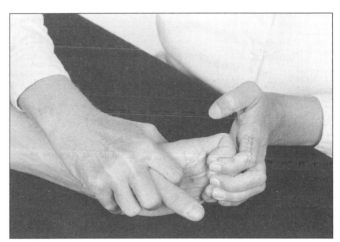

Figure 5-67. Lumbricales on stretch.

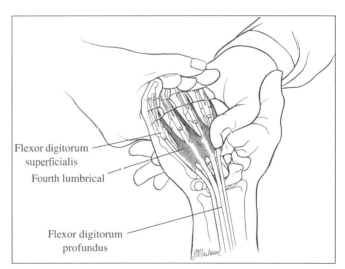

Figure 5-68. Wrist extension, MCP joint extension, and IP joint flexion to place lumbricales on stretch.

▼ MUSCLE STRENGTH ASSESSMENT (TABLES 5-4 AND 5-5)

T_{ABLE}
5-4 ▼ MUSCLE ACTIONS, ATTACHMENTS, AND NERVE SUPPLY: THE WRIST AND FINGERS[9]

Muscle	Primary Muscle Action	Muscle Origin	Muscle Insertion	Peripheral Nerve	Nerve Root
Flexor carpi radialis	Wrist flexion Wrist radial deviation	Common flexor origin on the medial epicondyle of the humerus	Palmar surface of the base of the second metacarpal and a slip to the base of the third metacarpal	Median	C67
Palmaris longus	Anchors palmar skin and fascia Wrist flexion	Common flexor origin on the medial epicondyle of the humerus	Distal palmar aspect of the flexor retinaculum; the palmar aponeurosis; skin and fascia of distal palm and webs of fingers	Median	C78
Flexor carpi ulnaris	Wrist flexion Wrist ulnar deviation	a. Humeral head: common flexor origin on the medial epicondyle of the humerus b. Ulnar head: medial margin of the olecranon process and by an aponeurosis on the upper two thirds of the posterior border of the ulna	Pisiform bone; sends slips to the hook of the hamate (pisohamate ligament), base of the fifth metacarpal (pisometacarpal ligament), and flexor retinaculum	Ulnar	C78T1
Extensor carpi radialis longus	Wrist extension Wrist radial deviation	Lower one third of the lateral supracondylar ridge of the humerus; common extensor origin on the lateral epicondyle of the humerus	Dorsal surface of the base of the second metacarpal bone	Radial	C67

Muscle	Primary Muscle Action	Muscle Origin	Muscle Insertion	Peripheral Nerve	Nerve Root
Extensor carpi radialis brevis	Wrist extension Wrist radial deviation	Common extensor origin on the lateral epicondyle of the humerus; radial collateral ligament of the elbow joint	Dorsal surface of the base of the third metacarpal bone	Posterior interosseous (radial)	C78
Extensor carpi ulnaris	Wrist extension Wrist ulnar deviation	Common extensor origin on the lateral epicondyle of the humerus; aponeurosis on the posterior border of the ulna	Tubercle on the ulnar aspect of the base of the fifth metacarpal bone	Posterior interosseous	C78
Flexor digitorum superficialis	Finger PIP flexion	a. Humeroulnar head: common flexor origin on the medial epicondyle of the humerus, the anterior band of the ulnar collateral ligament, and the medial aspect of the coronoid process b. Radial head: anterior border of the radius from the radial tuberosity to the insertion of pronator teres	Anterior surface of the middle phalanges of the index, middle, ring and little fingers	Median	C8T1
Flexor digitorum profundus	Finger DIP flexion	Upper three fourths of the anterior and medial aspects of the ulna; medial aspect of the coronoid process; by an aponeurosis on the upper three fourths of the posterior border of the ulna; anterior surface of the medial half of the interosseous membrane	Palmar aspect of the bases of the distal phalanges of the index, middle, ring, and little fingers	a. Lateral portion of muscle—anterior interosseus branch of median b. Medial portion of muscle—ulnar	C8T1

WRIST AND HAND

Muscle	Primary Muscle Action	Muscle Origin	Muscle Insertion	Peripheral Nerve	Nerve Root
Extensor digitorum communis	Finger MCP extension	Common extensor origin on the lateral epicondyle of the humerus	Dorsal surfaces of the bases of the distal and middle phalanges of the index, middle, ring, and little fingers	Posterior interosseous	C78
Extensor indicis proprius	Index finger MCP extension	Posterior surface of the ulna distal to the origin of extensor pollicis longus; posterior aspect of the interosseous membrane	Ulnar side of the extensor digitorum tendon to the index finger at the level of the second metacarpal head	Posterior interosseous	C78
Extensor digiti minimi	Fifth finger MCP extension	Common extensor origin on the lateral epicondyle of the humerus	Dorsal digital expansion of the fifth digit	Posterior interosseous	C78
Interosseous a. Dorsal	Finger MCP abduction	a. First: adjacent sides of the first and second metacarpal bones b. Second: adjacent sides of the second and third metacarpal bones c. Third: adjacent sides of the third and fourth metacarpal bones d. Fourth: adjacent sides of the fourth and fifth metacarpal bones	All insert into the dorsal digital expansions of either the index, middle, or ring fingers a. First: radial aspect of the base of the proximal phalanx of the index finger b. Second and third: radial and ulnar aspects respectively, of the base of the proximal phalanx of the middle finger c. Fourth: ulnar aspect of the base of the proximal phalanx of the ring finger	Ulnar	C8T1

Muscle	Primary Muscle Action	Muscle Origin	Muscle Insertion	Peripheral Nerve	Nerve Root
b. Palmar	Finger MCP adduction	a. First: ulnar side of the base of the first metacarpal bone b. Second; ulnar side of the palmar aspect of the second metacarpal bone c. Third: radial side of the palmar aspect of the fourth metacarpal bone d. Fourth: radial side of the palmar aspect of the fifth metacarpal bone	All insert into the dorsal digital expansions of either the thumb, index, ring, or little fingers The first also inserts into the sesamoid bone on the ulnar side of the base of the proximal phalanx of the thumb and into the phalanx The fourth also inserts into the radial side of the base of the proximal phalanx of the little finger	Ulnar	C8T1
Lumbricales	Finger MCP flexion and IP extension	Tendons of flexor digitorum profundus: a. First and second lumbricales: radial sides and palmar surfaces of the tendons of the index and middle fingers b. Third: adjacent sides of the tendons of the middle and ring fingers c. Fourth: adjacent sides of the tendons of the ring and little fingers	Radial aspect of the dorsal digital expansion of the corresponding index, middle, ring, and little fingers	a. Medial two lumbricales —ulnar b. Lateral two lumbricales —median	C8T1 C8T1
Abductor digiti minimi	Little finger MCP abduction	Pisiform bone; pisohamate ligament; tendon of flexor carpi ulnaris	Ulnar aspect of the base of the proximal phalanx of the little finger; dorsal digital expansion of the little finger	Ulnar	C8T1

WRIST AND HAND

Muscle	Primary Muscle Action	Muscle Origin	Muscle Insertion	Peripheral Nerve	Nerve Root
Opponens digiti minimi	Little finger opposition (flexion, and internal rotation of the 5th metacarpal bone)	Hook of hamate; flexor retinaculum	Ulnar and adjacent palmar surface of the fifth metacarpal bone	Ulnar	C8T1
Flexor digiti minimi	Little finger MCP flexion	Hook of hamate; flexor retinaculum	Ulnar aspect of the base of the proximal phalanx of the little finger	Ulnar	C8T1

Muscle	Primary Muscle Action	Muscle Origin	Muscle Insertion	Peripheral Nerve	Nerve Root
Flexor pollicis longus	Thumb IP joint flexion	Anterior surface of the radius between the bicipital tuberosity and the pronator quadratus; anterior surface of the lateral half of the interosseous membrane; lateral aspect of the coronoid process and the medial epicondyle of the humerus	Palmar aspect of the base of the distal phalanx of the thumb	Anterior interosseous branch of median	C7**8**
Flexor pollicis brevis	Thumb MCP joint flexion	a. Superficial head: flexor retinaculum and the tubercle of the trapezium bone b. Deep head: capitate and trapezoid bones and the palmar ligaments of the distal row of carpal bones	The radial side of the base of the proximal phalanx of the thumb	a. Superficial head—median b. Deep head—ulnar	C8T**1**
Extensor pollicis longus	Thumb IP joint extension	Middle third of the posterolateral aspect of the ulna; posterior surface of the interosseous membrane	Dorsal aspect of the base of the distal phalanx of the thumb	Posterior interosseous	C7**8**
Extensor pollicis brevis	Thumb MCP joint extension	Posterior aspect of the radius below the abductor pollicis longus; posterior surface of the interosseous membrane	Dorsal aspect of the base of the proximal phalanx of the thumb	Posterior interosseous	C7**8**

WRIST AND HAND

TABLE
5-5

▼ MUSCLE ACTIONS, ATTACHMENTS, AND NERVE SUPPLY: THE THUMB[9] *Continued*

Muscle	Primary Muscle Action	Muscle Origin	Muscle Insertion	Peripheral Nerve	Nerve Root
Abductor pollicis longus	Thumb radial abduction	Posterior aspect of the shaft of the ulna distal to the insertion of anconeus; posterior aspect of the shaft of the radius distal to the insertion of supinator; posterior aspect of the interosseous membrane	Radial aspect of the base of the first metacarpal bone; the trapezium bone	Posterior interosseous	C78
Abductor pollicis brevis	Thumb palmar abduction	Flexor retinaculum; tubercles of the scaphoid and trapezium bones; tendon of abductor pollicis longus	Radial aspect of the base of the proximal phalanx of the thumb; dorsal digital expansion of the thumb	Median	C8T1
Adductor pollicis	Thumb adduction	a. Oblique head: capitate bone and the palmar surfaces of the bases of the second and third metacarpal bones b. Transverse head: distal two thirds of the palmar surface of the shaft of the third metacarpal bone	Ulnar aspect of the base of the proximal phalanx of the thumb; dorsal digital expansion of the thumb	Ulnar	C8T1
Opponens pollicis	Thumb opposition (abduction, flexion, and internal rotation of the first metacarpal bone)	Flexor retinaculum; tubercle of the trapezium bone	Lateral surface and lateral aspect of the palmar surface of the first metacarpal bone	Median	C8T1

WRIST FLEXION AND RADIAL DEVIATION

Against Gravity: Flexor Carpi Radialis

Accessory muscles: flexor carpi ulnaris and palmaris longus.

• **Start Position.** The patient is sitting or supine. If sitting, the forearm is supinated and supported on a table. The wrist is extended and in ulnar deviation and the fingers and thumb are relaxed (Fig. 5-69).

• **Stabilization.** The therapist stabilizes the forearm proximal to the wrist.

• **Movement.** The patient flexes and radially deviates the wrist (Fig. 5-70). The patient should be instructed to keep the fingers and thumb relaxed.

• **Palpation.** Anterolateral aspect of the wrist in line with the second web space, on the radial side of palmaris longus.

• **Substitution/Trick Movement.** The patient may flex the wrist with palmaris longus and flexor carpi ulnaris. Using flexor carpi ulnaris alone, the patient will flex with ulnar deviation. If the patient flexes the fingers the flexor digitorum superficialis and profundus may substitute for the wrist flexors when movement is initiated.[19]

• **Resistance Location.** Applied distal to the wrist over the thenar eminence or the lateral aspect of the palm (Figs. 5-71 and 5-72).

• **Resistance Direction.** Wrist extension and ulnar deviation.

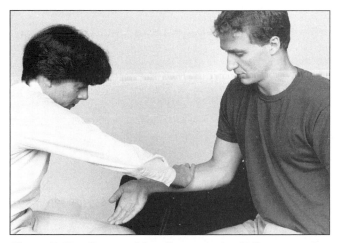

Figure 5-69.   Start position: flexor carpi radialis.

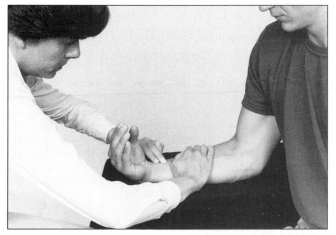

Figure 5-70.   Screen position: flexor carpi radialis.

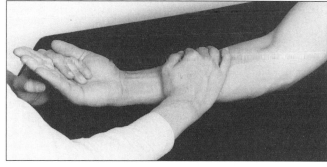

Figure 5-71.   Resistance: flexor carpi radialis.

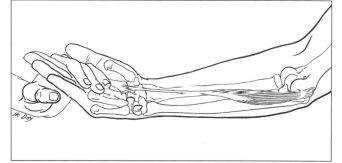

Figure 5-72.   Flexor carpi radialis.

WRIST AND HAND

Gravity Eliminated: Flexor Carpi Radialis

• **Start Position.** The patient is sitting or supine. The forearm is in slight pronation and supported on a table or powder board. The wrist is extended and in ulnar deviation and the fingers and thumb are relaxed (Fig. 5-73).

• **Stabilization.** The therapist stabilizes the forearm proximal to the wrist.

• **End Position.** The patient flexes and radially deviates the wrist through full ROM (Fig. 5-74).

• **Substitution/Trick Movement.** Flexor carpi ulnaris, palmaris longus, and flexor digitorum superficialis and profundus. As the patient flexes the wrist from the anatomical position, forearm pronation and thumb abduction through the action of abductor pollicis longus may be attempted.

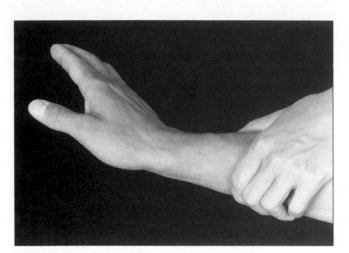

Figure 5-73. Start position: flexor carpi radialis.

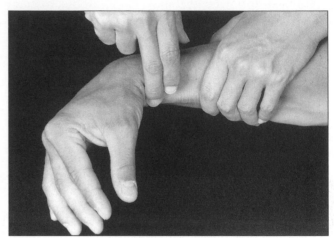

Figure 5-74. End position: flexor carpi radialis.

WRIST FLEXION AND ULNAR DEVIATION

Against Gravity: Flexor Carpi Ulnaris

Accessory muscles: flexor carpi radialis and palmaris longus.

• **Start Position.** The patient is sitting or supine. If sitting, the forearm is supinated and supported on a table. The wrist is extended and in radial deviation and the fingers and thumb are relaxed (Fig. 5-75).

• **Stabilization.** The therapist stabilizes the forearm proximal to the wrist.

• **Movement.** The patient flexes and ulnarly deviates the wrist through full ROM (Fig. 5-76).

• **Palpation.** Anteromedial aspect of the wrist proximal to the pisiform bone.

• **Substitution/Trick Movement.** Flexor carpi radialis, palmaris longus, and flexor digitorum superficialis and profundus. Using flexor carpi radialis alone, the patient will flex with radial deviation.

• **Resistance Location.** Applied over the hypothenar eminence (Figs. 5-77 and 5-78).

• **Resistance Direction.** Wrist extension and radial deviation.

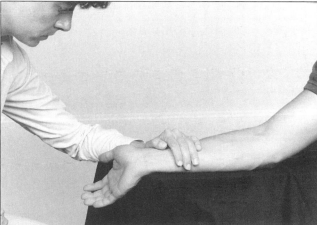

Figure 5-75.   Start position: flexor carpi ulnaris.

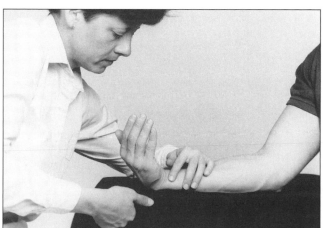

Figure 5-76.   Screen position: flexor carpi ulnaris.

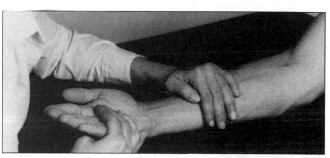

Figure 5-77.   Resistance: flexor carpi ulnaris.

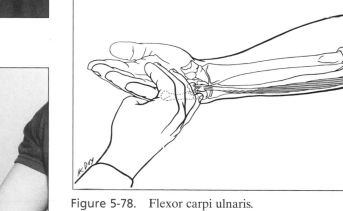

Figure 5-78.   Flexor carpi ulnaris.

Gravity Eliminated: Flexor Carpi Ulnaris

• **Start Position.** The patient is sitting or supine. The forearm is in slight supination and supported on a table or powder board. The wrist is extended and in radial deviation and the fingers and thumb are relaxed (Fig. 5-79).

• **Stabilization.** The therapist stabilizes the forearm proximal to the wrist.

• **End Position.** The patient flexes the wrist with ulnar deviation through full ROM (Fig. 5-80).

• **Substitution/Trick Movement.** Flexor carpi radialis, palmaris longus, and flexor digitorum superficialis and profundus.

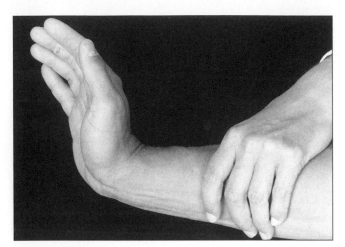

Figure 5-79.   Start position: flexor carpi ulnaris.

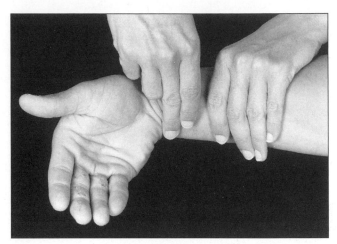

Figure 5-80.   End position: flexor carpi ulnaris.

WRIST FLEXION (NOT SHOWN)

Against Gravity: Flexor Carpi Radialis and Flexor Carpi Ulnaris

Accessory muscle: palmaris longus.

• **Start Position.** The patient is sitting or supine. If sitting, the forearm is supinated and supported on a table. The wrist is extended and the fingers and thumb are relaxed.

• **Stabilization.** The therapist stabilizes the forearm proximal to the wrist.

• **Movement.** The patient flexes the wrist through full ROM.

• **Palpation.** Flexor carpi radialis: Anterolateral aspect of the wrist in line with the second web space, on the radial side of palmaris longus. Flexor carpi ulnaris: anteromedial aspect of the wrist proximal to the pisiform bone.

• **Substitution/Trick Movement.** Flexor digitorum superficialis and profundus.

• **Resistance Location.** Applied over the palm of the hand.

• **Resistance Direction.** Wrist extension.

Gravity Eliminated: Flexor Carpi Radialis and Flexor Carpi Ulnaris

• **Start Position.** The patient is sitting or supine. The forearm is in midposition and supported on a table or powder board. The wrist is extended and the fingers and thumb are relaxed.

• **Stabilization.** The therapist stabilizes the forearm proximal to the wrist.

• **End Position.** The patient flexes the wrist through full ROM.

• **Substitution/Trick Movement.** Flexor digitorum superficialis and profundus.

Palmaris Longus. Palmaris longus is a weak flexor of the wrist and is not isolated for individual muscle testing. It can be palpated on the midline of the anterior aspect of the wrist during testing of flexor carpi radialis and ulnaris. Palmaris longus is a vestigial muscle in about 13% of subjects.[20] Its presence can be established through flexing the wrist and cupping the fingers and palm of the hand (Figs. 5-81 and 5-82). Its tendon stands out boldly when present.

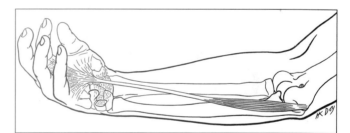

Figure 5-82.   Palmaris longus.

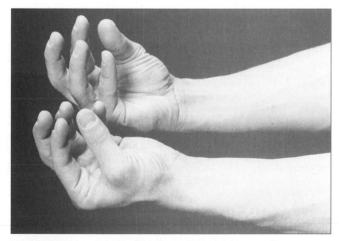

Figure 5-81.   Palmaris longus: the muscle is present in the right arm (observe the tendon at the wrist). The muscle is absent in the left arm.

WRIST EXTENSION AND RADIAL DEVIATION

Against Gravity: Extensor Carpi Radialis Longus and Extensor Carpi Radialis Brevis

Accessory muscle: extensor carpi ulnaris.

• **Start Position.** The patient is sitting or supine. In sitting, the forearm is pronated and supported on a table. The wrist is flexed and in ulnar deviation and the fingers and thumb are slightly flexed (Fig. 5-83).

• **Stabilization.** The therapist stabilizes the forearm proximal to the wrist.

• **Movement.** The patient extends and radially deviates the wrist through full ROM (Fig. 5-84). The patient should be instructed to keep the thumb and fingers relaxed.

• **Palpation.** Extensor carpi radialis longus: dorsal aspect of the wrist at the base of the second metacarpal. Extensor carpi radialis brevis: base of the third metacarpal.

• **Substitution/Trick Movement.** The patient may extend using extensor carpi ulnaris. Using only this muscle, the patient will extend with ulnar deviation.

• **Resistance Location.** Applied on the dorsal aspect of the hand over the second and third metacarpals (Figs. 5-85 and 5-86).

• **Resistance Direction.** Wrist flexion and ulnar deviation.

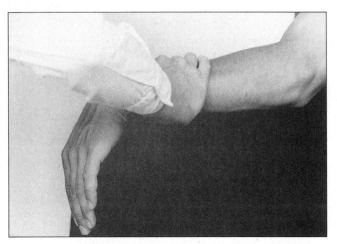

Figure 5-83.   Start position: extensor carpi radialis longus and brevis.

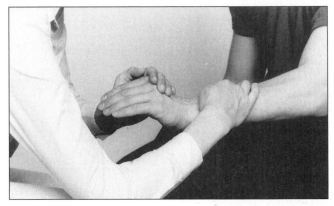

Figure 5-85.   Resistance: extensor carpi radialis longus and brevis.

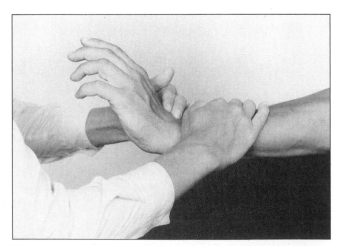

Figure 5-84.   Screen position: extensor carpi radialis longus and brevis.

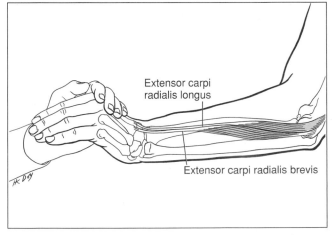

Extensor carpi radialis longus

Extensor carpi radialis brevis

Figure 5-86.   Extensor carpi radialis longus and brevis.

Gravity Eliminated: Extensor Carpi Radialis Longus and Extensor Carpi Radialis Brevis

• **Start Position.** The patient is sitting or supine. The forearm is in slight supination and supported on a table or powder board. The wrist is flexed in ulnar deviation. The fingers and thumb are slightly flexed (Fig. 5-87).

• **Stabilization.** The therapist stabilizes the forearm proximal to the wrist.

• **End Position.** The patient extends the wrist with simultaneous radial deviation through full ROM (Fig. 5-88).

• **Substitution/Trick Movement.** Extensor carpi ulnaris.

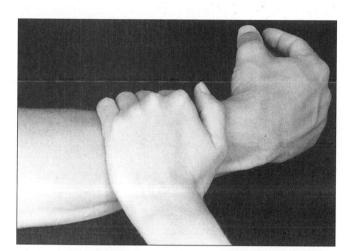

Figure 5-87. Start position: extensor carpi radialis longus and brevis.

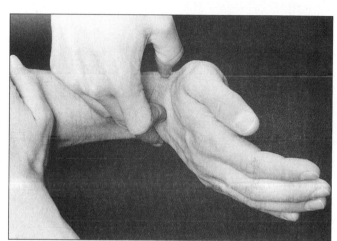

Figure 5-88. End position: extensor carpi radialis longus and brevis.

WRIST EXTENSION AND ULNAR DEVIATION

Against Gravity: Extensor Carpi Ulnaris

Accessory muscles: extensor carpi radialis longus and brevis.

• **Start Position.** The patient is sitting or supine. If sitting, the forearm is pronated and supported on a table. The wrist is flexed and in radial deviation and the fingers and thumb are slightly flexed (Fig. 5-89).

• **Stabilization.** The therapist stabilizes the forearm proximal to the wrist.

• **Movement.** The patient extends and ulnarly deviates the wrist through full ROM (Fig. 5-90). The patient should be instructed to keep the fingers relaxed.

• **Palpation.** On the dorsal aspect of the wrist proximal to the fifth metacarpal and distal to the ulnar styloid process.

• **Substitution/Trick Movement.** The patient may extend and radially deviate the wrist through the action of extensor carpi radialis longus and brevis.

• **Resistance Location.** Applied on the dorsal aspect of the hand over the fourth and fifth metacarpals (Figs. 5-91 and 5-92).

• **Resistance Direction.** Wrist flexion and radial deviation.

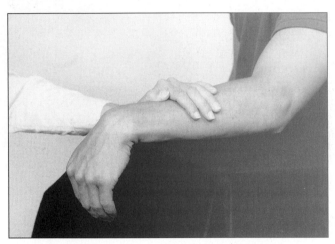

Figure 5-89. Start position: extensor carpi ulnaris.

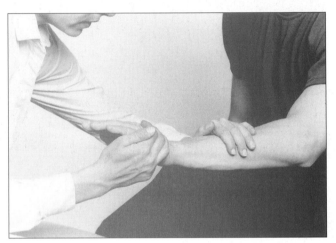

Figure 5-91. Resistance: extensor carpi ulnaris.

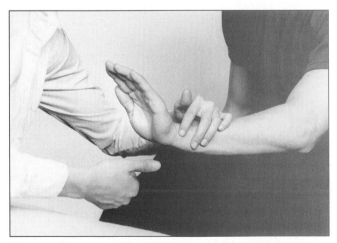

Figure 5-90. Screen position: extensor carpi ulnaris.

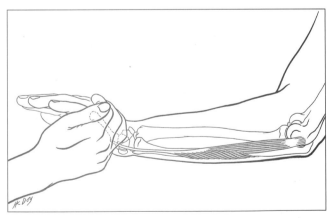

Figure 5-92. Extensor carpi ulnaris.

Gravity Eliminated: Extensor Carpi Ulnaris

• **Start Position.** The patient is sitting or supine. The forearm is in slight pronation and supported on a table or powder board. The wrist is flexed in radial deviation. The fingers and thumb are flexed (Fig. 5-93).

• **Stabilization.** The therapist stabilizes the forearm proximal to the wrist.

• **End Position.** The patient extends the wrist with simultaneous ulnar deviation through full ROM (Fig. 5-94).

• **Substitution/Trick Movement.** Extensor carpi radialis longus and brevis.

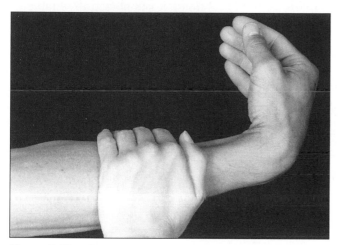

Figure 5-93. Start position: extensor carpi ulnaris.

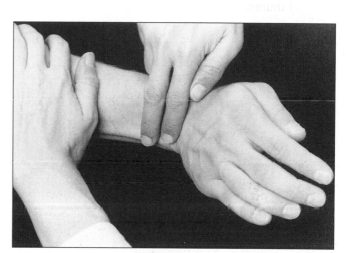

Figure 5-94. End position: extensor carpi ulnaris.

WRIST EXTENSION (NOT SHOWN)

Against Gravity: Extensor Carpi Radialis Longus, Extensor Carpi Radialis Brevis, and Extensor Carpi Ulnaris

• Start Position. The patient is sitting or supine. If sitting, the forearm is pronated and supported on a table. The wrist is flexed and the fingers and thumb are relaxed.

• Stabilization. The therapist stabilizes the forearm proximal to the wrist.

• Movement. The patient extends the wrist through full ROM. The patient should be instructed to keep the thumb and fingers relaxed.

• Palpation. Extensor carpi radialis longus: dorsal aspect of the wrist at the base of the second metacarpal. Extensor carpi radialis brevis: base of the third metacarpal. Extensor carpi ulnaris: on the dorsal aspect of the wrist proximal to the fifth metacarpal and distal to the ulnar styloid process.

• Substitution/Trick Movement. Extensor digitorum, extensor digiti minimi, and extensor indicis if the fingers are extended.

• Resistance Location. Applied on the dorsal aspect of the hand over the metacarpals.

• Resistance Direction. Wrist flexion.

Gravity Eliminated: Extensor Carpi Radialis Longus, Extensor Carpi Radialis Brevis, and Extensor Carpi Ulnaris

• Start Position. The patient is sitting or supine. The forearm is in midposition and supported on a table or powder board. The wrist is flexed, and the fingers and thumb are relaxed.

• Stabilization. The therapist stabilizes the forearm proximal to the wrist.

• End Position. The patient extends the wrist through full ROM.

• Substitution/Trick Movement. Extensor digitorum, extensor digiti minimi, extensor indicis.

▼ FINGER AND THUMB MUSCLES

Gravity is not considered to be a factor in manual muscle testing of the fingers and thumb because the weight of the part is small in comparison to the strength of the muscle.[19] Refer to Chapter 1 for grading parameters.

FINGER METACARPOPHALANGEAL EXTENSION (EXTENSOR DIGITORUM COMMUNIS, EXTENSOR INDICIS PROPRIUS, AND EXTENSOR DIGITI MINIMI)

• **Start Position.** The patient is sitting or supine. The forearm is pronated, the wrist is in a neutral position, and the fingers are flexed (Fig. 5-95).

• **Stabilization.** The therapist stabilizes the metacarpals.

• **Movement.** The patient extends all four MCP joints while maintaining flexion at the IP joints (Fig. 5-96).

• **Palpation** (Fig. 5-97). Extensor digitorum: the tendons to each finger can be palpated on the dorsum of the hand proximal to each metacarpal head. Extensor indicis: medial to the extensor digitorum tendon to the index finger. Extensor digiti minimi: lateral to the extensor digitorum tendon to the little finger.

• **Substitution/Trick Movement.** Stabilization of the wrist prevents the tenodesis effect of wrist flexion and subsequent MCP extension.[16,18]

• **Resistance Location.** Dorsal aspect of the proximal phalanx of each finger (Figs. 5-98 and 5-99).

• **Resistance Direction.** MCP flexion.

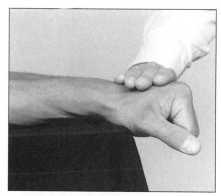

Figure 5-95. Start position: extensor digitorum, extensor indicis proprius, and extensor digiti minimi.

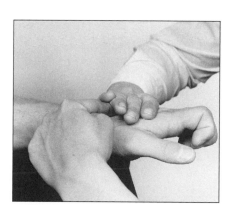

Figure 5-96. Screen position: extensor digitorum, extensor indicis, and extensor digiti minimi.

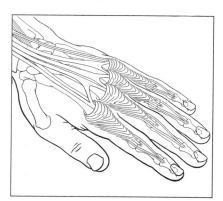

Figure 5-97. Extensor expansion.

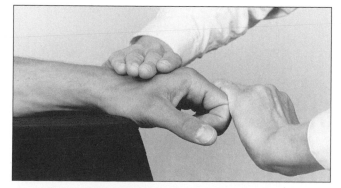

Figure 5-98. Resistance: extensor digitorum, extensor indicis, and extensor digiti minimi.

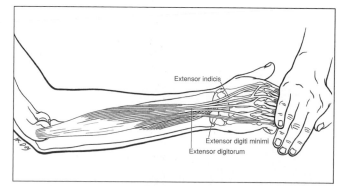

Figure 5-99. Extensor digitorum, extensor indicis, and extensor digiti minimi.

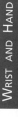

METACARPOPHALANGEAL ABDUCTION (DORSAL INTEROSSEI AND ABDUCTOR DIGITI MINIMI)

• **Start Position.** The patient is sitting or supine. Dorsal interossei (Fig. 5-100): the forearm is pronated and supported on a table, the wrist is in neutral, and the fingers are extended and adducted. Abductor digiti minimi (Fig. 5-101): the forearm is supinated.

• **Stabilization.** Dorsal interossei: the therapist stabilizes the dorsum of the hand over the metacarpal bones and wrist. Abductor digiti minimi: the therapist stabilizes the wrist and lateral three metacarpals.

• **Movement.** Dorsal interossei (Fig. 5-102): the patient abducts the index finger toward the thumb, the middle finger toward the index finger and then ring finger, and the ring finger toward the little finger. To prevent assistance from an adjacent finger, the non-test digits may require stabilization. Abductor digiti minimi (Fig. 5-103): the patient abducts the little finger.

• **Palpation.** The first dorsal interosseous is palpated on the radial aspect of the second metacarpal (see Fig. 5-102). The remaining interossei cannot be palpated. Abductor digiti minimi is palpated on the ulnar aspect of the fifth metacarpal (see Fig. 5-103).

• **Substitution/Trick Movement.** Maintain the MCP joints in neutral position to avoid finger abduction through contraction of the extensor digitorum communis.

• **Resistance Location.** Against the proximal phalanx of the digit being tested. The therapist resists on the radial side of the index and middle fingers and the ulnar side of the middle, ring, (Figs. 5-104 and 5-105), and little fingers (Figs. 5-106 and 5-107).

• **Resistance Direction.** Adduction.

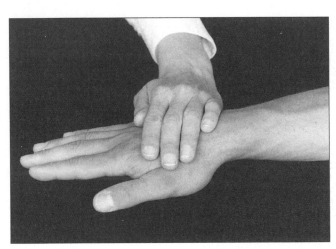

Figure 5-100.   Start position: dorsal interossei.

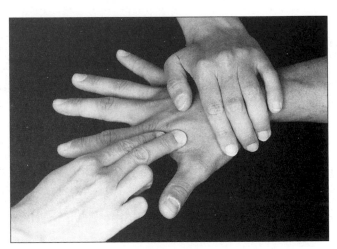

Figure 5-102.   Screen position: dorsal interossei.

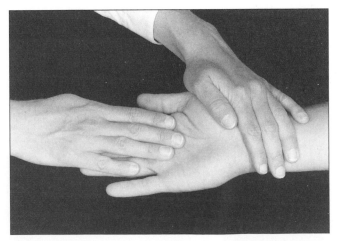

Figure 5-101.   Start position: abductor digiti minimi.

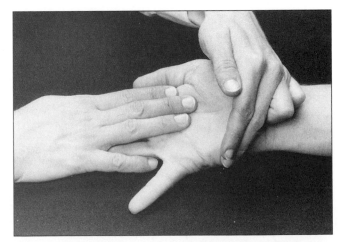

Figure 5-103.   Screen position: abductor digiti minimi.

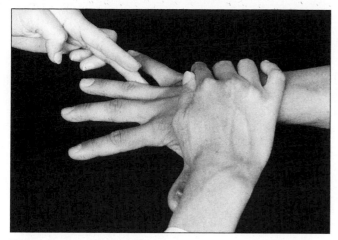

Figure 5-104. Resistance: fourth dorsal interosseous.

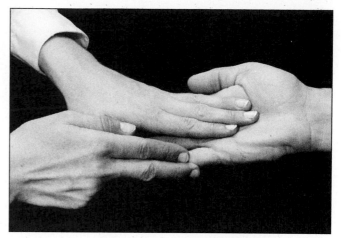

Figure 5-106. Resistance: abductor digiti minimi.

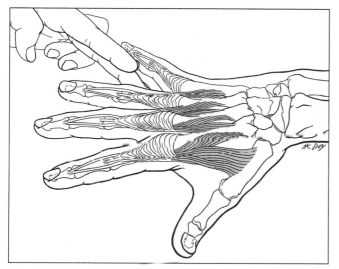

Figure 5-105. Dorsal interossei.

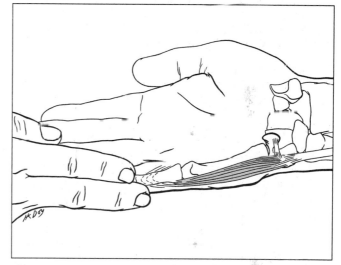

Figure 5-107. Abductor digiti minimi.

WRIST AND HAND

METACARPOPHALANGEAL ADDUCTION (PALMAR INTEROSSEI)

• Start Position. The patient is sitting or supine. If sitting, the forearm is supinated and supported on a table, the wrist is in neutral, and the fingers are abducted (Fig. 5-108).

• Stabilization. The therapist stabilizes the metacarpal bones and wrist.

• Movement. The patient adducts the index, ring, and little finger toward the middle finger (Fig. 5-109).

• Palpation. These muscles cannot be palpated.

• Substitution/Trick Movement. None.

• Resistance Location. Against the proximal phalanx of the digit being tested (Figs. 5-110 and 5-111). The therapist resists on the ulnar aspect of the index finger and on the radial aspect of the ring and fifth fingers.

• Resistance Direction. Abduction.

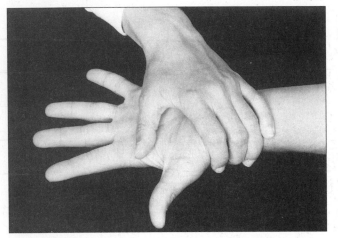

Figure 5-108.   Start position: palmar interossei.

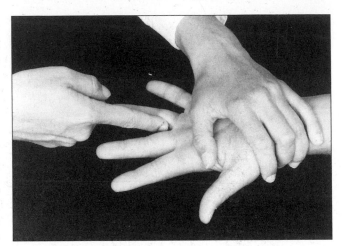

Figure 5-110.   Resistance: third palmar interosseous.

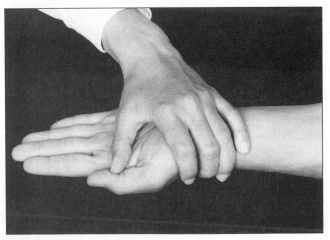

Figure 5-109.   Screen position: palmar interossei.

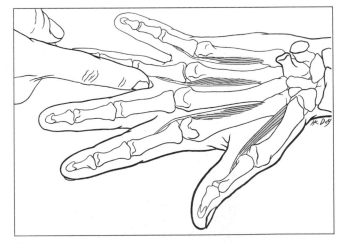

Figure 5-111.   Palmar interossei.

FINGER METACARPOPHALANGEAL FLEXION AND INTERPHALANGEAL EXTENSION (LUMBRICALES)

The interossei muscles also flex the MCP joints and simultaneously extend the IP joints. They have been isolated for testing as abductors and adductors. Should the interossei be strong, weakness elicited in this muscle test may be attributed to lumbricales. Accessory muscle: flexor digiti minimi (MCP joint flexion).

• **Start Position.** The patient is sitting or supine. The forearm is supinated or in midposition, supported on a table. The wrist is in a neutral position, the MCP joints are extended and adducted, and the IP joints are slightly flexed (Fig. 5-112).

• **Stabilization.** The therapist stabilizes the metacarpals.

• **Movement.** The patient flexes the MCP joints while simultaneously extending the IP joints (Fig. 5-113). The fingers are allowed to abduct to prevent assistance from adjacent fingers in static adduction.

• **Palpation.** The lumbricales cannot be palpated.

• **Substitution/Trick Movement.** Extensor digitorum communis.

• **Resistance Location.** Applied on the volar surface of the proximal phalanx and the dorsal surface of the middle phalanx (Figs. 5-114 and 5-115).

• **Resistance Direction.** MCP extension and IP flexion.

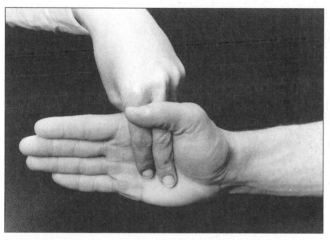

Figure 5-112. Start position: lumbricales.

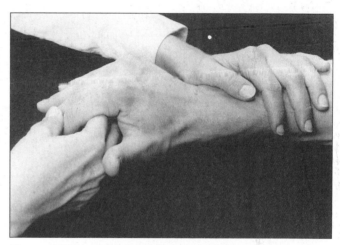

Figure 5-114. Resistance: first lumbricalis.

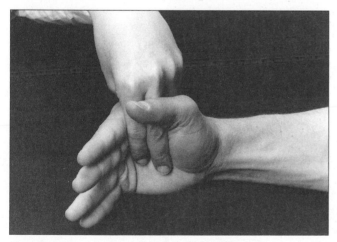

Figure 5-113. Screen position: lumbricales.

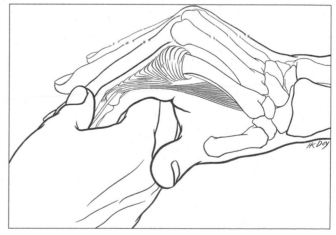

Figure 5-115. First lumbricalis.

FIFTH FINGER METACARPOPHALANGEAL FLEXION (FLEXOR DIGITI MINIMI)

Accessory muscles: fourth lumbricalis, fourth palmar interosseous, and abductor digiti minimi.

• **Start Position.** The patient is sitting or supine. If sitting, the forearm is supinated and supported on a table. The wrist is in a neutral position and the fingers are extended (Fig. 5-116).

• **Stabilization.** The therapist stabilizes the metacarpals.

• **Movement.** The patient flexes the MCP joint of the little finger while maintaining IP joint extension (Fig. 5-117).

• **Palpation.** On the hypothenar eminence medial to abductor digiti minimi.

• **Substitution/Trick Movement.** The patient may attempt to use flexor digitorum superficialis and profundus. Ensure that no flexion of the IP joints occurs. If flexion cannot be initiated, the patient may abduct the little finger through the action of abductor digiti minimi.

• **Resistance Location.** Applied on the volar aspect of the proximal phalanx of the little finger (Figs. 5-118 and 5-119).

• **Resistance Direction.** Extension.

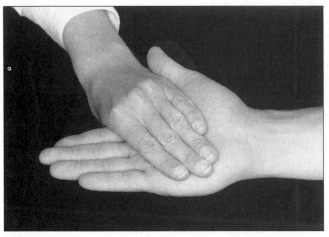

Figure 5-116.   Start position: flexor digiti minimi.

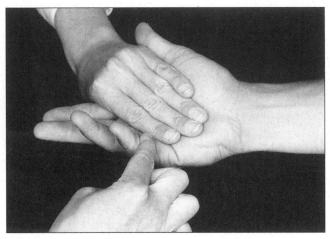

Figure 5-118.   Resistance: flexor digiti minimi.

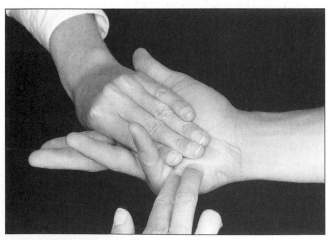

Figure 5-117.   Screen position: flexor digiti minimi.

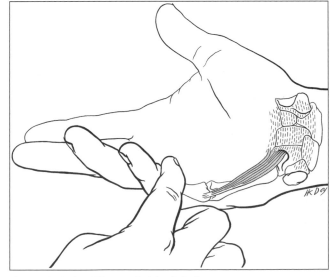

Figure 5-119.   Flexor digiti minimi.

FINGER PROXIMAL INTERPHALANGEAL FLEXION (FLEXOR DIGITORUM SUPERFICIALIS)

Accessory muscle: flexor digitorum profundus.

• **Start Position.** The patient is sitting or supine. In sitting, the forearm is supinated and supported on a table. The wrist is in a neutral position or slight extension and the fingers are extended. To rule out the contribution of flexor digitorum profundus, the fingers not being tested may be held in extension[21] (Fig. 5-120).

• **Stabilization.** The therapist stabilizes the metacarpals and the proximal phalanx of the finger being tested.

• **Movement.** The patient flexes the PIP joint of each finger while maintaining DIP joint extension (Fig. 5-121). The little finger is not isolated for testing and may flex with the ring finger. Isolated action of the little finger superficialis is not always possible.[22]

• **Palpation.** On the volar surface of the wrist between the palmaris longus and flexor carpi ulnaris tendons or on the proximal phalanx.

• **Substitution/Trick Movement.** Flexor digitorum profundus. The flexor digitorum profundus tendons to the ulnar three fingers often originate from a common muscle belly; thus, the action of the profundus is interdependent in these fingers.[23] Therefore, holding the nontest fingers in extension eliminates normal function of the profundus tendon of the test finger.

• **Resistance Location.** Applied on the volar surface of the middle phalanx (Figs. 5-122 and 5-123).

• **Resistance Direction.** Extension.

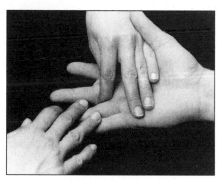

Figure 5-120.   Start position: flexor digitorum superficialis.

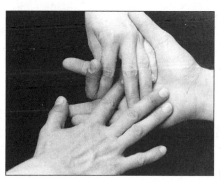

Figure 5-121.   Screen position: flexor digitorum superficialis.

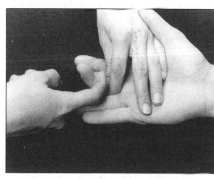

Figure 5-122.   Resistance: flexor digitorum superficialis.

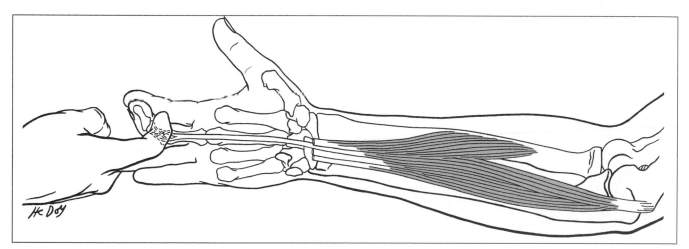

Figure 5-123.   Flexor digitorum superficialis.

FINGER DISTAL INTERPHALANGEAL FLEXION
(FLEXOR DIGITORUM PROFUNDUS)

• **Start Position.** The patient is sitting or supine. If sitting, the forearm is supinated and supported on a table. The wrist is in a neutral position or slight extension and the test finger is in extension (Fig. 5-124).

• **Stabilization.** The therapist stabilizes the proximal and middle phalanges of the test finger.

• **Movement.** The patient flexes the DIP joint through full ROM (Fig. 5-125).

The flexor digitorum profundus tendons to the ulnar three fingers often originate from a common muscle belly; thus, the action of the profundus is interdependent in these fingers and the nontest fingers should be held in slight flexion during testing.[23]

• **Palpation.** On the volar surface of the middle phalanx.

• **Resistance Location.** Applied on the volar aspect of the distal phalanx (Figs. 5-126 and 5-127).

• **Resistance Direction.** Extension.

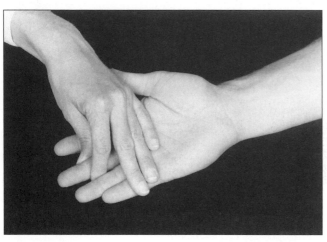

Figure 5-124.   Start position: flexor digitorum profundus.

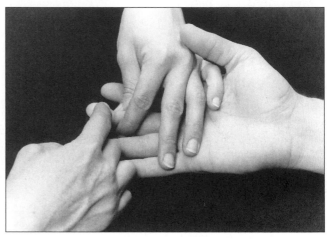

Figure 5-126.   Resistance: flexor digitorum profundus.

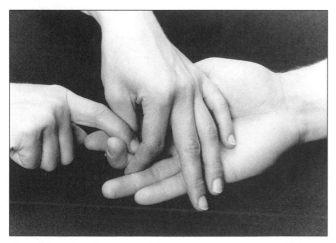

Figure 5-125.   Screen position: flexor digitorum profundus.

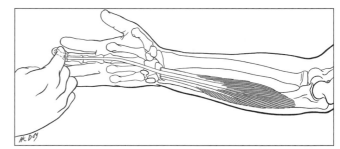

Figure 5-127.   Flexor digitorum profundus.

THUMB INTERPHALANGEAL FLEXION (FLEXOR POLLICIS LONGUS)

• **Start Position.** The patient is sitting or supine. The forearm is supinated, the wrist is in a neutral position, and the thumb is extended (Fig. 5-128).

• **Stabilization.** The therapist stabilizes the wrist, the thumb metacarpal, and proximal phalanx.

• **Movement.** The patient flexes the IP joint through full ROM (Fig. 5-129).

• **Palpation.** Volar aspect of the proximal phalanx.

• **Substitution/Trick Movement.** The relaxation of the thumb following extension of the IP joint may give the appearance of contraction of flexor pollicis longus.

• **Resistance Location.** Applied on the volar surface of the distal phalanx (Figs. 5-130 and 5-131).

• **Resistance Direction.** Extension.

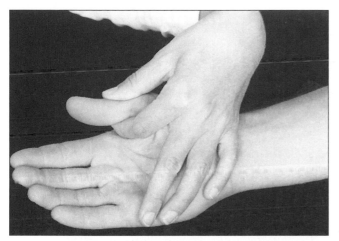

Figure 5-128.   Start position: flexor pollicis longus.

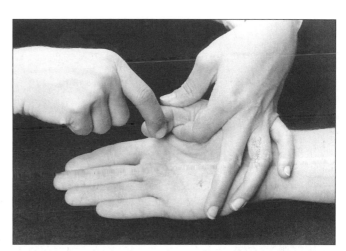

Figure 5-130.   Resistance: flexor pollicis longus.

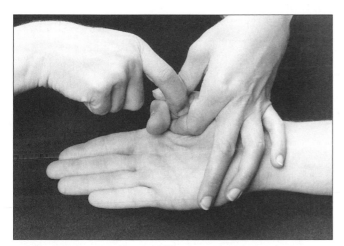

Figure 5-129.   Screen position: flexor pollicis longus.

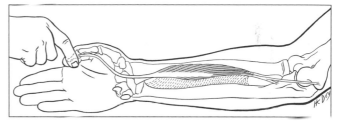

Figure 5-131.   Flexor pollicis longus.

THUMB METACARPOPHALANGEAL FLEXION (FLEXOR POLLICIS BREVIS)

Accessory muscle: flexor pollicis longus.

• **Start Position.** The patient is sitting or supine. The forearm is supinated, the wrist is in a neutral position, and the thumb is extended and adducted (Fig. 5-132).

• **Stabilization.** The therapist stabilizes the wrist and thumb metacarpal.

• **Movement.** The patient flexes the MCP joint while maintaining extension of the IP joint to minimize the action of flexor pollicis longus (Fig. 5-133).

• **Palpation.** Proximal to the MCP joint on the middle of the thenar eminence, medial to abductor pollicis brevis.

• **Substitution/Trick Movement.** Flexor pollicis longus.

• **Resistance Location.** Applied on the volar aspect of the proximal phalanx (Figs. 5-134 and 5-135).

• **Resistance Direction.** Extension.

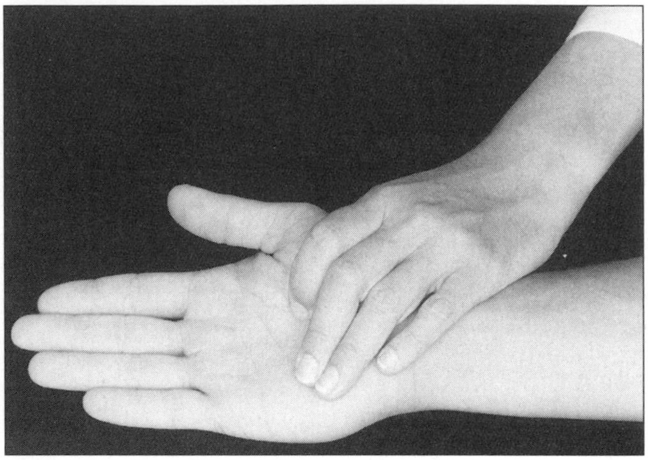

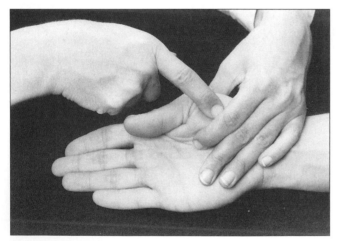

Figure 5-132. Start position: flexor pollicis brevis.

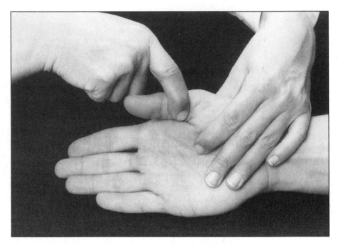

Figure 5-134. Resistance: flexor pollicis brevis.

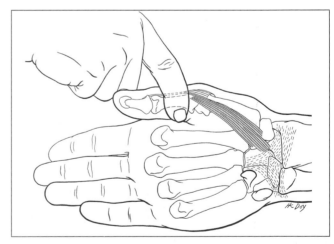

Figure 5-133. Screen position: flexor pollicis brevis.

Figure 5-135. Flexor pollicis brevis.

THUMB INTERPHALANGEAL EXTENSION (EXTENSOR POLLICIS LONGUS)

• **Start Position.** The patient is sitting or supine. The forearm is in midposition or slight pronation and the wrist is in a neutral position. The thumb is adducted with the MCP joint extended and the IP joint flexed (Fig. 5-136).

• **Stabilization.** The therapist stabilizes the thumb metacarpal and proximal phalanx.

• **Movement.** The patient extends the IP joint through full ROM (Fig. 5-137).

• **Palpation.** On the dorsal surface of the proximal phalanx or on the ulnar border of the anatomical snuff box (see Fig. 5-137).

• **Substitution/Trick Movement.** Positioning of the thumb in adduction limits the extensor action of abductor pollicis brevis and flexor pollicis brevis.[21] Rebound of contraction of flexor pollicis longus.

• **Resistance Location.** Applied on the dorsal aspect of the distal phalanx (Figs. 5-138 and 5-139).

• **Resistance Direction.** Flexion.

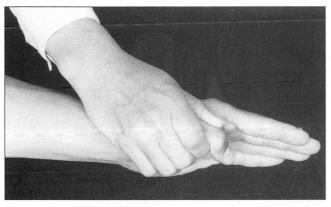

Figure 5-136.   Start position: extensor pollicis longus.

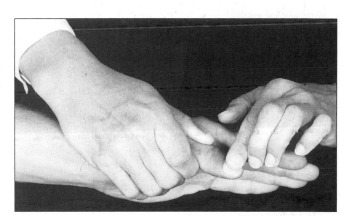

Figure 5-138.   Resistance: extensor pollicis longus.

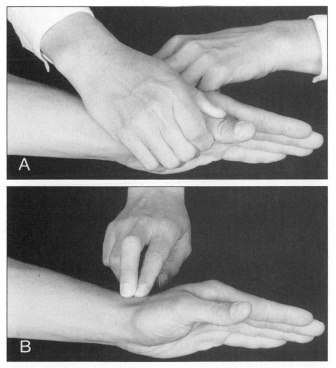

Figure 5-137.   (*A*) Screen position: extensor pollicis longus. (*B*) Palpation: extensor pollicis longus.

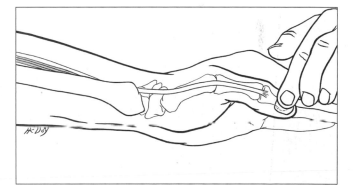

Figure 5-139.   Extensor pollicis longus.

THUMB METACARPOPHALANGEAL EXTENSION (EXTENSOR POLLICIS BREVIS)

Accessory muscle: extensor pollicis longus.

• **Start Position.** The patient is sitting or supine. The forearm is in midposition or slightly pronated and the wrist is in a neutral position. The thumb MCP and IP joints are flexed (Fig. 5-140).

• **Stabilization.** The therapist stabilizes the first metacarpal.

• **Movement.** The patient extends the MCP joint of the thumb while maintaining slight flexion of the IP joint (Fig. 5-141).

• **Palpation.** On the dorsoradial aspect of the wrist at the base of the shaft of the thumb metacarpal. It forms the radial border of the anatomical snuff box and is medial to the tendon of abductor pollicis longus (see Fig. 5-141).

• **Substitution/Trick Movement.** Extensor pollicis longus.

• **Resistance Location.** Applied on the dorsal surface of the proximal phalanx (Figs. 5-142 and 5-143).

• **Resistance Direction.** Flexion.

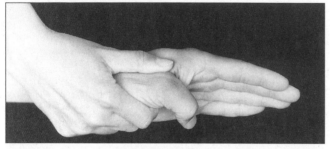

Figure 5-140.   Start position: extensor pollicis brevis.

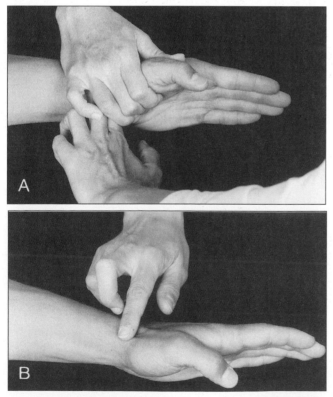

Figure 5-141.   (*A*) Screen position: extensor pollicis brevis. (*B*) Palpation: extensor pollicis brevis.

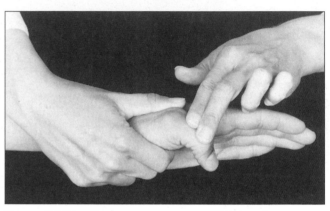

Figure 5-142.   Resistance: extensor pollicis brevis.

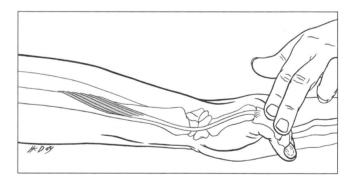

Figure 5-143.   Extensor pollicis brevis.

THUMB RADIAL ABDUCTION (ABDUCTOR POLLICIS LONGUS)

- **Start Position.** The patient is sitting or supine. The forearm is in supination and the wrist is in neutral. The thumb is adducted against the volar aspect of the index finger (Fig. 5-144).

- **Stabilization.** The therapist stabilizes the wrist and second metacarpal.

- **Movement.** The patient abducts the thumb in a radial direction through full ROM (Fig. 5-145). The thumb is taken away from the index finger at an angle of 45°[21] toward extension.

- **Palpation.** On the lateral aspect of the wrist at the base of the thumb metacarpal, and on the radial side of extensor pollicis brevis.

- **Substitution/Trick Movement.** Palmar abduction may be attempted through the action of abductor pollicis brevis.[24]

- **Resistance Location.** Applied on the lateral aspect of the thumb metacarpal (Figs. 5-146 and 5-147).

- **Resistance Direction.** Adduction and flexion.

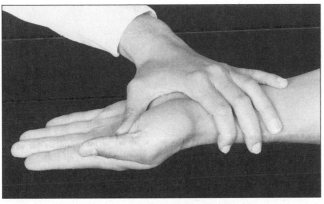

Figure 5-144.   Start position: abductor pollicis longus.

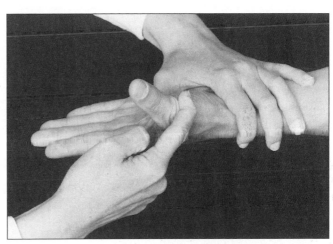

Figure 5-146.   Resistance: abductor pollicis longus.

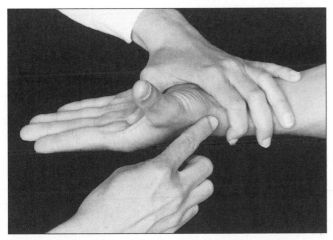

Figure 5-145.   Screen position: abductor pollicis longus.

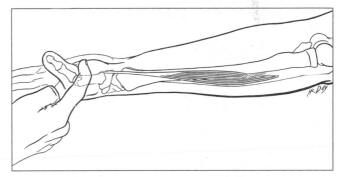

Figure 5-147.   Abductor pollicis longus.

THUMB PALMAR ABDUCTION (ABDUCTOR POLLICIS BREVIS)

• **Start Position.** The patient is sitting or supine. The forearm is in supination and the wrist is in a neutral position. The thumb is adducted against the volar aspect of the index finger (Fig. 5-148).

• **Stabilization.** The therapist stabilizes the wrist and the second metacarpal.

• **Movement.** The patient abducts the thumb through full ROM (Fig. 5-149). The thumb is taken away at a right angle to the index finger.[21]

• **Palpation.** On the lateral aspect of the thumb metacarpal.

• **Substitution/Trick Movement.** Radial abduction may be attempted through the action of abductor pollicis longus.[24]

• **Resistance Location.** Applied on the lateral aspect of the proximal phalanx (Figs. 5-150 and 5-151).

• **Resistance Direction.** Adduction.

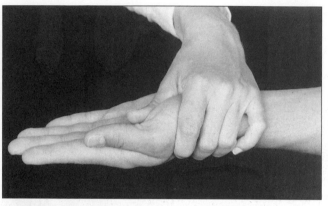

Figure 5-148.   Start position: abductor pollicis brevis.

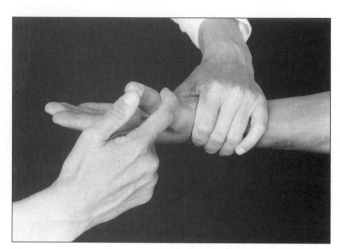

Figure 5-150.   Resistance: abductor pollicis brevis.

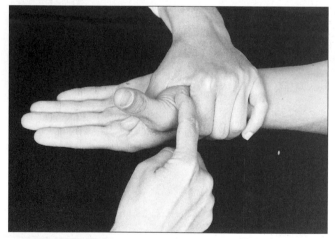

Figure 5-149.   Screen position: abductor pollicis brevis.

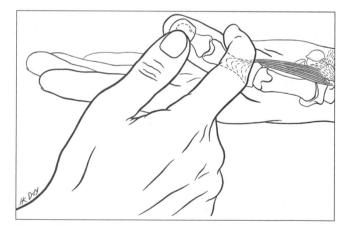

Figure 5-151.   Abductor pollicis brevis.

THUMB ADDUCTION (ADDUCTOR POLLICIS)

Accessory muscle: flexor pollicis brevis.

• **Start Position.** The patient is sitting or supine. The forearm is supinated. The wrist is in a neutral position and the fingers are extended. The MCP and IP joints of the thumb are flexed and the thumb is in palmar abduction (Fig. 5-152).

• **Stabilization.** The therapist stabilizes the wrist and the second through fifth metacarpals.

• **Movement.** The patient adducts the thumb while maintaining flexion of the MCP and IP joints (Fig. 5-153). If the patient has difficulty maintaining flexion, the MCP and IP joints may be held in extension.

• **Palpation.** On the palmar surface of the hand between the first and second metacarpals.

• **Substitution/Trick Movement.** Flexor pollicis longus and extensor pollicis longus.[18,21]

• **Resistance Location.** Applied on the medial aspect of the proximal phalanx (Figs. 5-154 and 5-155).

• **Resistance Direction.** Palmar abduction.

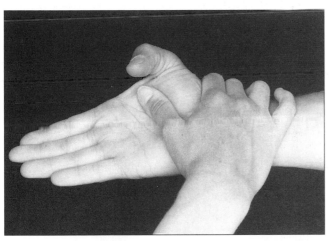

Figure 5-152.   Start position: adductor pollicis.

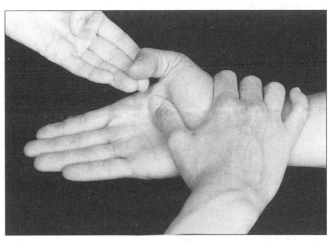

Figure 5-154.   Resistance: adductor pollicis.

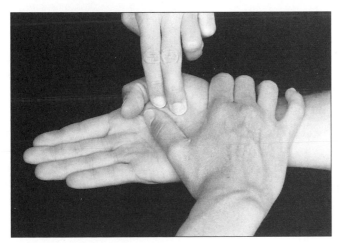

Figure 5-153.   Screen position: adductor pollicis.

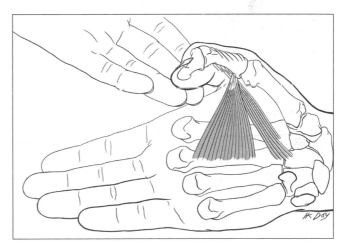

Figure 5-155.   Adductor pollicis.

OPPOSITION OF THE THUMB AND FIFTH FINGER (OPPONENS POLLICIS AND OPPONENS DIGITI MINIMI)

Accessory muscles: abductor pollicis brevis, adductor pollicis brevis, and flexor pollicis brevis.

• **Start Position.** The patient is sitting or supine. The forearm is supinated and the wrist is in a neutral position (Fig. 5-156). The fingers are extended and the MCP and IP joints of the thumb are extended. The thumb is in palmar abduction because the opponens pollicis cannot oppose effectively until the thumb is abducted.[21]

• **Stabilization.** The therapist stabilizes the distal forearm. The thumb may be supported in abduction if the abductor pollicis brevis is weak.

• **Movement.** The patient flexes and medially rotates the thumb metacarpal toward the little finger and the little finger flexes and rotates toward the thumb so that the pads of the finger and thumb touch (Fig. 5-157). The distal phalanges remain in extension throughout movement.

• **Palpation.** Opponens pollicis: lateral to abductor pollicis brevis on the radial aspect of the shaft of the thumb metacarpal. Opponens digiti minimi: on the volar surface of the shaft of the fifth metacarpal (see Fig. 5-157).

• **Substitution/Trick Movement.** Toward the end of range, the patient may flex the distal joints of the thumb and finger to give the appearance of full opposition. This substitution is absent if, in full opposition, the thumbnail is observed to lie in a plane parallel to the plane of the palm.

• **Resistance Location.** Both movements are resisted simultaneously and resistance is applied on the volar surfaces of the thumb metacarpal and fifth metacarpal (Figs. 5-158 and 5-159).

• **Resistance Direction.** Extension, adduction, and lateral rotation.

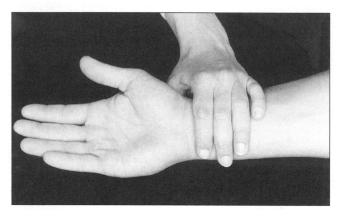

Figure 5-156. Start position: opponens pollicis and opponens digiti minimi.

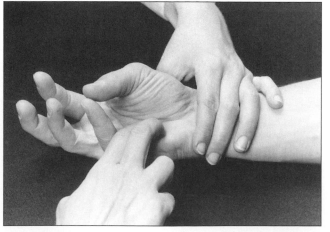

Figure 5-157. Screen position: opponens pollicis and opponens digiti minimi.

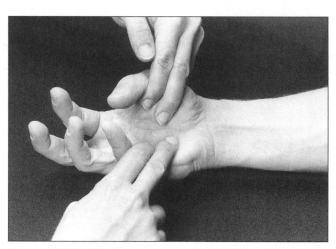

Figure 5-158. Resistance: opponens pollicis and opponens digiti minimi.

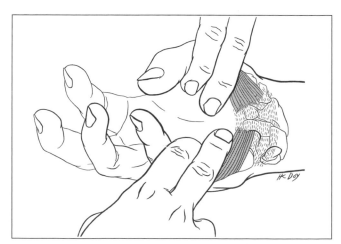

Figure 5-159. Opponens pollicis and opponens digiti minimi.

JOINT FUNCTION: WRIST

The wrist optimizes the function of the hand to touch, grasp, or manipulate objects. Wrist motion positions the hand in space relative to the forearm.[25] As a consequence of wrist motion and static positioning, the wrist serves to control the length-tension relations of the extrinsic muscles of the hand.

FUNCTIONAL RANGE OF MOTION: WRIST

Wrist extension and ulnar deviation are the most important positions or movements[26] for activities of daily living (ADL). Two approaches have been used to determine the wrist ROM required to perform ADL successfully.

In one approach, the wrist ROM was assessed as normal subjects performed ADL. Brumfield and Champoux[27] evaluated 15 ADL and found the normal functional range of wrist motion for most activities was between 10° flexion and 35° extension. Palmer and coworkers,[28] evaluating 52 standardized tasks, found comparable required ranges of 5° flexion and 30° extension. Normal functional range for radial deviation was 10° and 15° for ulnar deviation.[28]

Higher values (54° flexion, 60° extension, 40° ulnar deviation, and 17° radial deviation) for the maximum wrist motion required for ADL were reported by Ryu and colleagues[26] in evaluating 31 activities. The authors suggested differing methods of data analysis and the design and application of the goniometer as possible reasons for these values being higher compared to other studies.

More specific ROM requirements, for feeding activities, (ie, drinking from a cup or glass, eating using a fork or spoon, and cutting using a knife) are approximately from 3° wrist flexion to 35° wrist extension[27,29] and from 20° ulnar deviation to 5° radial deviation.[29]

Using the second approach, wrist ROM was artificially restricted and the ability to complete ADL was assessed. Nelson[30] evaluated the ability to perform 125 ADL (activities of work or recreation were not included) with the wrist splinted to allow for only 5° flexion, 6° extension, 7° radial deviation, and 6° ulnar deviation. With the wrist splinted in this manner, 123 ADL could be completed. Therefore, marked loss of wrist ROM may not significantly hinder a patient's ability to carry out ADL.

JOINT FUNCTION: HAND

The hand has multiple functions associated with ADL. The primary functions are to grasp, manipulate objects, and receive sensory information from the environment. The grasping function is isolated for presentation in this section.

FUNCTIONAL RANGE OF MOTION: HAND

Hume and coworkers[31] reported the IP and MCP joint ROM needed to perform many ADL. No significant differences in the functional positions of the individual fingers were found; therefore, the finger positions were reported as one. The PIP and DIP joint ROM of the fingers were 36° to 86° flexion and 20° to 61° flexion, respectively. The ROM at the MCP joints of the fingers and thumb were 33° to 73° flexion and 10° to 32° flexion, respectively. The ROM of the IP joint of the thumb was 2° to 43° flexion.

TABLE
5-6 ▼ ARCHES OF THE HAND

Arch	Location	Keystone	Mobility
Carpal arch	Distal row of carpal bones Proximal row of carpal bones	Capitate –	Fixed Mobile
Metacarpal arch	Level of metacarpal heads	Third metacarpal head	Mobile
Longitudinal arches	Carpals and each of the five rays*	MCP joints	Mobile; fixed (index and middle metacarpal)

*Ray: the metacarpal and phalanges of one finger.
Adapted from Tubiana R, Thomine JM, Macklin E. *Examination of the Hand and Wrist,* 2nd ed. St. Louis: Mosby; 1996

ARCHES OF THE HAND

The arches of the hand are described in Table 5-6. The arches are observed with the forearm supinated and the hand resting on a table (Fig. 5-160).

The carpal arch, a relatively fixed segment, is covered by the flexor retinaculum. This arrangement functions to maintain the long finger flexors close to the wrist joint, thus reducing the ability of these muscles to produce wrist flexion and enhancing the synergistic action of the wrist flexors and extensors in power grip.[18]

In the relaxed position of the hand, a gently cupped concavity is normally observed. When the hand is opened fully, the palm flattens. When gripping or manipulating objects, the palmar concavity becomes deeper and more gutter shaped. The flattening of the palm and guttering results from the mobility available at the rays of the ring and little fingers and thumb. These rays flex, rotate, and move toward the center of the palm so that the pads of the fingers and thumb are positioned to meet. This motion occurs at the CM joints. The mobile peripheral rays move around the fixed metacarpals of the index and middle fingers.

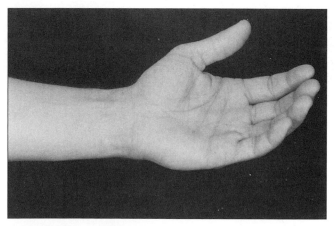

Figure 5-160. Palmar arches. Observe the transverse palmar concavities at the levels of the distal row of carpal bones and the metacarpal bones and the longitudinal concavities along the rays of each finger.

THE GRASPING FUNCTION OF THE WRIST AND HAND

The two terms that relate to the grasping function of the hand are prehension and grip. Tubiana and colleagues[18] point out that there is a fundamental difference in the meaning of the two terms. They define prehension as ". . . all the functions that are put into play when an object is grasped by the hands–intent, permanent sensory control, and a mechanism of grip."[18(p161)] Grip is defined as "the manual mechanical component of prehension."[18(p161)]

Napier[32] categorizes grip into two main gripping postures: precision grip and power grip. He emphasizes that these two postures provide the anatomical basis for all skilled or unskilled activities of the hand and that power and precision are the dominant characteristics in all prehensile activities. Power grips are used when power or force is required in a grasping activity. The object is held in a clamp, formed by the flexed fingers and the palm, with optional counterpressure on the object being applied by the thumb (Fig. 5-161).

When precision is required in an activity, the hand assumes a precision grip posture (Fig. 5-162). The object is pinched between the volar aspects of the fingers and the opposed thumb. Precision grip[32] involves stabilization of an object between the finger(s) and thumb. The function of precision grip is to secure the object so that the more proximal limb segments can move the object. An object may also be manipulated in the hand. Landsmeer[33] refers to this manipulation function as "precision handling."[33(p165)] The first phase is positioning the fingers and thumb to hold the object and the second phase is the actual manipulation or handling of the object.

The following description of wrist and hand function is limited to an analysis of power grip, precision grip, and precision handling. Emphasis is placed on the phases of the gripping process, movement patterns, static positioning, and muscle activity of the respective grip.

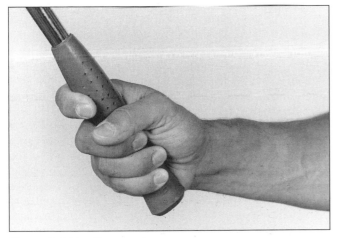

Figure 5-161.   Power grip.

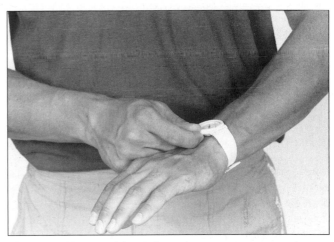

Figure 5-162.   Precision grip.

POWER GRIP

There are four phases of power grip: opening the hand, positioning the fingers, approaching the fingers or fingers and thumb to the object, and the actual grip.[33] Each phase is a prerequisite of effective grip.

Opening Phase (Fig. 5-163). Opening is an intuitive action and the amount is predetermined by an intent to grasp a specific object.[34] The hand assumes a posture that will accommodate the physical structure of the object. Full opening is not required for grasping tasks in daily self-care activities but may be required for grasp in leisure or occupational tasks.

The position of the wrist influences the fingers and thumb. Wrist flexion permits full extension of the fingers[18,35] to open the hand for grasp of large objects. In this position the tip of the thumb is level with the PIP joints of the fingers.[36] As the distance between the open hand's fingers and thumb encompasses excess space in relation to the object, the MCP joints of the fingers are often fully extended, whereas the IP joints are always flexed to a certain degree so that the gripping surfaces of the fingers face the object.[34]

The opening phase is a dynamic phase,[33] characterized by concentric muscle contraction. Active opening is achieved through the synergistic muscle action of the wrist flexors and the finger extensors.[8,12,35,36] The long extensors of the fingers extend the MCP joints and have a secondary wrist extensor action. To prevent the extensor action from occurring at the wrist, the wrist flexors function as counteracting synergists, keeping the wrist in a neutral position or flexion.[35] The integrity of extensor digitorum is essential for creating active finger opening.[34] The larger the object to be grasped, the more the fingers abduct and the thumb radially abducts and/or extends.

Finger and Thumb (Optional) Positioning Phase (see Fig. 5-163). The choice of finger position occurs in conjunction with the opening phase and adjustment to the desired position occurs at the MCP and IP joints.[33] The integrity of the activity of extensor digitorum in extending the MCP joints and lumbricales in creating a grip position is essential in this phase of grip.[34] When ulnar deviation of one or more MCP joints is a component of the intended grip, the interossei replace the lumbricales.[34]

Approach Phase (Fig. 5-164). The movement pattern identified for this phase is wrist extension, finger and thumb flexion, and adduction. As in the opening phase, the position of the wrist influences the fingers and thumb. Wrist extension permits full flexion of the fingers[18,35] as one grasps an object. As the object is approached the fingers usually flex simultaneously and close around the object[35] so the palm of the hand contacts the object. Flexor digitorum profundus is the critical muscle used in free closing of the hand.[37] The wrist extensors function to stabilize the wrist and prevent wrist flexion by profundus and superficialis.[35] The thenar muscles, when the thumb is involved, are active as the thumb approaches the object

for its final position of adduction and/or opposition. Both the position and muscle activity are influenced by the shape of the object to be grasped.

Static Grip Phase (Fig. 5-165). This phase is a power or stabilization phase and is characterized by isometric muscle contraction. The function of the hand complex is to stabilize an object so that it can be moved by the proximal limb segments[33] and contributes to the aggregate power of the arm.

The power grip has three significant characteristics: (1) the wrist is held in neutral or extension, (2) the fingers are maintained in flexion and abduction or adduction, and (3) the volar surfaces of the fingers and portions of the palm make forceful contact with the object. The thumb may or may not be included in the grip.[12] For example, in grasping a briefcase (Fig. 5-166) the thumb does not contribute to the grip and this grip is referred to as a hook grasp. In grasping a cylindrical object, such as a hammer or a cup (Fig. 5-167), the thumb does contribute to the grip. When included for force, the thumb may be flexed and adducted. When included for an element of precision, it is usually abducted and flexed.

The shape, size, and/or weight of the object influences the degree of finger flexion, the area of palmar contact, and thumb position. When grasping different sized cylinders, the DIP joint angle remains constant and the fingers adjust to the new cylinder size through changes in the joint angles at the MCP and PIP joints.[38] It should also be noted that as the diameter of a cylindrical object increases the total grip strength has been shown to decrease.[39]

The ability of the two ulnar fingers to flex and rotate at the CM joints and flex beyond 90° at the MCP joints contributes to digitopalmar contact on the ulnar side of the hand. Research by Bendz[40] shows the hypothenar muscles, notably the flexor digiti minimi and the abductor digiti minimi, contract to flex the fifth metacarpal and proximal phalanx of the fifth digit. The abductor digiti minimi also rotates the fifth metacarpal. These muscles contract to provide strength to the grip, but for full strength the flexor carpi ulnaris is subsequently recruited to augment the contractions of the flexor and abductor digiti minimi via the common attachment of these muscles to the pisiform bone.[40] However, the ring and little finger can generate only 70% of the force of the index and middle fingers, so that power requirements fall to the radial fingers.[41] As increased force is required in the grasp, the wrist ulnarly deviates. The greatest force generated at the phalanges is obtained when the wrist is in ulnar deviation.[41] Within the general classification of Napier's[32] descriptors of power grip, various subgroups of postures can be identified. Kamakura and associates[42] identify five patterns of power grip. These patterns have the three general characteristics previously specified. Specific patterns may be differentiated according to the involvement of the thumb, degree of range of movement, finger position, and/or the amount of digitopalmar contact area. Sollerman and Sperling[43] developed a code system that classifies hand grips according to the participation of the various parts of the hand, the positioning of the fingers and the joints, the contact surfaces, and the relationship between the longitudinal axis of the object and the hand. The postural details described in both studies illustrate the immense variety of ways that one can grasp an object and the concomitant muscle activity that may exist in these postures.

Long and associates[37] present electromyographic data of intrinsic-extrinsic muscle activity involved in five classifications of power grip: simple squeeze, hammer squeeze, screwdriver squeeze, disc grip, and spherical grip. The following summary of their findings provides insight into the muscle activity patterns involved in the static grip phase of hand posture.

The extrinsic finger flexors provide the major gripping force. Flexor digitorum profundus and superficialis both contribute to power grip with superficialis increasing its participation as force requirements increase. The major intrinsic participation is provided through the interossei. They abduct or adduct the proximal phalanx to align the fingers with the object so that the extrinsic flexors can provide the gripping power. The interossei also provide gripping power as they flex the metacarpophalangeal joints.

When the thumb is adducted and flexed in power grip, the muscle power is provided through the isometric contraction of adductor pollicis[12,36,37,44] and flexor pollicis longus.[12,36] Flexor pollicis brevis contributes to the stability required in a firm grasp.[36,44]

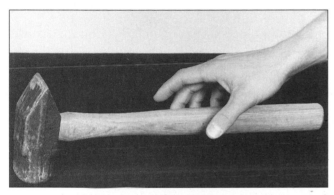

Figure 5-163.   Power grip: opening phase and finger/optional thumb positioning phase.

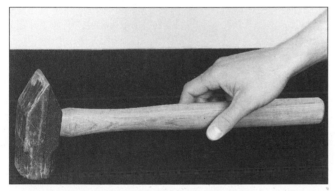

Figure 5-164.   Power grip: approach phase.

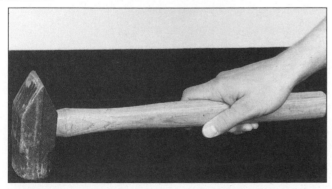

Figure 5-165.   Power grip: static grip phase.

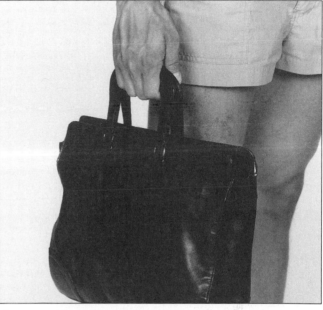

Figure 5-166.   Power grip without the involvement of the thumb.

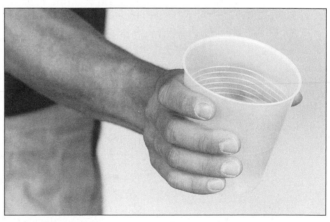

Figure 5-167.   Power grip with the thumb contributing to the grip.

PRECISION GRIP AND PRECISION HANDLING

Three common phases can be identified for precision grip and handling: opening the hand, positioning the fingers and thumb, and approaching the fingers and thumb to the object. The last phase in precision grip is static grip. The last phase in precision handling is manipulation of the object.

Opening Phase (Fig. 5-168). The amount of opening and number of fingers involved varies with the shape and purpose of the object. The wrist position also varies with the purpose of the object or task to be performed and location of the object. The elected opening posture is that which positions the wrist, fingers, and thumb for the subsequent function of stabilization or manipulation. Because of the infinite number of ways that an object can be stabilized or manipulated, the range of movement and muscle activity is more variable than power grip. The same pattern of movement is evident but as more precision is demanded, finer motor control is required.

Finger and Thumb Positioning Phase (see Fig. 5-168). As indicated in power grip, adjustment of the fingers and thumb to the object occurs concurrently with the opening phase with many positions possible through the positioning of the MCP and IP joints. However, in precision grip or handling the thumb is always involved and is positioned to achieve opposition to bring it into pad-to-pad contact with the finger or fingers.

Approach Phase (Fig. 5-169). The movement pattern and muscular requirements of the wrist are similar to power grip. The wrist can either move into extension while the MCP joints flex or remain in flexion with the MCP joints flexing. The MCP joints of the index, middle, and ring fingers usually flex in precision grip and precision handling. The MCP joint of the little finger may be flexed or extended. The position is influenced by its function. When the little finger is involved in com-

pression on the object or against the other fingers, it will be flexed. When an object is being pinched or manipulated with the other three fingers, the little finger may be extended to provide tactile input to the hand or to contribute to stabilization of the hand on a working surface. There is no deviation at the wrist.[32] In addition to finger MCP flexion, there is abduction or adduction of one or more fingers. The proximal PIP joint(s) of the finger(s) flex or extend.[45] Although IP flexion is required for subsequent manipulation, flexion or extension may be required in precision grip. The DIP joints may be flexed or extended. As in power grip, the integrity of the flexor digitorum profundus is critical to approaching an object in a flexion pattern. Lumbrical activity is a prerequisite to the initiation of an extension approach.[46]

The approach of the thumb incorporates the movement of opposition as the function of the thumb is to oppose the fingers. Opposition is a sequential movement incorporating abduction, flexion, and adduction of the first metacarpal, with simultaneous rotation.[12] Thenar muscle control occurs through opponens pollicis, flexor pollicis brevis, abductor pollicis brevis, and adductor pollicis.

Precision Grip (Fig. 5-170). When the fingers and thumb contact the object, the hand grips the object. Precision grip[32] involves stabilization of an object between the finger(s) and thumb. The function of precision grip is to secure an object so that the more proximal limb segments can move the object.

There are five hand postures that illustrate the characteristics of precision grip and are used frequently in ADL: pulp pinch (Fig. 5-171), lateral pinch (Fig. 5-172), tripod pinch (Fig. 5-173), five-pulp pinch (Fig. 5-174), and tip pinch (Fig. 5-175). They share the common characteristic of pinch between the thumb and one or more fingers. Sollerman and Sperling[47] report that of the hand postures used in ADL, the first four pinch postures are used 65% of the time. The specific posture assumed when pinching an object is influenced by the purpose of the object.[32,48] Pulp pinch and lateral pinch are isolated for analysis of posture and muscular activity.

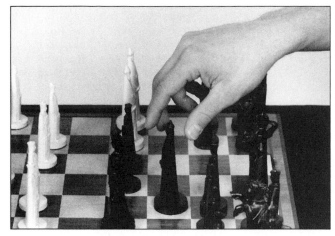

Figure 5-168. Precision grip or handling: opening phase and finger and thumb positioning phase.

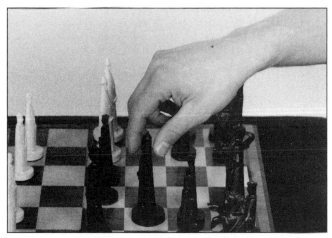

Figure 5-169. Precision grip or handling: approach phase.

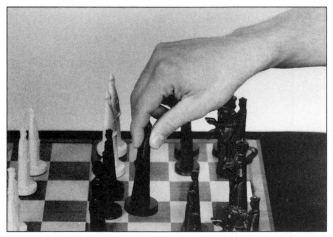

Figure 5-170. Precision grip: static grip phase.

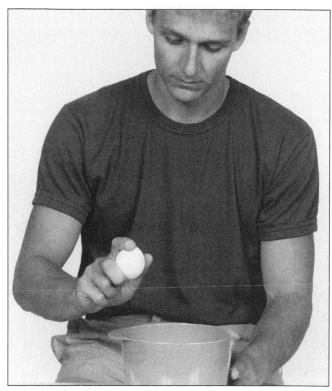

Figure 5-171. Pulp pinch.

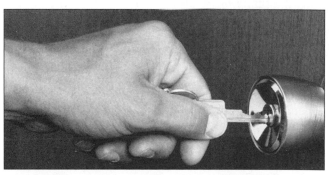

Figure 5-172. Lateral pinch.

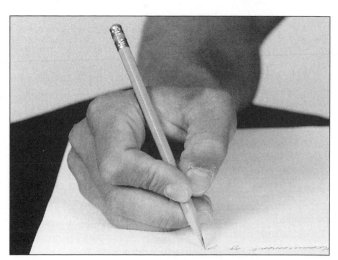

Figure 5-173. Tripod pinch.

• Pulp Pinch (see Figs. 5-171, 5-173, and 5-174). The object is pinched between the pulp of the thumb and the pulp of one or more fingers. The thumb and finger(s) are opposed to each other. The most commonly used fingers are the index finger and/or middle finger. The index finger is of significant value in activities. It is strong, can abduct, has relative independence of its musculature, and has proximity to the thumb.[18] The middle finger adds an element of strength to precision grip (tripod pinch). The ring and little fingers contribute to five-pulp pinch.

The thumb assumes a position of CM flexion, abduction, and rotation. The MCP joints and IP joints can be flexed or fully extended. The compression force for stabilization of the object is achieved through the muscular contraction of opponens pollicis, adductor pollicis, and flexor pollicis brevis.[37] The adductor pollicis increases its contribution as increased pressure is required. The flexor pollicis longus contributes to distal phalanx compression when the distal phalanx is flexed.[12,44]

The radial three fingers are normally flexed at the MCP joint. The little finger may be flexed or extended. The DIP joints of the fingers may be flexed or extended. When flexed, the flexor digitorum profundus plays a key role in the compression. When the distal joint is extended, flexor digitorum superficialis is the muscle recruited for maintenance of position. These extrinsic muscles contribute to the power in pinch with assistance being provided by the first palmar and dorsal interosseous and first lumbricalis.[37] It has been suggested by Maier and colleagues[49] that the intrinsic muscles may even play a primary role in production of low isometric forces in precision grip.

• Lateral Pinch (see Fig. 5-172). The difference between this form of pinch and pulp pinch is that the thumb pulp stabilizes an object against the side of the index finger with counterpressure being provided by the index finger. The thumb is more adducted and not as rotated. The muscle activity is the same as pulp pinch except that the palmar interosseous and lumbricalis reduce their activity and the first dorsal interosseous is very active in providing index finger abduction force to stabilize the object.[37] The index finger is flexed at the MCP joint and may be flexed or extended at the PIP and DIP joints.[45] Although flexion of the proximal phalanx is the most commonly used posture, extension may be the desired posture in precision grip of objects with flat surfaces such as a plate, book, or magazine. The lumbricales and dorsal interosseous muscles are active in the extension posture.[45]

Precision Handling (see Fig. 5-175). This term refers to manipulation of an object using the fingers and thumb.[33] The dominant characteristic in precision handling is manipulation through concentric muscle contraction. The static phase is very brief and pressure applied to the object is light. In most daily activities the wrist usually assumes a position of extension for the purposes of stabilization of the hand and flexion of the distal joints. However in the performance of perineal

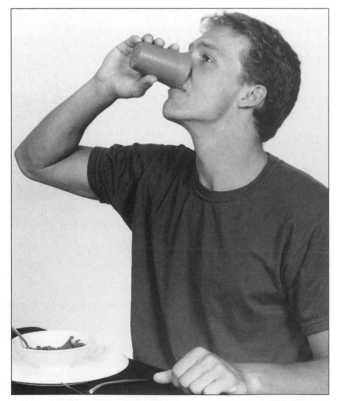

Figure 5-174. Five-pulp pinch.

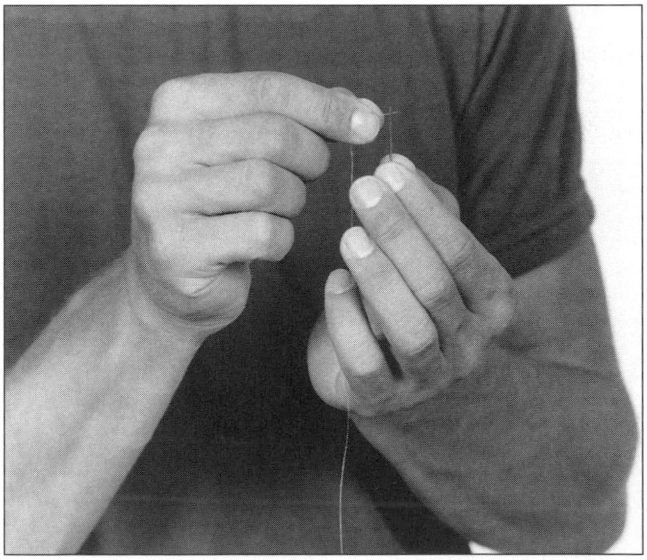

Figure 5-175. Tip pinch of a needle with precision handling of the thread.

hygiene activities and dressing activities at the back, the wrist assumes a flexed posture. The finger and thumb position is partly determined by the size and shape of the object but the major determinant is that the object requires a change in position.[37]

Long and associates[37] describe two types of manipulation that characterize precision handling with involvement of the thumb and radial two fingers: translation and rotation. In translation the object is pushed away from or returned to the palm by the fingertips. There is a handling phase and return phase for each motion sequence. Translation toward the palm involves the motion sequences of flexion at the MCP and IP joints (handling phase) and extension of the IP joints (return phase). Translation toward the palm is under the control of the extrinsic flexors and interossei in the handling phase and lumbricales in the return phase. Translation away from the palm involves the motion sequences of flexion at the MCP joints with extension of the IP joints (handling phase) and flexion at the MCP and IP joints (return phase). The interossei and lumbrical muscles are dominant in translation away from the palm.

In rotation, the object is rotated in a clockwise or counter-clockwise direction. The rotation of the object is accomplished through the interossei muscles as they abduct and adduct. The lumbrical muscles function to extend the IP joints and are active in both rotations.

During precision handling the thenar triad of flexor pollicis brevis, opponens pollicis, and abductor pollicis brevis are active. Adductor pollicis only becomes active when force is required against the index finger.

Precision handling usually involves the radial two fingers and thumb. However, the remaining two fingers may be involved in manipulation or stabilization. The hypothenar muscles are active when the little finger is flexed and abducted through the activity of abductor digit minimi, opponens digiti minimi, and flexor digiti minimi.[44]

REFERENCES

1. Kellor M, Frost J, Silberberg N, Iverson I, Cummings R. Hand strength and dexterity. *Am J Occup Ther.* 1971; 25:77–83.
2. Weiss MW, Flatt AE. A pilot study of 198 normal children: pinch strength and hand size in the growing hand. *Am J Occup Ther.* 1971;25:10–12.
3. Mathiowetz V, Wiemer DM, Federman SM. Grip and pinch strengths: norms for 6- to 19-year olds. *Am J Occup Ther.* 1986;40:705–711.
4. Bohannon RW. Handgrip dynamometers: issues relevant to application. *J Hum Muscle Perform.* 1991;1:16–36.
5. Mathiowetz V. Reliability and validity of grip and pinch strength measurements. *Critical Reviews in Physical and Rehabilitation Medicine.* 1991;2:201–212.
6. Balogun JA, Adenlola SA, Akinloye AA. Grip strength normative data for the Harpenden dynamometer. *J Orthop Sports Phys Ther.* 1991;14:155–160.
7. Dunn W. Grip strength in children aged 3 to 7 years using a modified sphygmomanometer: comparison of typical children and children with rheumatic disorders. *Am J Occup Ther.* 1993;47:421–428.
8. Kapandji IA. *The Physiology of the Joints.* Vol 1. 5th ed. New York: Churchill Livingstone; 1982.
9. Soames RW, ed. Skeletal system. Salmons S, ed. Muscle. *Gray's Anatomy.* 38th ed. New York: Churchill Livingstone; 1995.
10. Norkin CC, White DJ. *Measurement of Joint Motion: A Guide to Goniometry.* 2nd ed. Philadelphia: FA Davis; 1995.
11. Daniels L, Worthingham C. *Muscle Testing: Techniques of Manual Examination.* 5th ed. Philadelphia: WB Saunders; 1986.
12. Norkin CC, Levangie PK. *Joint Structure & Function: A Comprehensive Analysis.* 2nd ed. Philadelphia: FA Davis; 1992.
13. Cyriax J. *Textbook of Orthopaedic Medicine, vol 1. Diagnosis of Soft Tissue Lesions.* 8th ed. London: Bailliere Tindall; 1982.
14. Magee DJ. *Orthopedic Physical Assessment.* 3rd ed. Philadelphia: WB Saunders; 1997.
15. American Academy of Orthopaedic Surgeons. *Joint Motion: Method of Measuring and Recording.* Chicago: Author; 1965.
16. Scott AD, Trombly CA. Evaluation. In: Trombly CA. *Occupational Therapy for Physical Dysfunction.* 2nd ed. Baltimore: Williams & Wilkins; 1983.
17. Swanson AB, Goran-Hagert C, DeGroot Swanson G. Evaluation of impairment of hand function. In: Hunter JM, Schneider LH, Mackin EJ, Bell JA. *Rehabilitation of the Hand.* St. Louis: CV Mosby; 1978.
18. Tubiana R, Thomine JM, Macklin E. *Examination of the Hand and Wrist.* 2nd ed. St. Louis: Mosby; 1996.
19. Kendall FP, McCreary EK, Provance PG. *Muscles Testing and Function.* 4th ed. Baltimore: Williams & Wilkins; 1993.
20. Woodburne RT. *Essentials of Human Anatomy.* 5th ed. London: Oxford University Press; 1973.
21. Wynn Parry CB. *Rehabilitation of the Hand.* 4th ed. London: Butterworths; 1981.
22. Baker DS, Gaul JS, Williams VK, Graves M. The little finger superficialis—clinical investigation of its anatomic and functional shortcomings. *J Hand Surg.* 1981;6: 374–378.
23. Aulincino PL. Clinical examination of the hand. In: Hunter JM, Macklin EJ, Callahan AD. *Rehabilitation of the Hand: Surgery and Therapy.* 4th ed. St. Louis: Mosby; 1995.
24. Pedretti LW. Evaluation of muscle strength. In: Pedretti LW. *Occupational Therapy Practice Skills for Physical Dysfunction.* 2nd ed. St. Louis: CV Mosby; 1985.
25. Nordin M, Frankel VH. *Basic Biomechanics of the Musculoskeletal System.* 2nd ed. Philadelphia: Lea & Febiger; 1989.
26. Ryu J, Cooney WP, Askew LJ, An K-N, Chao EYS. Functional ranges of motion of the wrist joint. *J Hand Surg.* 1991;16A:409–419.
27. Brumfield RH, Champoux JA. A biomechanical study of normal functional wrist motion. *Clin Orthop.* 1984; 187:23–25.
28. Palmer AK, Werner FW, Murphy DM, Glisson R. Functional wrist motion: a biomechanical study. *J Hand Surg.* 1985;10A:39–46.
29. Safaee-Rad R, Shwedyk E, Quanbury AO, Cooper JE. Normal functional range of motion of upper limb joints during performance of three feeding activities. *Arch Phys Med Rehabil.* 1990;71:505–509.
30. Nelson DL. Functional wrist motion. *Hand Clin.* 1997; 13:83–92.

31. Hume MC, Gellman H, McKellop H, Brumfield RH. Functional range of motion of the joints of the hand. *J Hand Surg.* 1990;15A:240–243.
32. Napier JR. The prehensile movements of the human hand. *J Bone Joint Surg.* 1956;38B:902–913.
33. Landsmeer JMF. Power grip and precision handling. *Ann Rheum Dis.* 1962;21:164–169.
34. Benz P. The motor balance of the fingers of the open hand. *Scand J Rehabil Med.* 1980;12:115–121.
35. Smith LK, Weiss EL, Lehmkuhl LD. *Brunnstrom's Clinical Kinesiology.* 5th ed. Philadelphia: FA Davis; 1996.
36. Tubiana R. Architecture and functions of the hand. In: Tubiana R, Thomine JM, Mackin E. *Examination of the Hand & Upper Limb.* Philadelphia: WB Saunders; 1984.
37. Long C, Conrad PW, Hall EA, Furler SL. Intrinsic-extrinsic muscle control of the hand in power grip and precision handling. *J Bone Joint Surg.* 1970;52A:853–867.
38. Lee JW, Rim K. Measurement of finger joint angles and maximum finger forces during cylinder grip activity. *J Biomed Eng.* 1991;13:152–162.
39. Radhakrishnan S, Nagaravindra M. Analysis of hand forces in health and disease during maximum isometric grasping of cylinders. *Med Biol Eng Comput.* 1993; 31:372–376.
40. Bendz P. The functional significance of the fifth metacarpus and hypothenar in two useful grips of the hand. *Am J Phys Med Rehabil.* 1993;72:210–213.
41. Hazelton FT, Smidt GL, Flatt AE, Stephens RI. The influence of wrist position on the force produced by the finger flexors. *J Biomech.* 1975;8:301–306.
42. Kamakura N, Matsuo M, Ishii H, Mitsuboshi F, Miura Y. Patterns of static prehension in normal hands. *Am J Occup Ther.* 1980;34:437–445.
43. Sollerman C, Sperling L. Evaluation of ADL function–especially hand function. *Scand J Rehabil Med.* 1978; 10:139–143.
44. Basmajian JV, DeLuca CJ. *Muscles Alive: Their Function Revealed by Electromyography.* 5th ed. Baltimore: Williams & Wilkins; 1985.
45. Benz P. Systemization of the grip of the hand in relation to finger motor systems. *Scand J Rehabil Med.* 1974; 6: 158–165.
46. Benz P. Motor balance in formation and release of the extension grip. *Scand J Rehabil Med.* 1980;12:155–160.
47. Sollerman C, Sperling L. Classification of the hand grip: a preliminary study. *Am J Occup Med.* 1976;18:395–398.
48. Sperling L, Jacobson-Sollerman C. The grip pattern of the healthy hand during eating. *Scand J Rehabil Med.* 1977;9:115–121.
49. Maier MA, Hepp-Reymond M-C. EMG activation patterns during force production in precision grip. *Exp Brain Res.* 1995;103:108–122.

CHAPTER 6

HIP

▼ SURFACE ANATOMY (Figs. 6-1, 6-2, and 6-3)

Structure	Location
1. Iliac crest	A convex bony ridge on the upper border of the ilium; the top of the iliac crest is level with the space between the spines of L4 and L5.
2. Anterior superior iliac spine (ASIS)	Round bony prominence at the anterior end of the iliac crest.
3. Tubercle of the ilium	Approximately 5 cm above and lateral to the ASIS along the lateral lip of the iliac crest.
4. Posterior superior iliac spine (PSIS)	Round bony prominence at the posterior end of the iliac crest, felt subcutaneously at the bottom of the dimples on the proximal aspect of the buttocks; the spines are at the level of the spine of S2.
5. Ischial tuberosity	With the hip passively flexed, this large bony prominence is lateral to the midline of the body and just proximal to the gluteal fold (the deep transverse groove between the buttock and the posterior aspect of the thigh).
6. Greater trochanter	With the tip of the thumb on the lateral aspect of the iliac crest, the tip of the third digit placed distally on the lateral aspect of the thigh locates the upper border of the greater trochanter.
7. Adductor tubercle	Medial projection at the distal end of the femur at the proximal portion of the medial epicondyle.
8. Lateral epicondyle of the femur	Small bony prominence on the lateral condyle of the femur.
9. Patella	Large triangular sesamoid bone on the anterior aspect of the knee. The base is proximal and the apex distal.

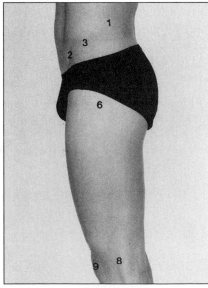

Figure 6-1. Lateral aspect of the trunk and thigh.

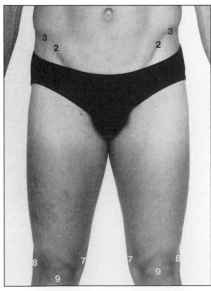

Figure 6-2. Anterior aspect of the trunk and thigh.

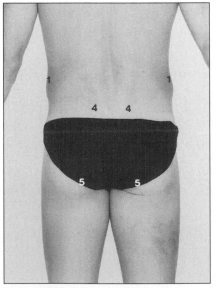

Figure 6-3. Posterior aspect of the trunk and thigh.

▼ ASSESSMENT PROCESS: THE HIP

1. The therapist observes:
   a. Function
   b. Posture, body symmetry, atrophy, and skin condition
   c. Active range of motion (AROM) at the trunk, hip, knee, and ankle joints
2. The therapist assesses passive range of motion (PROM) by:
   a. Estimating joint PROM
   b. Determining the end feels at the joint
   c. Establishing the presence or absence of pain
   d. Determining the presence of a capsular or noncapsular pattern
3. The therapist measures PROM through goniometry.
4. The therapist assesses muscle strength through manual muscle testing.

	Flexion	Extension	Abduction	Adduction	Internal Rotation	External Rotation
Articulation[1,2]	Hip	Hip	Hip	Hip	Hip	Hip
Plane	Sagittal	Sagittal	Frontal	Frontal	Horizontal	Horizontal
Axis	Frontal	Frontal	Sagittal	Sagittal	Longitudinal	Longitudinal
Normal limiting factors[1, 3–6]	Soft tissue apposition of the anterior thigh and the abdomen (knee is flexed); tension in the posterior hip joint capsule and gluteus maximus	Tension in the anterior joint capsule, the iliofemoral, ischiofemoral, and pubofemoral ligaments and iliopsoas	Tension in pubofemoral and ischiofemoral ligaments, the inferior band of the iliofemoral ligament, the inferior joint capsule, and hip adductor muscles	Soft tissue apposition of the thighs. With the contralateral leg in abduction or flexion: tension in the iliotibial band, the superior joint capsule, superior band of the iliofemoral ligament, the ischiofemoral ligament, and hip abductor muscles	Tension in the ischiofemoral ligament, the posterior joint capsule, and the external rotator muscles	Tension in the iliofemoral and pubofemoral ligaments, the anterior joint capsule, and the medial rotator muscles
Normal end feel[3,7,8]	Soft/firm	Firm	Firm	Soft/firm	Firm	Firm
Normal AROM[9]	0–120°	0–30°	0–45°	0–30°	0–45°	0–45°

Capsular pattern:[7,8] The order of restriction may vary: flexion, abduction, and internal rotation

▼ RANGE OF MOTION ASSESSMENT AND MEASUREMENT

The articulations and joint axes of the hip are illustrated in Figures 6-4, 6-5, and 6-6. The structure of the hip joint is described in Table 6-1.

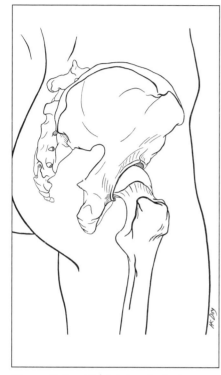

Figure 6-4.   Hip joint articulation.

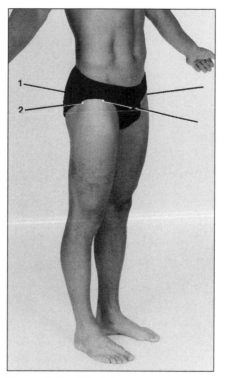

Figure 6-5.   Hip joint axes:
(*1*) abduction–adduction;
(*2*) flexion–extension.

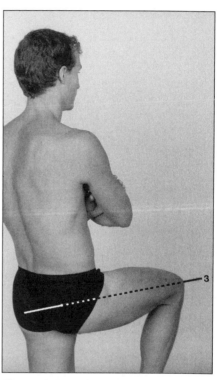

Figure 6-6.   Hip joint axis:
(*3*) internal–external rotation.

GENERAL SCAN: LOWER EXTREMITY ACTIVE RANGE OF MOTION

The AROM of the lower extremity joints is scanned, starting with the patient in the supine position with the legs in the anatomical position. In the supine-lying position, the patient extends the toes, dorsiflexes the ankle, and brings the heel toward the contralateral hip (Fig. 6-7). The therapist observes the AROM of hip flexion, abduction, external rotation, knee flexion, an-kle dorsiflexion, and toe extension. As the patient attempts to touch the contralateral hip, the level reached by the heel may be used as a guide of AROM of the hip and knee joints.

The patient flexes the toes, plantarflexes the ankle, extends the knee, adducts, internally rotates and extends the hip to move the great toe toward the corner on the other side of the plinth as illustrated in Figure 6-8. The therapist observes the AROM of hip adduction, internal rotation, knee extension, ankle plantarflexion, and toe flexion.

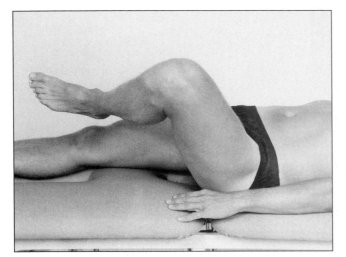

Figure 6-7.   Scan of AROM of the lower extremity.

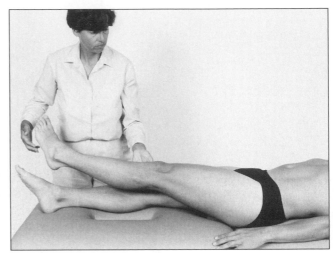

Figure 6-8.   Scan of AROM of the lower extremity.

HIP FLEXION

AROM Assessment

• **Substitution/Trick Movement.** Posterior pelvic tilt and flexion of the lumbar spine.

PROM Assessment

• **Start Position.** The patient is supine. The hip and knee on the test side are in the neutral position. The other hip may be flexed or extended (Fig. 6-9).

• **Stabilization.** The therapist stabilizes the pelvis. The trunk is stabilized through body positioning.

• **Therapist's Distal Hand Placement.** The therapist raises the lower extremity off the plinth and grasps the posterior aspect of the distal femur.

• **End Position.** While maintaining pelvic stabilization, the therapist applies slight traction to move the femur anteriorly to the limit of hip flexion (Fig. 6-10).

• **End Feel.** Hip flexion—soft.

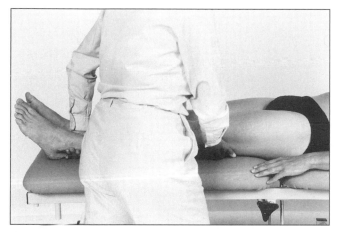

Figure 6-9.   Start position: hip flexion.

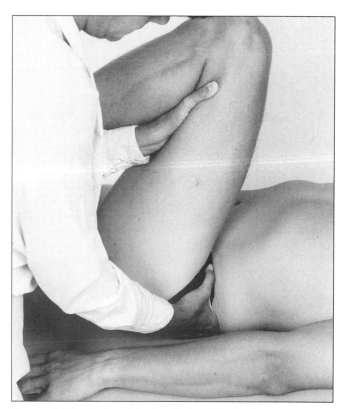

Figure 6-10.   Soft end feel at limit of hip flexion.

Measurement: Universal Goniometer

• **Start Position.** The patient is supine. The hip and knee on the test side are in the neutral position. The contralateral hip may be flexed or extended (Fig. 6-11).

• **Stabilization.** The trunk is stabilized through body positioning, and the therapist stabilizes the pelvis.

• **Goniometer Axis.** The axis is placed over the greater trochanter of the femur.

• **Stationary Arm.** Parallel to the midaxillary line of the trunk.

• **Movable Arm.** Parallel to the longitudinal axis of the femur, pointing toward the lateral epicondyle.

• **End Position.** The hip is flexed to the limit of motion (120°) while flexing the knee (Fig. 6-12).

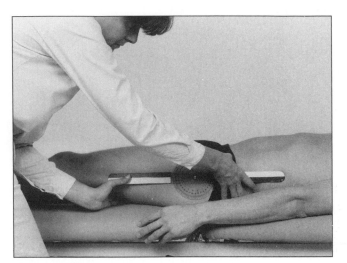

Figure 6-11.   Start position: hip flexion.

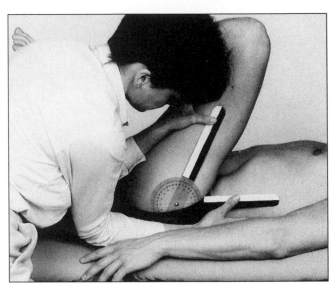

Figure 6-12.   End position: hip flexion.

HIP EXTENSION

AROM Assessment

• **Substitution/Trick Movement.** Anterior pelvic tilt and extension of the lumbar spine.

PROM Assessment

• **Start Position.** The patient is prone. Both hips and knees are in the neutral position. The feet are over the end of the plinth (Fig. 6-13).

• **Stabilization.** The therapist stabilizes the pelvis.

• **Therapist's Distal Hand Placement.** The therapist grasps the anterior aspect of the distal femur.

• **End Position.** The therapist applies slight traction to and moves the femur posteriorly to the limit of hip extension (Fig. 6-14).

• **End Feel.** Hip extension—firm.

Measurement: Universal Goniometer

• **Start Position.** The patient is prone. The hips and knees are in the neutral position. The feet are over the end of the plinth (Fig. 6-15).

• **Stabilization.** The pelvis is stabilized through strapping.

• **Goniometer Axis.** The axis is placed over the greater trochanter of the femur.

• **Stationary Arm.** Parallel to the midaxillary line of the trunk.

• **Movable Arm.** Parallel to the longitudinal axis of the femur, pointing toward the lateral epicondyle.

• **End Position.** The patient's knee is maintained in extension. The hip is extended to the limit of motion (30°) (Fig. 6-16).

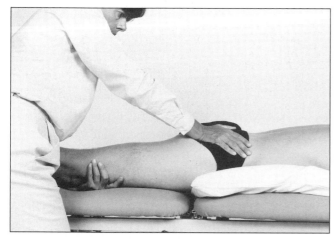

Figure 6-13.   Start position: hip extension.

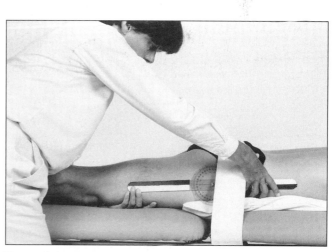

Figure 6-15.   Start position: hip extension.

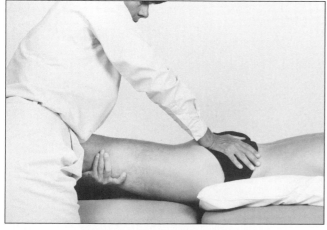

Figure 6-14.   Firm end feel at limit of hip extension.

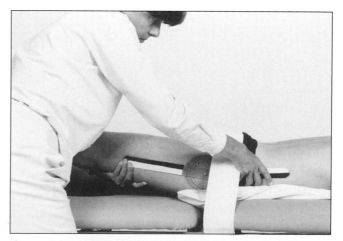

Figure 6-16.   End position: hip extension.

HIP ABDUCTION

AROM Assessment

• **Substitution/Trick Movement.** External rotation and flexion of the hip, hiking of the ipsilateral pelvis.

PROM Assessment

• **Start Position.** The patient is supine; the pelvis is level and the lower extremities are in the anatomical position (Fig. 6-17).

• **Stabilization.** The therapist stabilizes the pelvis. If additional stabilization of the trunk and pelvis is re-quired, the contralateral lower extremity may be positioned in hip abduction with the knee flexed over the edge of the plinth and the foot supported on a stool (see Fig. 6-21).

• **Therapist's Distal Hand Placement.** The therapist grasps the medial aspect of the distal femur.

• **End Position.** The therapist applies slight traction to and moves the femur to the limit of hip abduction motion (Fig. 6-18).

• **End Feel.** Hip abduction—firm.

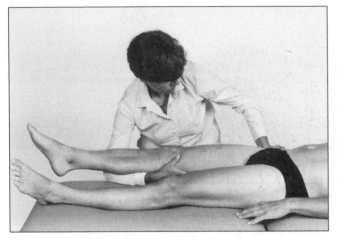

Figure 6-17. Start position for hip abduction.

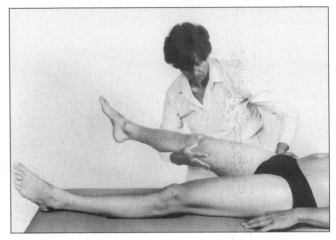

Figure 6-18. Firm end feel at the limit of hip abduction.

Measurement: Universal Goniometer

- **Start Position.** The patient is supine with the lower extremities in the anatomical position (Fig. 6-19A). Ensure the pelvis is level.

- **Goniometer Axis.** The axis is placed over the ASIS on the side being measured (Fig. 6-19B).

- **Stationary Arm.** Along a line between the two ASISs.

- **Movable Arm.** Parallel to the longitudinal axis of the femur. In the start position described, the goniometer will indicate 90°. This is recorded as 0°. For example, if the goniometer reads 90° at the start position for hip abduction and 60° at the end position, hip abduction PROM would be 30°.

- **End Position.** The hip is abducted to the limit of motion (45°) (Fig. 6-20).

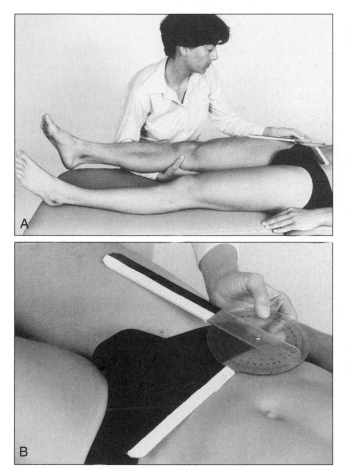

Figure 6-19. (*A*) Start position: hip abduction. (*B*) Goniometer alignment.

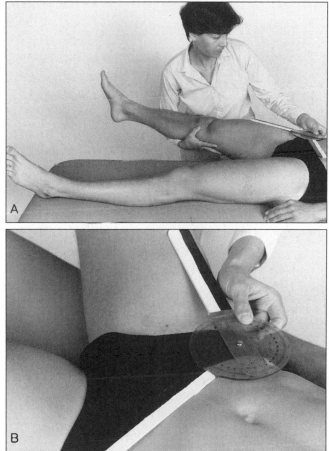

Figure 6-20. (*A*) End position: hip abduction. (*B*) Goniometer alignment.

HIP ADDUCTION

AROM Assessment

• **Substitution/Trick Movement.** Hip internal rotation, hiking of the contralateral pelvis.

PROM Assessment

• **Start Position.** The patient is supine, the pelvis is level and the lower extremity is in the anatomical position. The hip on the nontest side is abducted to allow full ROM in adduction on the test side (Fig. 6-21).

• **Stabilization.** The therapist stabilizes the pelvis.

• **Therapist's Distal Hand Placement.** The therapist grasps the distal femur.

• **End Position.** The therapist applies slight traction and moves the femur to the limit of hip adduction ROM (30°) (Fig. 6-22).

• **End Feel.** Hip adduction—soft or firm.

Measurement: Universal Goniometer

• **Start Position.** The patient is supine with the lower extremity in the anatomical position. The hip on the nontest side is abducted to allow full range of hip adduction on the test side (see Fig. 6-21). The pelvis is level.

• **Goniometer Axis.** The axis is placed over the ASIS on the side being measured. The goniometer is aligned the same as for hip abduction ROM measurement (see Fig. 6-19).

• **Stationary Arm.** Along a line between the two ASISs.

• **Movable Arm.** Parallel to the longitudinal axis of the femur. In the start position described, the goniometer will indicate 90°. This is recorded as 0°. For example, if the goniometer reads 90° at the start position for hip adduction and 105° at the end position, hip adduction PROM would be 15°.

• **End Position.** The hip is adducted to the limit of motion (30°) (Fig. 6-23).

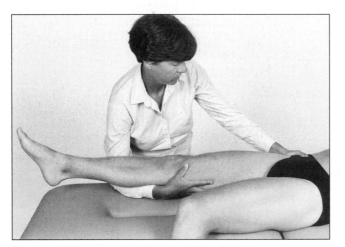

Figure 6-21. Start position: hip adduction.

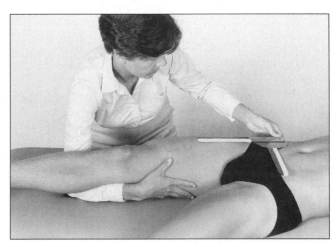

Figure 6-23. End position: universal goniometer measurement for hip adduction.

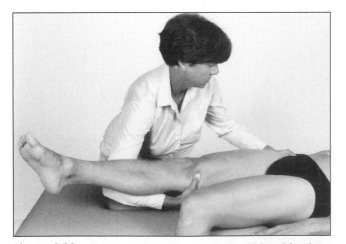

Figure 6-22. Soft or firm end feel at limit of hip adduction.

HIP INTERNAL AND EXTERNAL ROTATION

AROM Assessment

• **Substitution/Trick Movement.** Lateral tilting of the pelvis. In sitting, the patient shifts body weight to raise the pelvis and lift the buttocks off the sitting surface.

PROM Assessment

• **Start Position.** The patient is sitting or supine with the hip and knee flexed to 90° (Fig. 6-24).

• **Stabilization.** The pelvis is stabilized through body positioning. The therapist maintains the position of the femur, without restricting movement.

• **Therapist's Distal Hand Placement.** The therapist grasps the distal tibia and fibula.

• **End Position.** The therapist applies slight traction to the distal femur, then moves the tibia and fibula in a lateral direction to the limit of hip internal rotation (Fig. 6-25) and in a medial direction the limit of hip external rotation (Fig. 6-26).

• **End Feel.** Hip internal rotation—firm; hip external rotation—firm.

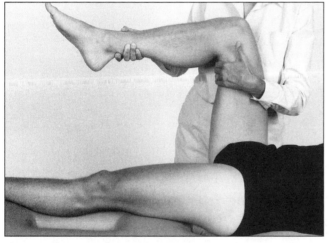

Figure 6-24. Start position: hip internal and external rotation.

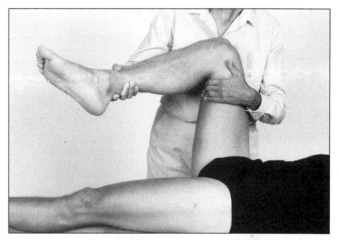

Figure 6-26. Firm end feel at the limit of hip external rotation.

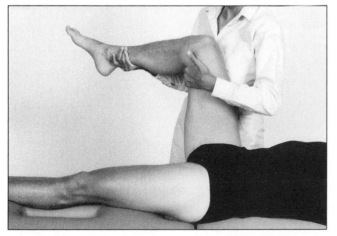

Figure 6-25. Firm end feel at the limit of hip internal rotation.

Hip

Measurement: Universal Goniometer

• **Start Position.** The patient is sitting. In sitting, the hip being measured is in 90° of flexion and neutral rotation with the knee flexed to 90°. A pad is placed under the distal thigh to keep the thigh in a horizontal position. The contralateral hip is abducted and the foot is supported on a stool (Fig. 6-27).

   Alternative starting positions are supine with the lower extremities in anatomical position or prone (not shown). In prone, the pelvis is stabilized through strapping (see Fig. 6-31).

• **Stabilization.** In sitting, the pelvis is stabilized through body positioning and the the patient grasps the edge of the plinth. The therapist maintains the position of the femur, without restricting movement.

• **Goniometer Axis.** The axis is placed over the midpoint of the patella (Fig. 6-28).

• **Stationary Arm.** Perpendicular to the floor.

• **Movable Arm.** Parallel to the anterior midline of the tibia.

• **End Position.** Internal rotation (Fig. 6-29): The hip is internally rotated to the limit of motion (45°) to move the leg and foot in a lateral direction. External rotation (Figs. 6-30 and 6-31): The hip is externally rotated to the limit of motion (45°) to move the leg and foot in a medial direction.

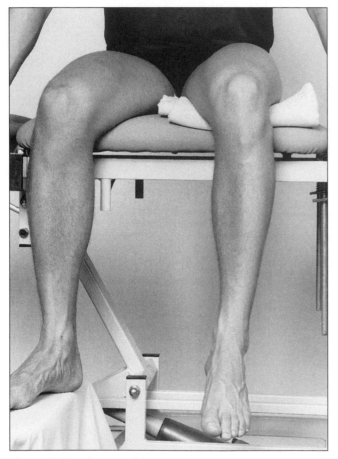

Figure 6-27. Start position: hip internal and external rotation.

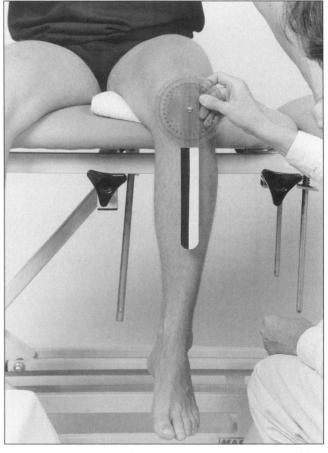

Figure 6-28. Start position: goniometer placement for hip internal and external rotation.

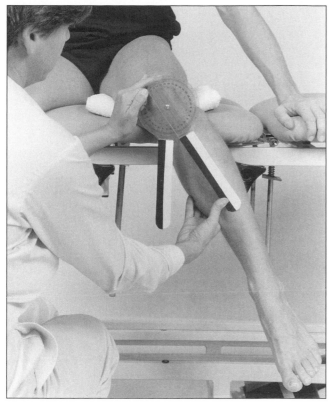

Figure 6-29. End position: internal rotation.

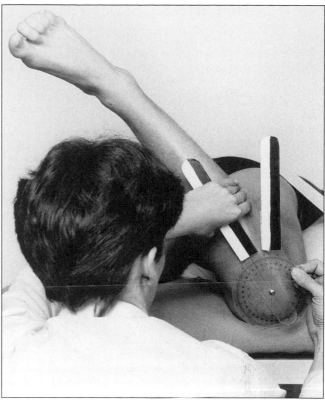

Figure 6-31. Alternate end position: external rotation.

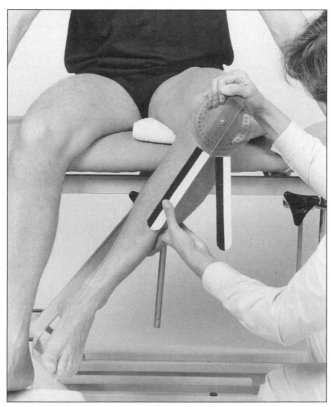

Figure 6-30. End position: external rotation.

MEASUREMENT OF MUSCLE LENGTH: HAMSTRINGS (SEMITENDINOSUS, SEMIMEMBRANOSUS, BICEPS FEMORIS)

• **Start Position.** The patient is supine with the lower extremities in the anatomical position (Fig. 6-32).

• **Stabilization.** It is difficult to stabilize the pelvis when performing passive straight leg raise (SLR) and pelvic rotation is not eliminated from the movement.[10]

To stabilize the pelvis, the contralateral thigh is held on the plinth with the use of a strap (see Fig. 6-32) or by the therapist placing one knee over the anterior surface of the thigh (not shown). When interpreting test results, the therapist should consider that changes in passive SLR may also result from changes in the degree of pelvic rotation.[11]

• **Goniometer Placement.** The goniometer is placed the same as for hip flexion.

• **End Position.** The hip is flexed to the limit of motion while maintaining knee extension, so that the biceps femoris, semitendinosus, and semimembranosus are put on full stretch (see Figs. 6-33 and 6-34). The ankle is relaxed in plantarflexion during the test.

• **End Feel.** Hamstrings on stretch—firm.

• **Measurement.** The therapist uses a goniometer to measure and record the available hip flexion PROM (Figs. 6-33, 6-34, and 6-35). A restriction of less than 80° for SLR in normal subjects is generally imposed by lack of extensibility of hamstrings.[12] Normal ROM of hamstring length is about 80° hip flexion.[13]

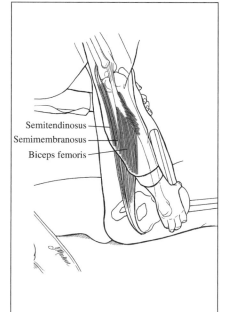

Figure 6-32. Start position: length of hamstrings.

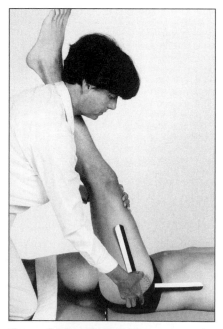

Figure 6-33. End position: universal goniometer measurement of hamstrings length.

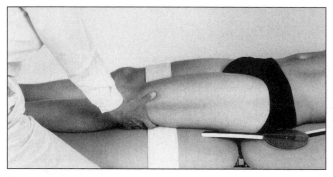

Semitendinosus
Semimembranosus
Biceps femoris

Figure 6-34. Hamstring muscles on stretch.

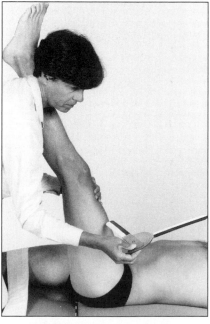

Figure 6-35. Reading goniometer: hamstrings length.

MEASUREMENT OF MUSCLE LENGTH: HIP ADDUCTORS
(ADDUCTOR LONGUS, ADDUCTOR BREVIS, ADDUCTOR MAGNUS, PECTINEUS, AND GRACILIS)

• **Start Position.** The patient is supine with the lower extremity in the anatomical position. On the nontest side, the hip is abducted, the knee is flexed, and the foot rests on a stool beside the plinth (Fig. 6-36).

• **Stabilization.** The therapist stabilizes the pelvis.

• **Goniometer Placement.** The goniometer is placed the same as for hip abduction.

• **End Position.** The hip is abducted to the limit of motion so that the hip adductor muscles are put on full stretch (Fig. 6-37).

• **End Feel.** Hip adductors on stretch—firm.

• **Measurement.** If the hip adductors are shortened, hip abduction PROM will be restricted proportional to the decrease in muscle length. The therapist uses a goniometer to measure and record the available hip abduction ROM (Figs. 6-38 and 6-39).

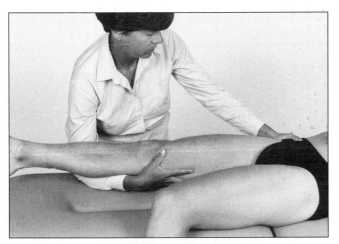

Figure 6-36.   Start position: length of hip adductors.

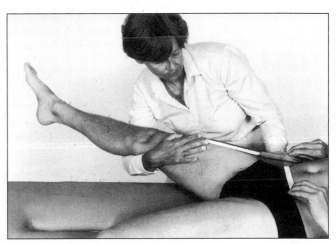

Figure 6-38.   Goniometer measurement: length of hip adductors.

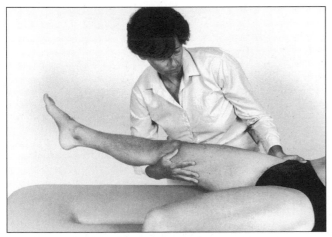

Figure 6-37.   Hip adductors on stretch.

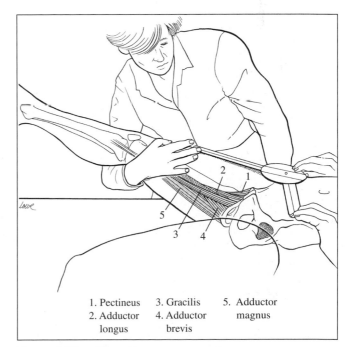

1. Pectineus   3. Gracilis   5. Adductor
2. Adductor   4. Adductor   magnus
   longus   brevis

Figure 6-39.   Hip adductors on stretch.

MEASUREMENT OF MUSCLE LENGTH: HIP FLEXORS (ILIACUS AND PSOAS MAJOR)—THOMAS TEST

• **Start Position.** The patient is supine, and using both hands, holds the hips and knees in flexion to flatten the lumbar spine (Fig. 6-40). Care should be taken to avoid flexion of the lumbar spine due to excessive hip flexion ROM.

• **Stabilization.** The therapist stabilizes the pelvis.

• **Goniometer Placement.** The same as for hip flexion with the axis over the greater trochanter of the femur.

• **End Position.** The test leg is allowed to fall toward the plinth (Fig. 6-41). The therapist applies slight overpressure on the anterior aspect of the thigh to passively move the femur posteriorly to the limit of movement. With shortness of the hip flexors, the angle between the midaxillary line of the trunk and longitudinal axis of the femur represents the degree of hip flexion contracture (Figs. 6-42 and 6-43). Note that a flexion deformity at the hip can be obscured by an increased lumbar lordosis.[14] It is also necessary to ensure that lack of knee extension ROM does not cause the hip to be maintained in a flexed posture in the absence of hip flexor contracture.

• **End Feel.** Iliacus and psoas major on stretch—firm.

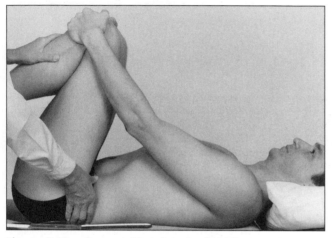

Figure 6-40. Start position: length of hip flexors.

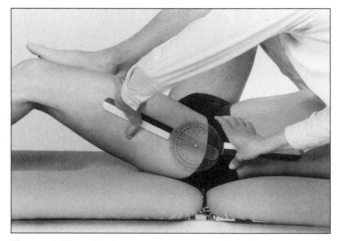

Figure 6-42. Goniometer measurement: length of hip flexors.

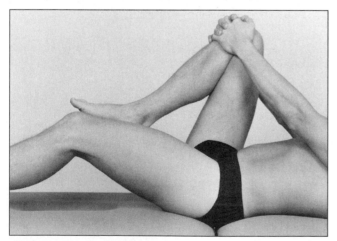

Figure 6-41. Restricted hip extension due to shortened hip flexors.

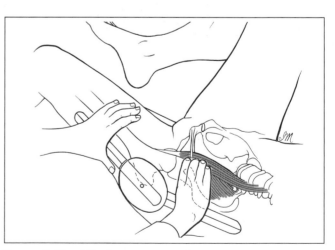

Figure 6-43. Hip flexors on stretch.

ASSESSMENT OF MUSCLE LENGTH: TENSOR FASCIA LATAE (ILIOTIBIAL BAND)— OBER'S TEST

• **Start Position.** The patient is in the side-lying position on the nontest side and holds the nontest leg in hip and knee flexion. The therapist stands behind and against the patient's buttocks to maintain the side-lying position. The therapist positions the hip in abduction and extension to stretch the iliotibial band over the greater trochanter. The hip is in neutral rotation and the knee is positioned in 90° flexion (Fig. 6-44).

• **Stabilization.** The position of the nontest leg stabilizes the pelvis and lumbar spine; the therapist stabilizes the lateral pelvis at the superior aspect of the iliac crest.

• **End Position.** The test leg is allowed to fall toward the plinth. The therapist may apply slight overpressure on the lateral aspect of the thigh to passively adduct the

hip to the limit of movement (not shown). With shortness of the tensor fascia latae, the hip remains abducted (Figs. 6-45 and 6-46). If the leg cannot be passively adducted to the horizontal, there is maximal tightness; if the horizontal position is reached, there is moderate tightness; and if the leg falls below horizontal but does not completely reach the plinth, there is minimal tightness.[15]

Note that a tightness of tensor fascia latae at the hip can be obscured by a downward lateral tilt of the pelvis on the test side that may be accompanied by trunk side flexion on the opposite side. The position of the test leg must be carefully maintained in hip extension and neutral or slight external rotation to perform an accurate test of tensor fascia latae tightness.

If the rectus femoris muscle is tight or there is need to decrease stress in the region of the knee, the Ober's test may be modified and performed with the knee in extension[13] (not shown).

• **End Feel.** Tensor fascia latae (iliotibial band) on stretch—firm.

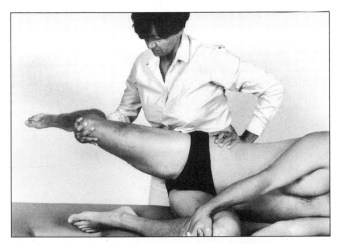

Figure 6-44.   Start position: length of tensor fascia latae.

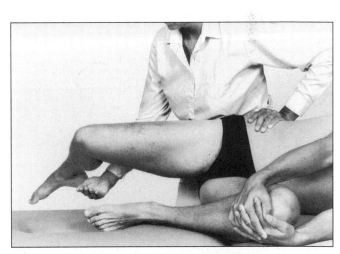

Figure 6-45.   End position: tensor fascia latae on stretch.

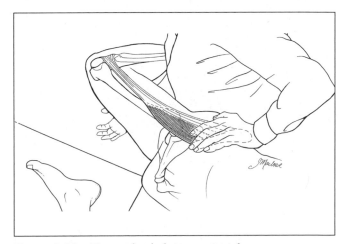

Figure 6-46.   Tensor fascia latae on stretch.

TABLE 6-2 ▼ MUSCLE ACTIONS, ATTACHMENTS, AND NERVE SUPPLY: THE HIP[2]

Muscle	Primary Muscle Action	Muscle Origin	Muscle Insertion	Peripheral Nerve	Nerve Root
Psoas major	Hip flexion	Anterior aspects of the transverse processes of all of the lumbar vertebrae; sides of the bodies and intervertebral discs of T12 and all of the lumbar vertebrae	Lesser trochanter of the femur	Ventral rami of the lumbar	L123
Iliacus	Hip flexion	Superior two thirds of the iliac fossa, inner lip of the iliac crest; the ventral sacroiliac and iliolumbar ligaments; and the upper surface of the lateral aspect of the sacrum	Lateral side of the tendon of psoas major; and into the lesser trochanter	Femoral	L23
Sartorius	Hip flexion, abduction, and external rotation Knee flexion	ASIS and the upper one half of the notch below it	Upper part of the medial surface of the tibia (anterior to gracilis and semitendinosus)	Femoral	L23
Obturator internus	Hip external rotation	Pelvic surface of the inferior ramus of the pubis and ischium and the superior ramus of the pubis; the pelvic surface of the obturator membrane; above and behind the obturator foramen, as far as the upper part of the greater sciatic foramen	Anterior impression on the medial aspect of the greater trochanter of the femur, superior and anterior to the trochanteric fossa (after passing through the lesser sciatic notch)	Nerve to obturator internus	L5S1

TABLE
6-2

▼ MUSCLE ACTIONS, ATTACHMENTS, AND NERVE SUPPLY: THE HIP[2] *Continued*

Muscle	Primary Muscle Action	Muscle Origin	Muscle Insertion	Peripheral Nerve	Nerve Root
Gemellus superior	Hip external rotation	Dorsal aspect of the spine of the ischium	Medial aspect of the greater trochanter along with obturator internus	Nerve to obturator internus	L5S1
Gemellus inferior	Hip external rotation	Superior aspect of the tuberosity of the ischium	Medial aspect of the greater trochanter along with obturator internus	Nerve to quadratus femoris	L5S1
Obturator externus	Hip external rotation	Superior and inferior pubic ramus and the inferior ramus of the ischium; medial two thirds of the outer surface of the obturator membrane; medial side of the obturator foramen	Trochanteric fossa of the greater trochanter of the femur	Obturator	L34
Quadratus femoris	Hip external rotation	Upper portion of the external aspect of the ischial tuberosity	Quadrate tubercle and area of bone just below it on the femur	Nerve to quadratus femoris	L5S1
Pectineus	Hip adduction	Pecten pubis between the iliopectineal eminence and the pubic tubercle	Line between the lesser trochanter and the linea aspera	Femoral	L23
Adductor longus	Hip adduction	Front of the pubis in the angle between the crest and the symphysis	Middle third of the linea aspera of the femur	Obturator	L234
Adductor brevis	Hip adduction	External surface of the inferior pubic ramus between gracilis and obturator externus	Line between lesser trochanter and linea aspera; upper part of linea aspera	Obturator	L23
Gracilis	Hip adduction	Lower half of the body of the pubis; the inferior ramus of the pubis and ischium	Upper part of the medial surface of the tibia (between sartorius and semitendinosus)	Obturator	L23

TABLE 6-G

▼ MUSCLE ACTIONS, ATTACHMENTS, AND NERVE SUPPLY: THE HIP[2] *Continued*

Muscle	Primary Muscle Action	Muscle Origin	Muscle Insertion	Peripheral Nerve	Nerve Root
Adductor magnus	Hip adduction	External surface of the inferior ramus of the pubis adjacent to the ischium; the external surface of the inferior ramus of the ischium; and the inferolateral aspect of the ischial tuberosity	Medial margin of the gluteal tuberosity of the femur; medial lip of the linea aspera; and the medial supracondylar line; adductor tubercle	Obturator, Sciatic (tibial division)	L234
Piriformis	Hip external rotation	Pelvic surface of the sacrum between the second to fourth sacral foramina, and gluteal surface of the ilium adjacent to the posterior inferior iliac spine	Medial aspect of the upper border of the greater trochanter of the femur (after passing through the greater sciatic foramina)		L5S12
Gluteus maximus	Hip extension	Posterior gluteal line of the ilium and the iliac crest above and behind the line; aponeurosis of the erector spinae; dorsal surface of the lower part of the sacrum and the side of the coccyx; and sacrotuberous ligament	Iliotibial tract and gluteal tuberosity	Inferior gluteal	L5S12
Tensor fascia latae	Hip flexion, abduction, and internal rotation (through the iliotibial tract—knee extension)	Anterior aspect of the outer lip of the iliac crest; the outer surface and notch below the ASIS; and the deep surface of the fascia lata	Iliotibial tract	Superior gluteal	L45S1

TABLE
6-2

▼ **MUSCLE ACTIONS, ATTACHMENTS, AND NERVE SUPPLY: THE HIP[2]** *Continued*

Muscle	Primary Muscle Action	Muscle Origin	Muscle Insertion	Peripheral Nerve	Nerve Root
Gluteus medius	Hip abduction and internal rotation	Outer surface of the ilium between the iliac crest and posterior gluteal line above and the anterior gluteal line below	Oblique ridge, downwards and forwards, on the lateral surface of the greater trochanter	Superior gluteal	L**45**S1
Gluteus minimus	Hip abduction and internal rotation	Outer surface of the ilium between the anterior and inferior gluteal lines and the margin of the greater sciatic notch	Anterolateral aspect of the greater trochanter	Superior gluteal	L**45**S1

HIP

HIP FLEXION

Against Gravity: Iliopsoas

Accessory muscles: rectus femoris, sartorius, tensor fascia latae, and pectineus.

• **Start Position.** The patient is sitting. The lower leg is off the plinth with the knee flexed and foot unsupported. The contralateral foot is supported on a stool (Fig. 6-47).

• **Alternate Start Position.** The patient is supine. The hip and knee are in the anatomical position. The leg not being tested is flexed at the hip and knee (Fig. 6-48). This start position may be contraindicated with low back pain.

• **Stabilization.** The therapist stabilizes the pelvis by placing the hand over the ipsilateral iliac crest. If sitting, the patient grasps the edge of the plinth to stabilize the proximal body segments.

• **Movement.** The patient flexes the hip through full ROM. The knee is allowed to flex (Fig. 6-49). In the supine position, the hip and knee are flexed (Fig. 6-50). Beyond 90° gravity assists motion and the therapist can add resistance.

• **Palpation.** Iliacus and psoas major are not easily palpated.

• **Substitution/Trick Movement.** Substitution by the accessory muscles can be observed through additional movement patterns: abduction and external rotation through sartorius; abduction and internal rotation through tensor fascia latae.[4]

• **Resistance Location.** Applied over the anterior aspect of the thigh proximal to the knee joint (Figs. 6-51, 6-52, and 6-53).

• **Resistance Direction.** Hip extension.

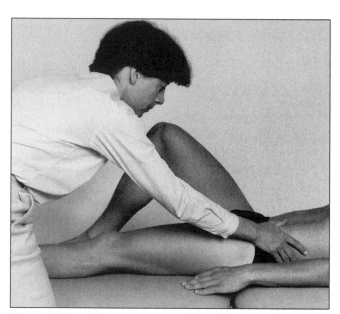

Figure 6-48.   Alternate start position: iliopsoas.

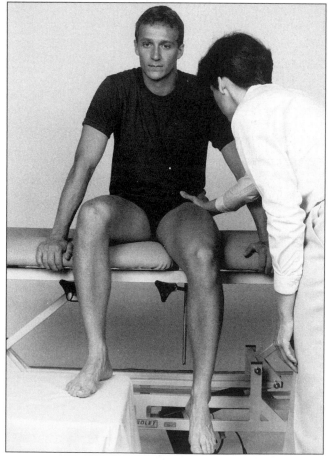

Figure 6-47.   Start position: iliopsoas.

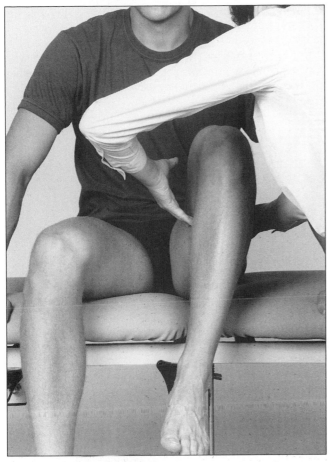

Figure 6-49.   Screen position: iliopsoas.

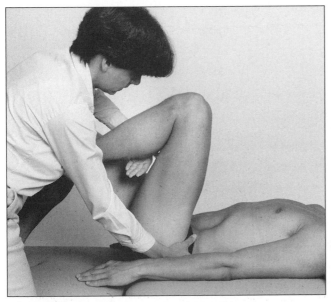

Figure 6-50.   Alternate screen position: iliopsoas.

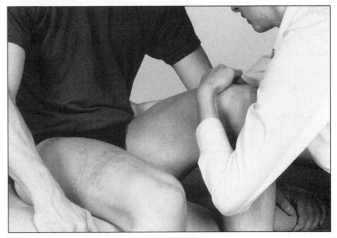

Figure 6-51.   Resistance: iliopsoas.

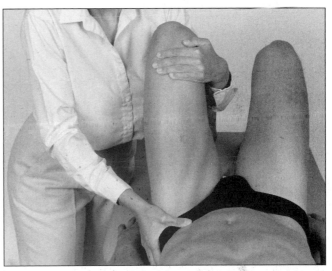

Figure 6-52.   Resistance in alternate test position: iliopsoas.

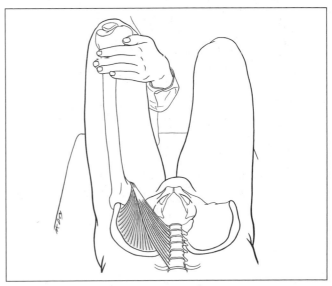

Figure 6-53.   Iliopsoas.

Gravity Eliminated: Iliopsoas

• **Start Position.** The patient is lying on the nontest side and the patient holds the nontest leg in maximal hip and knee flexion (Fig. 6-54). The therapist stands behind the patient to maintain the side-lying position and supports the weight of the lower extremity. The hip is extended and the knee is flexed. Knee flexion places the hamstrings on slack.

• **Stabilization.** The position of the nontest leg stabilizes the lumbar spine; the therapist stabilizes the pelvis.

• **End Position.** The patient flexes the hip through full ROM (Fig. 6-55).

• **Substitution/Trick Movement.** Hip abduction with hip external or internal rotation[4] and posterior pelvic tilt through the abdominal muscles.[16]

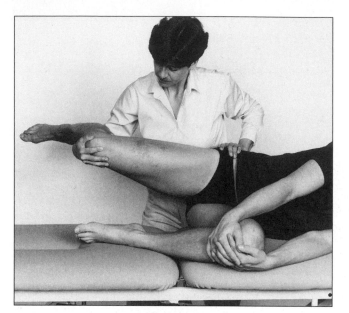

Figure 6-54.   Start position: iliopsoas.

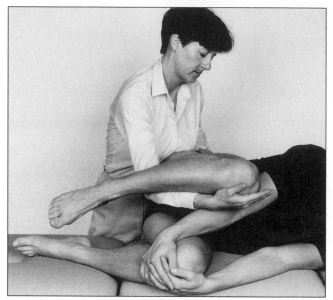

Figure 6-55.   End position: iliopsoas.

HIP FLEXION, ABDUCTION, AND EXTERNAL ROTATION WITH KNEE FLEXION

Against Gravity: Sartorius

Accessory muscles: iliopsoas, rectus femoris, and tensor fascia latae.

- **Start Position.** The patient is supine with both legs in the anatomical position (Fig. 6-56).

- **Stabilization.** The weight of the trunk.

- **Movement.** The patient flexes, abducts, and externally rotates the hip and flexes the knee (Fig. 6-57).

- **Palpation.** On the anterior aspect of the thigh medial to tensor fascia latae.

- **Substitution/Trick Movement.** Iliopsoas and rectus femoris. To ensure the correct movement, the heel of the test leg should pass just above and parallel to the shin of the contralateral leg. The activity in tensor fascia latae decreases when hip flexion is combined with external rotation.[17]

- **Resistance Locations.** Applied at the same time: (1) at the anterolateral aspect of the thigh proximal to the knee joint and (2) at the posterior aspect of the lower leg proximal to the ankle joint (Figs. 6-58 and 6-59).

- **Resistance Direction.** (1) Hip extension, adduction, and internal rotation; (2) knee extension.

Assisted Against Gravity: Sartorius. The test procedure is the same as described for the against gravity test. Assistance, equal to the weight of the limb, is provided throughout range.

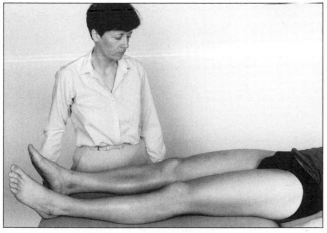

Figure 6-56.   Start position: sartorius.

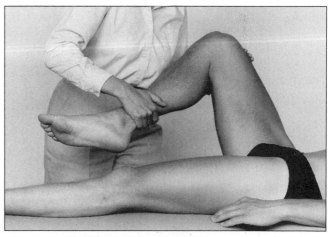

Figure 6-58.   Resistance: sartorius.

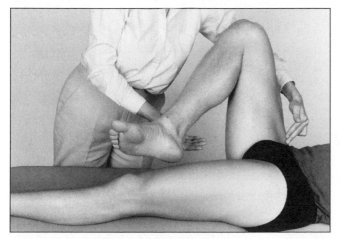

Figure 6-57.   Screen position: sartorius.

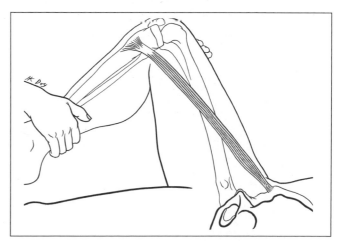

Figure 6-59.   Sartorius.

HIP EXTENSION

Against Gravity: Gluteus Maximus, Biceps Femoris, Semitendinosus, and Semimembranosus

Accessory muscles: adductor magnus, piriformis, and gluteus medius.

- **Start Position.** This position is indicated for testing patients with tight hip flexors (Fig. 6-60). The patient is standing with the trunk flexed and thorax resting on the plinth. The leg not being tested is placed under the table so that the hip and knee are flexed. The test leg hip is flexed and the knee is extended.

- **Alternate Start Position.** This position is indicated for elderly patients or those with generalized weakness (Fig. 6-61). The patient is prone with the legs in the anatomical position and two pillows are placed under the pelvis to flex the hips.

- **Stabilization.** The therapist or a pelvic strap stabilizes the pelvis. The patient grasps the edge of the plinth; the weight of the trunk offers stabilization.

- **Movement.** The patient extends the hip with the knee held in extension (Figs. 6-62 and 6-63). The patient is instructed to maintain external rotation to gain maximum contraction of the gluteus maximus. Extending the hip with the knee actively flexed places the hamstrings in a shortened position and this test position has been advocated for isolation of gluteus maximus.[4] Although some of the efficiency of hamstrings may be decreased when the knee is actively maintained in flexion,[5,18] the hamstrings are active in maintaining knee flexion and cannot be eliminated.[13,18] The therapist can passively hold the knee in flexion to isolate the gluteus maximus, but it is difficult to maintain the knee position while applying pressure to the thigh.[13]

- **Palpation.** Gluteus maximus: medial to its insertion on the gluteal tuberosity or adjacent to its origin from the posterior aspect of the ilium (see Fig. 6-68B).

- **Substitution/Trick Movement.** Lumbar spine extension.

- **Resistance Location.** Applied on the posterior aspect of the thigh proximal to the knee joint (Figs. 6-64, 6-65, and 6-66).

- **Resistance Direction.** Hip flexion.

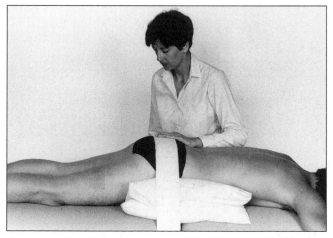

Figure 6-61.   Alternate start position: hip extensors.

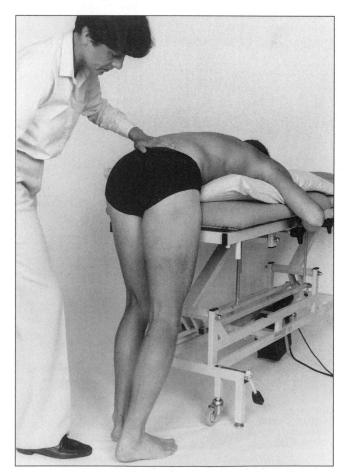

Figure 6-60.   Start position: hip extensors.

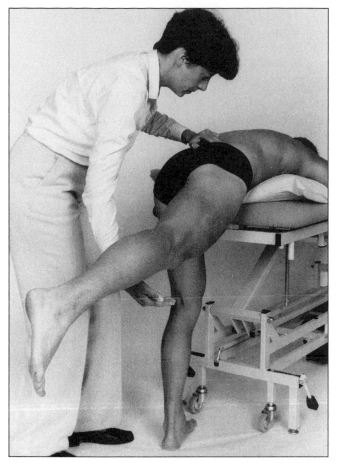

Figure 6-62. Screen position: hip extensors.

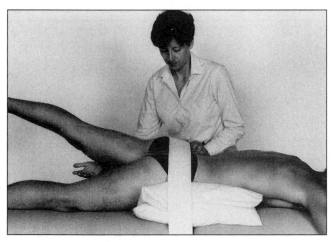

Figure 6-63. Alternate screen position: hip extensors.

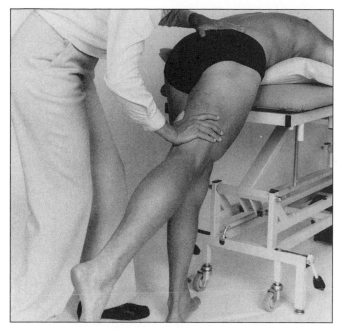

Figure 6-64. Resistance: hip extensors.

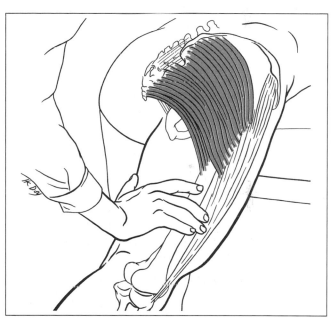

Figure 6-65. Gluteus maximus.

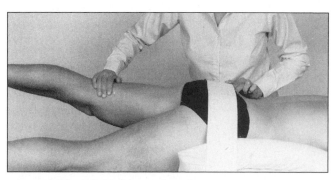

Figure 6-66. Resistance in alternate start position: hip extensors.

Gravity Eliminated: Gluteus Maximus, Biceps Femoris, Semitendinosus, and Semimembranosus

• **Start Position.** The patient is lying on the nontest side with the hip flexed and the knee passively flexed by the therapist (Fig. 6-67).

• **Stabilization.** The patient holds the nontest leg in maximal hip and knee flexion to stabilize the trunk and pelvis and prevent lumbar spine extension.

• **End Position.** The patient extends the hip through full ROM (Fig. 6-68). The knee is allowed to extend if tightness is present in rectus femoris.

• **Substitution/Trick Movement.** Hip abduction or adduction.

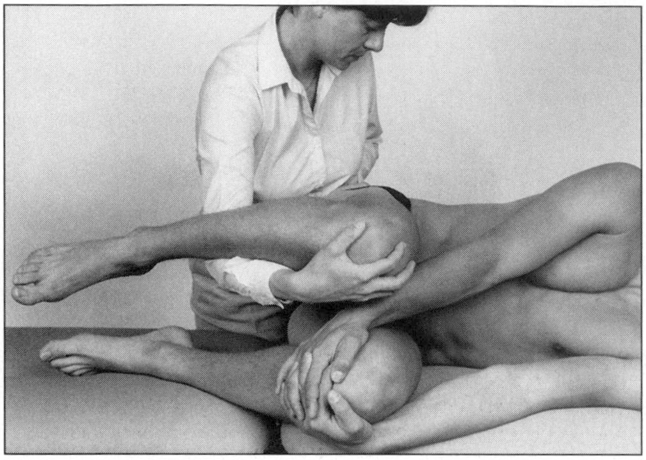

Figure 6-67.   Start position: hip extensors.

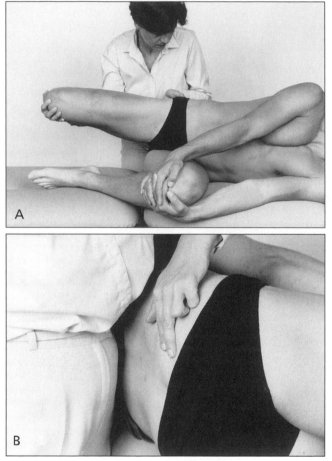

Figure 6-68.   (*A*) End position: hip extensors. (*B*) The therapist is palpating the gluteus maximus.

HIP ABDUCTION

Against Gravity: Gluteus Medius and Gluteus Minimus

Accessory muscles: tensor fascia latae and gluteus maximus (upper fibers).

• **Start Position.** The patient is lying on the nontest side with the hip and knee maintained in flexion by the patient to stabilize the trunk and pelvis (Fig. 6-69). The therapist stands behind and against the patient's buttocks to maintain the side-lying position. The hip of the leg to be tested is slightly extended and in neutral rotation.

• **Stabilization.** The position of the nontest leg offers stabilization; the therapist stabilizes the pelvis by placing the hand on the superior aspect of the iliac crest.

• **Movement.** The patient abducts the hip through full ROM. The patient is instructed to lead with the heel to prevent flexion of the hip (Fig. 6-70).

• **Palpation.** The gluteus medius is palpated just distal to the lateral lip of the iliac crest or proximal to the greater trochanter of the femur. Gluteus minimus lies deep to gluteus medius and is not palpable.

• **Substitution/Trick Movement.** Hip flexion through iliacus and psoas major, pelvic elevation through quadratus lumborum. The patient may abduct the leg with hip flexion and internal rotation through the action of tensor fascia latae.

• **Resistance Location.** Applied on the lateral aspect of the thigh proximal to the knee (Figs. 6-71, 6-72, and 6-73).

• **Resistance Direction.** Hip adduction.

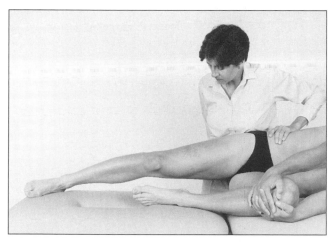

Figure 6-69. Start position: gluteus medius and gluteus minimus

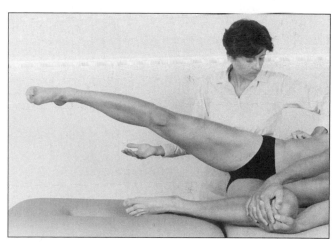

Figure 6-70. Screen position: gluteus medius and gluteus minimus.

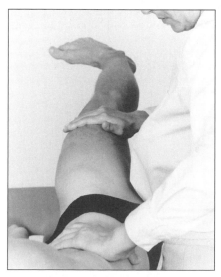

Figure 6-71. Resistance: gluteus medius and gluteus minimus.

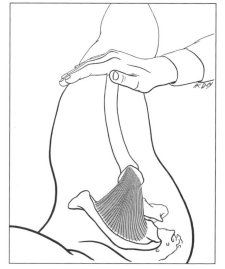

Figure 6-72. Gluteus medius.

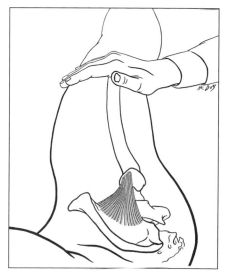

Figure 6-73. Gluteus minimus.

Gravity Eliminated: Gluteus Medius and Gluteus Minimus

- **Start Position.** The patient is supine with the lower extremity in the anatomical position (Fig. 6-74). The therapist supports the weight of the limb.

- **Stabilization.** The therapist stabilizes the pelvis.

- **End Position.** The patient abducts the hip through full ROM (Fig. 6-75).

- **Substitution/Trick Movement.** Hip flexion and pelvic elevation.

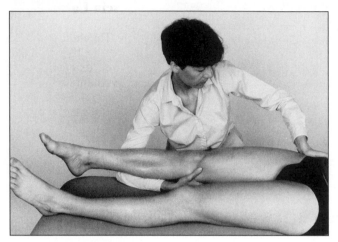

Figure 6-74.   Start position: gluteus medius and gluteus minimus.

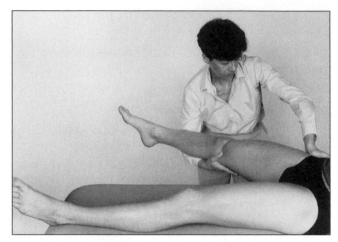

Figure 6-75.   End position: gluteus medius and gluteus minimus.

HIP ABDUCTION AND HIP FLEXION

Against Gravity: Tensor Fascia Latae

Accessory muscles: gluteus medius and gluteus minimus.

• **Start Position.** The patient is lying on the side not being tested and supports the leg in maximal hip and knee flexion (Fig. 6-76). The leg on the test side is placed in 10° to 20° of hip flexion and in internal rotation. The pelvis is rolled backward and the therapist stands behind and against the patient's buttocks to maintain this position in side-lying. The knee is in extension.

• **Stabilization.** The position of the nontest leg offers stabilization; the therapist stabilizes the pelvis by placing a hand on the superior aspect of the iliac crest.

• **Movement.** The patient abducts the hip through full ROM and slightly flexes the hip (Fig. 6-77).

• **Palpation.** Lateral to the upper portion of sartorius or distal to the greater trochanter on the iliotibial band.

• **Substitution/Trick Movement.** Quadratus lumborum (pelvic elevation), iliacus and psoas major (hip flexion), and gluteus medius and minimus (hip abduction).

• **Resistance Location.** Applied on the anterolateral aspect of the thigh proximal to the knee joint (Figs. 6-78 and 6-79).

• **Resistance Direction.** Hip adduction and extension.

Gravity Eliminated: Tensor Fascia Latae

• **Start Position.** The patient is supine. The therapist supports the weight of the lower extremity in 10° to 20° of hip flexion, internal rotation, and knee extension and maintains the support throughout movement (Fig. 6-80).

• **Stabilization.** The weight of the patient's trunk offers stabilization.

• **End Position.** The patient abducts the hip through full ROM and slightly flexes the hip (Fig. 6-81).

• **Substitution/Trick Movement.** Quadratus lumborum, iliacus, psoas major, and gluteus medius and minimus.

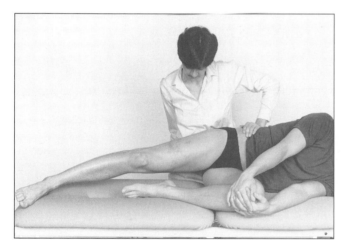

Figure 6-76.   Start position: tensor fascia latae.

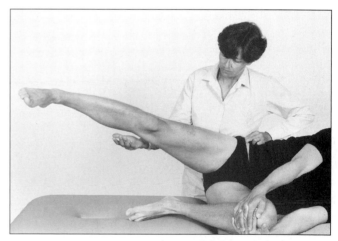

Figure 6-77.   Screen position: tensor fascia latae.

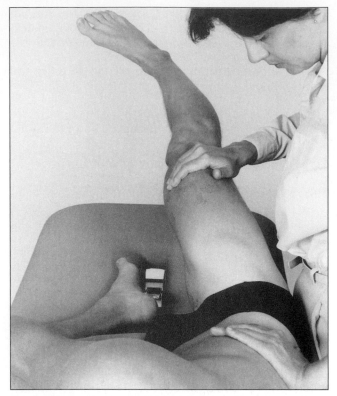

Figure 6-78.　Resistance: tensor fascia latae.

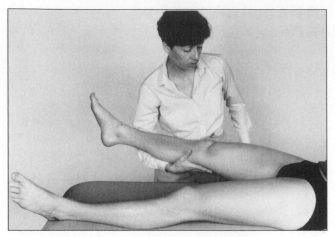

Figure 6-80.　Start position: tensor fascia latae.

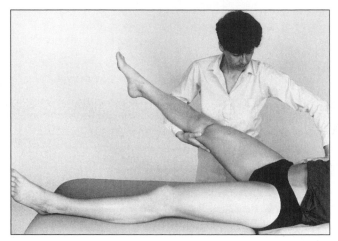

Figure 6-81.　End position: tensor fascia latae.

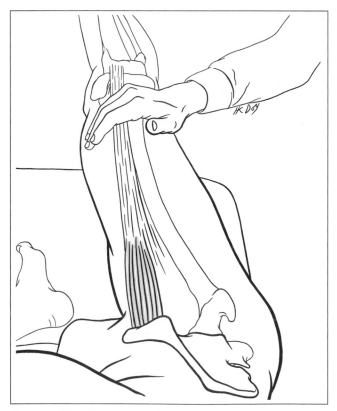

Figure 6-79.　Tensor fascia latae.

CLINICAL TEST: WEAKNESS OF HIP ABDUCTOR MECHANISM

The hip abductor muscles primarily function to maintain a level pelvis during unilateral stance.[18] Assumption of a unilateral stance occurs in walking when one leg is swinging forward and the other foot maintains contact with the ground. In standing with one foot off the ground, the weight of the head, arms, trunk, and ipsilateral limb rotate the pelvis in a downward direction on the unsupported side.[18] This downward rotation must be balanced around the femoral head by contraction of the hip abductors.[18] When weakness or paralysis of the abductors is present in the stance leg, the pelvis on the contralateral side will drop. Weakness or paralysis may be clinically detected through the Trendelenburg test.[5,14,19]

Trendelenburg Test. The patient is standing on the leg to be tested and places the hands lightly on a table to maintain balance (not shown). The contralateral hip and knee are flexed so that the foot clears the floor. The therapist stands behind the patient and observes the posture of the pelvis and trunk. A negative Trendelenburg sign (Fig. 6-82) indicates no abductor weakness. The PSISs are level or slightly inclined toward the unsupported side. A positive Trendelenburg sign (Fig. 6-83) indicates abductor weakness. The PSISs are not level and the pelvis drops on the unsupported side. As a compensatory balance mechanism for abductor weakness, the patient will shift the trunk over the involved side.

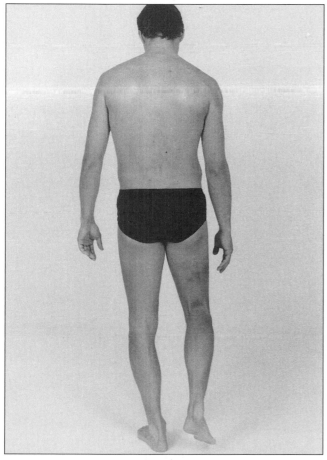

Figure 6-82.   Negative Trendelenburg sign.

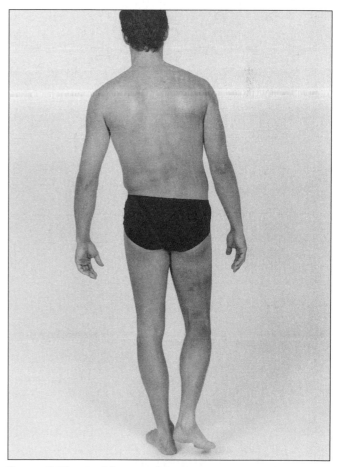

Figure 6-83.   Positive Trendelenburg sign.

HIP ADDUCTION

Resisted Gravity Eliminated and Gravity Eliminated: Adductor Longus, Adductor Brevis, Adductor Magnus, Pectineus, and Gracilis

• **Start Position.** A gravity eliminated test position is assumed. The patient is supine. The hip to be tested is in about 40° of abduction, neutral rotation, and extension. The knee is extended. The therapist supports the weight of the limb. The contralateral lower extremity remains on the plinth in extension (Fig. 6-84).

• **Stabilization.** The patient grasps the edge of the plinth. If additional stabilization of the trunk and pelvis is required, the contralateral lower extremity may be positioned in hip abduction with the knee flexed over the edge of the plinth and the foot supported on a stool (Fig. 6-85).

• **Movement.** The hip is adducted until it contacts the contralateral limb (Fig. 6-86). The patient is instructed to maintain neutral rotation.

• **Palpation.** The adductors are palpated as a group on the medial, proximal aspect of the thigh.

• **Resistance Location.** Applied on the medial aspect of the thigh proximal to the knee joint (Figs. 6-87 and 6-88).

• **Resistance Direction.** Hip abduction.

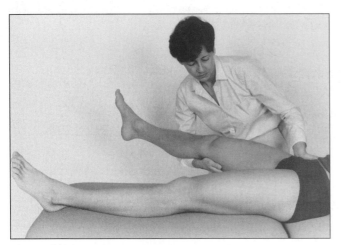

Figure 6-84.   Start position: hip adductors.

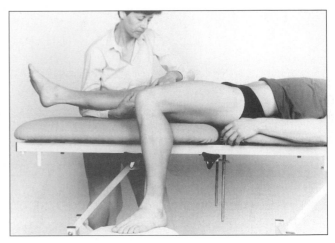

Figure 6-85.   Alternate stabilization position: hip adductors.

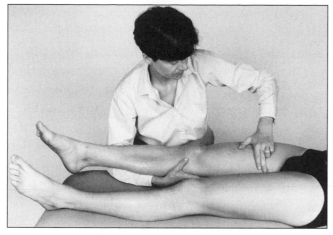

Figure 6-86.   Screen position: hip adductors.

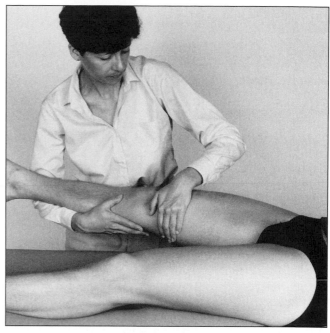

Figure 6-87.   Resistance: hip adductors.

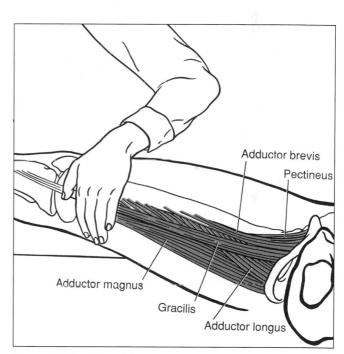

Figure 6-88.   Hip adductors.

HIP INTERNAL ROTATION

Against Gravity: Gluteus Medius, Gluteus Minimus, and Tensor Fascia Latae

Accessory muscle: adductor longus.

• **Start Position.** The patient is sitting (Fig. 6-89). The hip is in 90° of flexion and neutral rotation. A pad is placed under the distal thigh to keep the thigh in a horizontal position. The midpoint of the patella is aligned with the ASIS. The leg not being tested is abducted and the foot is supported on a stool.

• **Stabilization.** The weight of the trunk provides some stabilization. The patient grasps the edge of the plinth to stabilize the pelvis. The therapist places a hand on the medial aspect of the distal thigh to prevent adduction of the hip. The therapist maintains the position of the femur, without restricting movement.

• **Movement.** The patient internally rotates the hip through full ROM (Fig. 6-90).

• **Palpation.** Refer to previous test descriptions for palpation of gluteus medius, gluteus minimus, and tensor fascia latae.

• **Substitution/Trick Movement.** Pelvic elevation, contralateral trunk side flexion, and hip adduction.

• **Resistance Location.** Applied on the lateral aspect of the lower leg proximal to the ankle joint (Fig. 6-91). The application of resistance stresses the knee joint and caution should be exercised.

• **Resistance Direction.** Hip external rotation.

• **Alternate Test Position.** The patient is in a supine position with the hip extended. This position may be indicated when knee instability prevents application of resistance as described. In a supine position, resistance is applied proximal to the knee joint. The force exerted by the internal rotators is greater in hip flexion than extension.[20] For the purpose of interrater reliability, the hip position should be recorded.

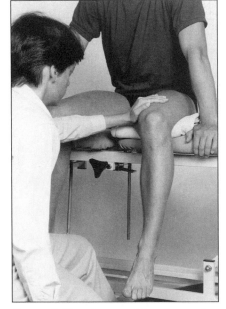

Figure 6-89. Start position: internal rotators.

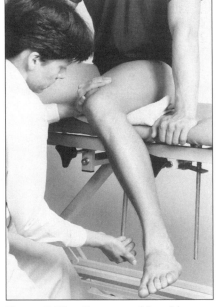

Figure 6-90. Screen position: hip internal rotators.

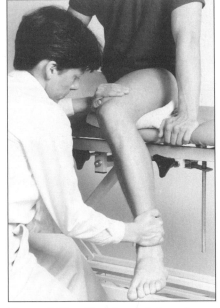

Figure 6-91. Resistance: internal rotators.

Gravity Eliminated: Gluteus Medius, Gluteus Minimus, and Tensor Fascia Latae

• **Start Position.** The patient is supine. The therapist supports the leg in a position of 90° of hip flexion, neutral rotation, and knee flexion (Fig. 6-92).

• **Stabilization.** The patient grasps the edge of the plinth for stabilization of the pelvis.

• **End Position.** The patient internally rotates the hip through full ROM (Fig. 6-93). The therapist's supporting hand on the medial aspect of the thigh should allow full rotation and prevent hip adduction. The movement is repeated and the therapist palpates the muscles.

• **Substitution/Trick Movement.** Hip adduction and knee flexion.

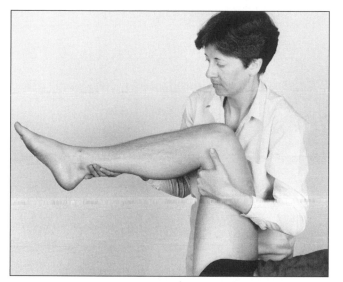

Figure 6-92.   Start position: internal rotators.

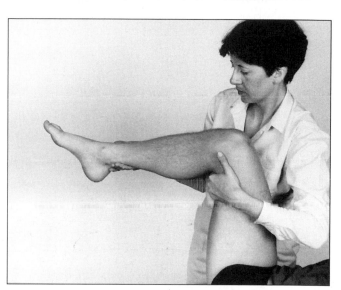

Figure 6-93.   End position: internal rotators.

HIP EXTERNAL ROTATION

Against Gravity: Piriformis, Obturator Externus, Gemellus Superior, Quadratus Femoris, Gemellus Inferior, and Obturator Internus

Accessory muscle: gluteus maximus in hip extension.

• **Start Position.** The patient is sitting (Fig. 6-94). The hip is in 90° of flexion and neutral rotation. A pad is placed under the distal thigh to keep the thigh in a horizontal position. The midpoint of the patella is aligned with the ASIS. With knee instability, the patient is in a supine position with the hip extended.

• **Stabilization.** The weight of the trunk provides some stabilization. The patient grasps the edge of the plinth to stabilize the pelvis. The therapist places a hand on the anterolateral aspect of the distal thigh to prevent hip abduction and flexion. The therapist maintains the position of the femur, without restricting movement.

• **Movement.** The patient externally rotates the hip through full ROM (Fig. 6-95).

• **Palpation.** The external rotators are too deep to palpate.

• **Substitution/Trick Movement.** Hip flexion and abduction; ipsilateral trunk side flexion.

• **Resistance Location.** Applied on the medial aspect of the lower leg proximal to the ankle joint (Figs. 6-96 and 6-97). Application of resistance stresses the knee joint and caution should be exercised. The alternate test position described for internal rotators may be used in the presence of knee instability.

• **Resistance Direction.** Internal rotation.

Gravity Eliminated: External Rotators

• **Start Position.** The position is the same as described for internal rotation.

• **End Position.** The patient externally rotates the hip through full ROM (Fig. 6-98).

• **Substitution/Trick Movement.** Hip flexion and abduction and knee flexion.

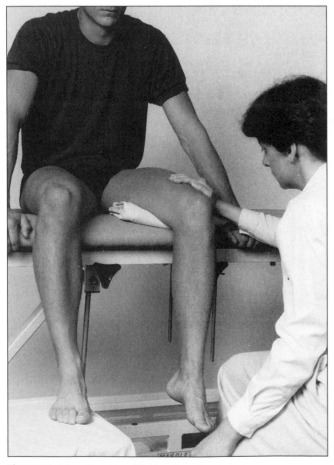

Figure 6-94.   Start position: external rotators.

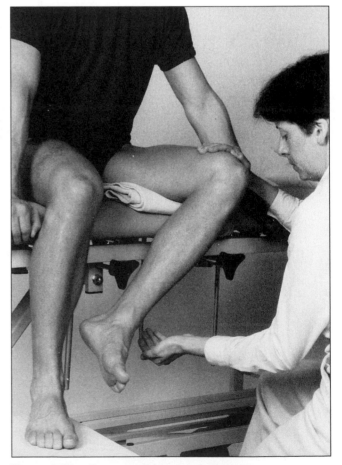

Figure 6-95.   Screen position: external rotators.

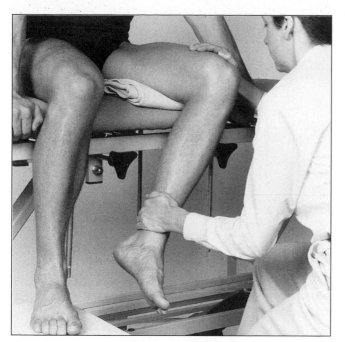

Figure 6-96. Resistance: external rotators.

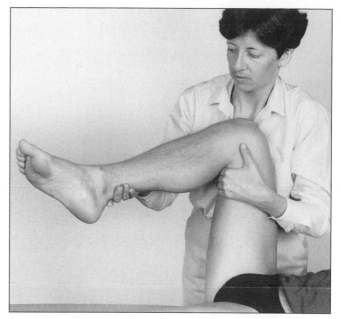

Figure 6-98. End position: external rotators.

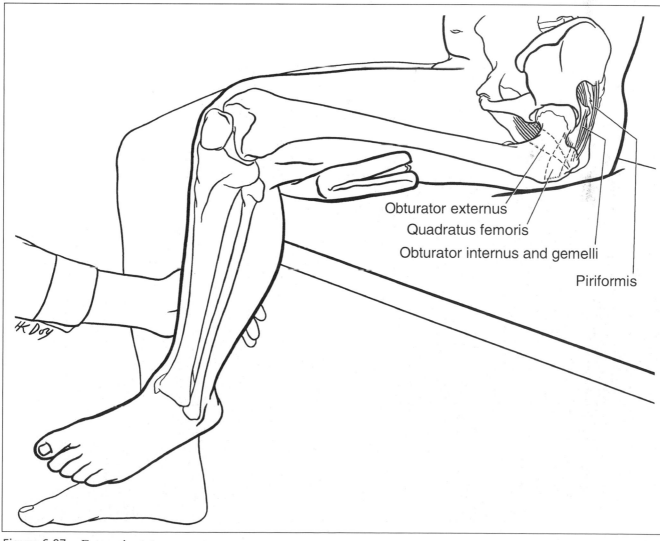

Obturator externus
Quadratus femoris
Obturator internus and gemelli
Piriformis

Figure 6-97. External rotators.

JOINT FUNCTION[18]

The hip joint transmits forces between the ground and the pelvis to support the body weight and acts as a fulcrum during single leg stance. Through hip movement the body may be moved closer to or farther away from the ground. The hip brings the foot closer to the trunk and positions the lower limb in space.

FUNCTIONAL RANGE OF MOTION

The hip joint may be flexed, extended, abducted, adducted, and internally and externally rotated. In performing functional activities, hip movements are accompanied at various points in the ROM by lumbar-pelvic motions.[21] These motions extend the functional range capabilities of the hip joint. The lumbar and pelvic motions are included in the following description of motion, with the purpose of explaining the interdependence of the components of the pelvic girdle and trunk throughout movement.

Hip Flexion and Extension

As in the shoulder joint, movement at the hip joint is augmented by motions occurring at the more central joints. Hip movement "may result from movement of the pelvis on the femur, from movement of the femur on the pelvis, or from a combination of pelvic and femoral motion."[5(p273)] As the femur moves on the pelvis to produce hip flexion, hip ROM is augmented by a posterior pelvic tilt (ie, the ASIS moves superiorly and posteriorly) and flexion of the lumbar spine. In hip extension, the movement is increased by an anterior pelvic tilt (ie, the ASIS moves inferiorly and anteriorly) and extension of the lumbar spine.

The normal AROM for hip flexion is 0° to 120° and extension is 0° to 30°.[9] Full hip flexion and extension ROMs are required for many activities of daily living (ADL). Standing requires 0° or slight hip extension.[22] Using electrogoniometric measures, it has been found that without using compensatory movement patterns at other joints, activities such as squatting to pick up an object from the ground, tying a shoelace with the foot on the ground (Fig. 6-99) or with the foot across the opposite thigh, and rising from a sitting position (Fig. 6-100) require an average of between 110° and 120° of hip flexion.[23]

Activities requiring less than 90° of hip flexion include ascending (Fig. 6-101) and descending stairs,[23,24] sitting in a chair of standard height,[23] and donning a pair of trousers (Fig. 6-102). Ascending stairs requires an average of 67° hip flexion and descending requires an average of 36° of hip flexion.[23] A maximum of about 1° to 2° hip extension may be required to ascend and descend stairs.[24]

The range required for sitting is determined by the height of the chair. To sit from standing requires an average of 104° hip flexion[23] and to rise from sitting requires an average of between 98° and 101° hip flexion ROM.[25] About 84° of hip flexion is required for sitting in a standard chair.[23] These ranges increase with decreased chair height and decrease with increased chair height.

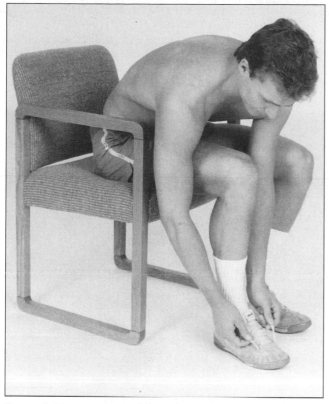

Figure 6-99. Tying a shoelace with the foot flat on the floor requires about 120° of hip flexion.[23]

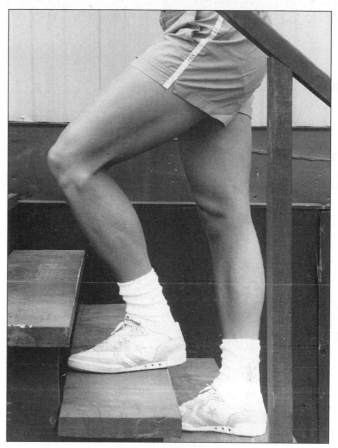

Figure 6-101. Ascending stairs.

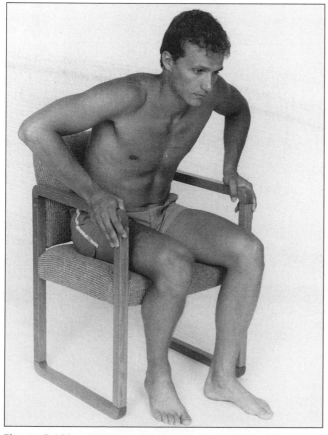

Figure 6-100. Rising from a sitting position requires at least 90° of hip flexion.[23]

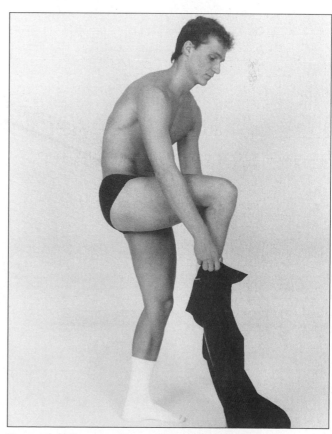

Figure 6-102. Donning a pair of trousers.

Hip Abduction and Adduction

The normal AROM at the hip for abduction is 0° to 45° and for adduction is 0° to 30°.[9] However, most daily functions do not require the full ranges of hip abduction and adduction. Many ADL can be performed within an arc of 0° to 20° of hip abduction.[23] Squatting to pick up an object and sitting with the foot across the opposite thigh (Fig. 6-103) are examples of activities performed within this ROM. Mounting a man's bicycle (Fig. 6-104) may require the full range of hip abduction. Hip adduction in ADL is illustrated when sitting with the thighs crossed and when standing on one leg; the stance leg adducts as a result of the pelvis dropping on the contralateral side.

Hip Internal and External Rotation

The AROM of hip internal and external rotation is 0° to 45° in both directions.[9] The extremes of these rotational motions are seldom used in ADL. Ranges of 0° to 20° external rotation are required for most ADL.[23] Mounting a bicycle (see Fig. 6-104), sitting on a chair with the foot across the opposite thigh to tie a shoelace, or visually observing the skin on the sole of the foot when performing foot hygiene activities illustrate the use of hip external rotation. Squatting to pick up an object from the floor is an example of a functional activity that requires 20° of hip internal rotation.[23]

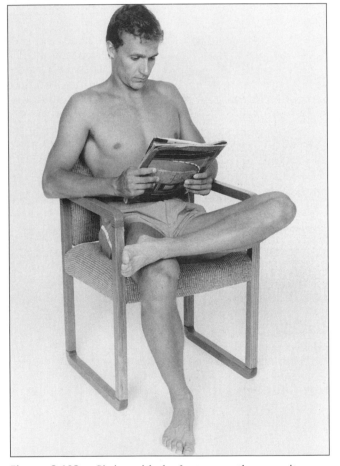

Figure 6-103. Sitting with the foot across the opposite thigh requires hip flexion, abduction, and external rotation.

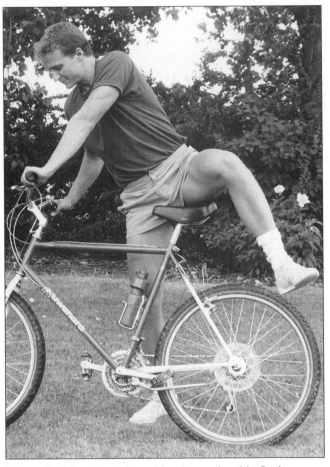

Figure 6-104. Mounting a bicycle requires hip flexion, abduction, and external rotation.

Gait

A normal walking pattern requires hip motion in the sagittal, frontal, and horizontal planes. In the sagittal plane, about 10° to 20° of hip extension is required at terminal stance and 30° of hip flexion is required at the end of swing phase and the beginning of stance phase as the limb is advanced forward to take the next step (from the Rancho Los Amigos gait analysis forms as cited in Norkin and Levangie[22]).

With the feet fixed on the ground, the femoral heads can act as fulcrums for the pelvis as it tilts anteriorly and posteriorly. The pelvis can also tilt laterally causing the iliac crests to move either superiorly or inferiorly. Lateral tilting of the pelvis occurs when one leg is off the ground, the hip joint of the supporting leg acts as a fulcrum, and the tilting results in relative abduction and adduction at the hip joints.[22] When walking there is a lateral tilt of the pelvis inferiorly on the unsupported side during the swing phase of the gait cycle. This dropping of the pelvis on the unsupported side results in abduction at the hip on the same side. As the pelvis drops, the inferior aspect of the pelvis moves toward the femur of the stance leg producing hip adduction on this side. About 7° of hip abduction is required at initial swing and 5° of hip adduction is required at the end of the stance phase of the gait cycle.[26]

Pelvic rotation occurs in the horizontal plane about a vertical axis. Rotations of the thigh occur relative to the pelvis. As the swinging leg advances during locomotion, the pelvis rotates forward on the same side. The fulcrum for this forward rotation of the pelvis is the head of the femur on the supporting leg. As the supporting or stance leg is fixed on the ground, the pelvis rotates around the femoral head resulting in internal rotation at the hip joint. As the pelvis moves forward on the swing side, the swinging leg moves forward in the sagittal plane in the line of progression, resulting in external rotation of the hip during the swing phase of the gait cycle. During the normal gait cycle about 5° of internal and 9° of external rotation are required at the hip joint.[26] External rotation occurs at the end of the stance phase and through most of the swing phase and internal rotation occurs at terminal swing before initial contact to the end of the stance phase.[26] Refer to Appendix D for further description and illustrations of the positions and motions at the hip joint during gait.

Hip flexion and extension ROM requirements for slow-paced (<8-minute mile) and fast-paced (>7.5-minute mile) running have been investigated and described by Pink et al.[27] Fast-paced running required averages of 31° maximum hip flexion at the end of middle swing and 11° maximum hip extension at toe off. Slower paced running required lower maximal ranges of hip flexion and extension than fast-paced running.

MUSCLE FUNCTION

Hip Extension

The hip extensor muscles are the gluteus maximus, semimembranosus, semitendinosus, biceps femoris, and adductor magnus.[28] The contribution of the five hip extensors in functional activities is partly determined by the position of the hip joint and the magnitude of the force required to perform hip extension. The hamstrings usually initiate the movement of hip extension[29] and the gluteus maximus contracts when the thigh moves beyond the anatomical position, into hyperextension, or when extension occurs against resistance.[29,30] The hamstrings produce motion at the hip and knee joints. According to Németh et al.,[31] the position of the knee has no effect on the strength of hip extension with the knee flexed between 0° and 90°. The adductor magnus acts as a hip extensor from 90° to 0° of hip flexion; its effect as a hip extensor is somewhat less in men in the final 30° of the extension motion as the anterior portion of the muscle becomes ineffective as an extensor.[28]

The action of the hip extensors is illustrated in activities where the body is raised,[32,33] such as getting up from sitting[34] (Fig. 6-105), climbing stairs (see Fig. 6-101), and jumping. The hip extensors contract in lifting activities performed with the knees and hips flexed[29,35,36] (see Fig. 7-38). The extensors control the forward movement of the pelvis when leaning forward in the sitting or standing positions and initiate and perform the posterior motion of the pelvis to sit or stand upright again.[18,35,37] The gluteus maximus contracts when one holds a crouch position[33] to change a car tire or look into a low cupboard.

In the standing position, thigh extension is performed by the hamstrings and when resistance is added to the movement the gluteus maximus assists to extend the hip.[30] Thus, the extensors contract to propel one forward when skating. The gluteus maximus contracts strongly to extend the thigh at the extreme of movement, as the hip is hyperextended.[29,33]

Hip Flexion

Iliacus and psoas major (often referred to as iliopsoas) are the primary flexors of the hip joint. Tensor fascia latae (anteromedial fibers),[38] rectus femoris, sartorius, gracilis, and the hip adductors assist the iliopsoas. The hip adductors assist in flexion when the hip is in an extended position.[18] Gracilis flexes the hip primarily in the initial stages of the motion[39] and with the knee in extension but not with the knee flexed.[30] The action of the adductors and gracilis in hip flexion is illustrated in the action of kicking

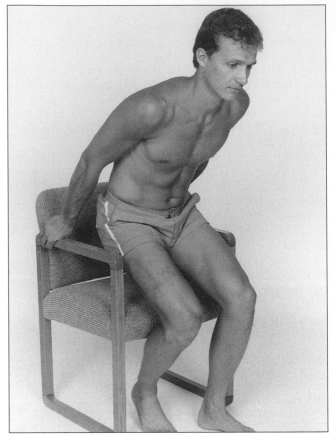

Figure 6-105. The hip extensors function when the body is raised when getting up from a chair.

a ball and swimming using the flutter kick. The action of sartorius as a hip flexor, abductor, external rotator, and knee flexor[40] is illustrated when positioning the foot across the thigh in sitting (see Fig. 6-103).

The iliopsoas is the only flexor effective in flexing the hip beyond 90° in the sitting position[18] in activities such as raising the lower limb to sit with the thighs crossed or with the foot on the opposite thigh (see Fig. 6-103) and pulling on a sock (see Fig. 7-41). The hip flexor muscles contract with the abdominals to raise the trunk when moving in bed from supine to sitting. The iliopsoas controls the movement of the trunk and pelvis as one leans backward in sitting[18] to look overhead or lowers the trunk to lie down in bed from a sitting position. Other activities that require contraction of the hip flexors include donning a pair of trousers (see Fig. 6-102), climbing a ladder, ascending stairs (see Fig. 6-101), and stepping in and out of the bathtub.

Hip Abduction

The muscles responsible for hip abduction are the gluteus medius, gluteus minimus, and tensor fascia latae. The upper fibers of the gluteus maximus assist with abduction when force is required.[41] The main function of the hip abductor muscles is to keep the pelvis level when one foot is off the ground. When standing on one leg, the hip joint of the supporting leg and the pelvis act as a first-class lever. The head of the femur represents the fulcrum and the pelvis the lever arm. With one foot off the ground the pelvis is unsupported and will drop down on the same side due to the torque created by the weight of the head, arms, trunk, and leg causing the pelvis to rotate around the head of the femur of the stance leg. The hip abductor muscles on the stance side contract with a reversed origin and insertion to pull the iliac crest (pelvis) down on the same side, causing the pelvis to rotate around the head of the femur and rise on the unsupported side. The pelvic leveling action of the hip abductors in single leg stance is illustrated in walking, running, and kicking a ball.

In single leg stance the hip abductors may not be required to contract to keep the pelvis level if the trunk is shifted over the supporting leg so that the line of gravity of the head, arms, and trunk falls through the hip joint.

If the pelvis is allowed to drop on the non–weight-bearing side when standing on one leg, the fascia latae and the iliotibial tract become taut on the weight-bearing side to maintain the posture of the pelvis and the hip abductors do not contract.[42]

The hip abductors may contract bilaterally in activities that require abduction of the non–weight-bearing extremity such as standing when mounting a bicycle (see Fig. 6-104) and karate (Fig. 6-106).

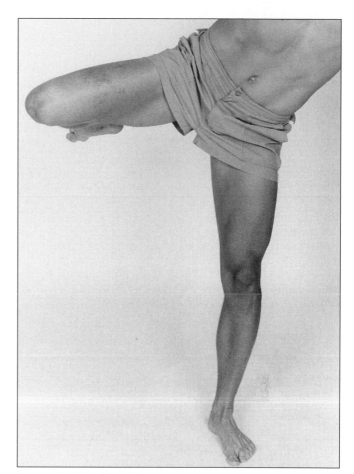

Figure 6-106.   Hip abductor muscle function.

Hip Adduction

Activities such as climbing a rope,[18] kicking a ball across the front of the body, and horseback riding require contraction of the hip adductors that includes the adductor magnus, adductor longus, adductor brevis, gracilis, and pectineus. Janda and Stara (cited in Basmajian and DeLuca[41]) suggest that the hip adductors function primarily as postural muscles in various activities rather than prime movers for hip adduction.

Hip Internal Rotation

The primary internal rotators of the hip include the tensor fascia latae, anterior fibers of the gluteus medius and minimus,[43] and the hip adductor muscles.[44,45] The semimembranosus and semitendinosus internally rotate the hip when the hip is in extension.[30] The internal rotators are active in walking or when pivoting on one foot in the standing position.[18]

Hip External Rotation

The piriformis, obturator internus, obturator externus, quadratus femoris, and gemellus superior and inferior, and sartorius externally rotate the hip joint. The piriformis and obturator internus function most effectively as external rotators when the thigh is extended and become less effective as the thigh is flexed.[43] The gluteus maximus and biceps femoris also rotate the hip externally when the hip is in extension.[30] Mounting a bicycle (see Fig. 6-104), performing karate (see Fig. 6-106), and positioning the foot across the opposite thigh to tie a shoelace (Fig. 6-107) require contraction of the external rotators of the hip.

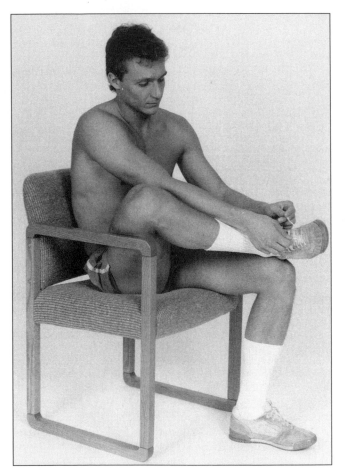

Figure 6-107. The hip external rotators contract to position the foot across the opposite thigh.

Standing Posture

The line of gravity shifts in relation to the hip joint and may pass either slightly anterior to, slightly posterior to, or through the hip joint in the sagittal plane.[46] Regardless of the exact location of the line of gravity, there is little muscular activity at the hip in symmetrical standing. Electromyography has shown no activity in the gluteus maximus, medius, and minimus in easy standing.[37] There appears to be variable activity in the iliopsoas muscles because Basmajian[47] recorded slight to moderate activity and Joseph and Williams[37] detected no activity in standing using electromyography.

Gait[48]

The hamstrings and gluteus maximus contract at the end of the swing phase and the beginning of the stance phase to decelerate the forward swinging extremity and to extend the hip at initial contact and loading response. The gluteus maximus inserts into the iliotibial band and as the muscle contracts it pulls the band posteriorly. The tensor fascia latae contracts at the beginning of the stance phase to prevent the posterior displacement of the iliotibial band. The hip abductors, gluteus medius and minimus, contract on the side of the weight-bearing extremity when the pelvis is unsupported on the contralateral side during the swing phase of the gait cycle. The contraction of the gluteus medius and minimus prevents the pelvis from dropping on the unsupported side during the swing phase. The hip flexors, iliopsoas and rectus femoris,[49] and tensor fascia latae contract at the end of the stance phase and early swing phase to initiate hip flexion. The activity of the hip adductors is variable, but these muscles are active during the swing phase of the gait cycle. The hip adductors contract to keep the extremity in the midline and may assist in maintaining hip flexion at the end of swing phase.[22]

Montgomery et al.[50] provide a description of the hip muscle activity during running.

REFERENCES

1. Kapandji IA. *The Physiology of the Joints.* Vol 2. 5th ed. New York: Churchill Livingstone; 1982.
2. Soames RW, ed. Skeletal system. Salmons S, ed. Muscle. *Gray's Anatomy.* 38th ed. New York: Churchill Livingstone; 1995.
3. Norkin CC, White DJ. *Measurement of Joint Motion: A Guide to Goniometry.* 2nd ed. Philadelphia: FA Davis; 1995.
4. Daniels L, Worthingham C. *Muscle Testing: Techniques of Manual Examination.* 5th ed. Philadelphia: WB Saunders; 1986.
5. Norkin CC, Levangie PK. *Joint Structure & Function: A Comprehensive Analysis.* Philadelphia: FA Davis; 1983.
6. Woodburne RT. *Essentials of Human Anatomy.* 5th ed. London: Oxford University Press; 1973.
7. Cyriax J. *Textbook of Orthopaedic Medicine, Vol 1. Diagnosis of Soft Tissue Lesions.* 8th ed. London: Bailliere Tindall; 1982.
8. Magee DJ. *Orthopedic Physical Assessment.* 3rd ed. Philadelphia: WB Saunders; 1997.
9. American Academy of Orthopaedic Surgeons. *Joint Motion: Method of Measuring and Recording.* Chicago: Author; 1965.
10. Bohannon RW. Cinematographic analysis of the passive straight-leg-raising test for hamstring muscle length. *Phys Ther.* 1982;62:1269–1274.
11. Bohannon R, Gajdosik R, LeVeau BF. Contribution of pelvic and lower limb motion to increases in the angle of passive straight leg raising. *Phys Ther.* 1985;65:474–476.
12. Göeken LN, Hof AtL. Instrumental straight-leg raising: results in healthy subjects. *Arch Phys Med Rehabil.* 1993;74:194–203.
13. Kendall FP, McCreary EK, Provance PG. *Muscles Testing and Function.* 4th ed. Baltimore: Williams & Wilkins; 1993.
14. Salter RB. *Textbook of Disorders and Injuries of the Musculoskeletal System.* 2nd ed. Baltimore: Williams & Wilkins; 1983.
15. Gose JC, Schweizer P. Iliotibial band tightness. *J Orthop Sports Phys Ther.* 1989;10:399–407.
16. Trombly CA. Evaluation of biomechanical and physiological aspects of motor performance. In: Trombly CA, ed. *Occupational Therapy for Physical Dysfunction.* 4th ed. Baltimore: Williams & Wilkins; 1995.
17. Carlsoo S, Fohlin L. The mechanics of the two-joint muscles rectus femoris, sartorius and tensor fascia latae in relation to their activity. *Scand J Rehabil Med.* 1969;1:107–111.
18. Smith LK, Weiss EL, Lehmkuhl LD. *Brunnstrom's Clinical Kinesiology.* 5th ed. Philadelphia: FA Davis; 1996.
19. Hoppenfeld S. *Physical Examination of the Spine and Extremities.* New York: Appleton-Century-Crofts; 1976.
20. Jarvis DK. Relative strength of the hip rotator muscle groups. *Phys Ther Rev.* 1952;32:500–503.
21. Cailliet R. *Low Back Pain Syndrome.* 2nd ed. Philadelphia: FA Davis; 1968.
22. Norkin CC, Levangie PK. *Joint Structure & Function: A Comprehensive Analysis.* 2nd ed. Philadelphia: FA Davis; 1992.
23. Johnston RC, Smidt GL. Hip motion measurements for selected activities of daily living. *Clin Orthop.* 1970;72:205–215.
24. Livingston LA, Stevenson JM, Olney SJ. Stairclimbing kinematics on stairs of differing dimensions. *Arch Phys Med Rehabil.* 1991;72:398–402.
25. Ikeda ER, Schenkman ML, Riley PO, Hodge WA. Influence of age on dynamics of rising from a chair. *Phys Ther.* 1991;71:473–481.
26. Johnston RC, Smidt GL. Measurement of hip-joint motion during walking: evaluation of an electrogoniometric method. *J Bone Joint Surg.* 1969;51A:1083–1094.
27. Pink M, Perry J, Houglum PA, Devine DJ. Lower extremity range of motion in the recreational sport runner. *Am J Sports Med.* 1994;22:541–549.
28. Németh G, Ohlsén H. In vivo moment arm lengths for hip extensor muscles at different angles of hip flexion. *J Biomech.* 1985;18:129–140.
29. Fischer FJ, Houtz SJ. Evaluation of the function of the gluteus maximus muscle. *Am J Phys Med.* 1968;47:182–191.
30. Wheatley MD, Jahnke WD. Electromyographic study of the superficial thigh and hip muscles in normal individuals. *Arch Phys Med.* 1951;32:508–515.
31. Németh G, Ekholm J, Arborelius UP, Harms-Ringdahl K, Schüldt K. Influence of knee flexion on isometric hip extensor strength. *Scand J Rehabil Med.* 1983;15:97–101.
32. Németh G, Ekholm J, Arborelius UP. Hip joint load and muscular activation during rising exercises. *Scand J Rehabil Med.* 1984;16:93–102.
33. Karlsson E, Jonsson B. Function of the gluteus maximus muscle. *Acta Morphol Neerl-Scand.* 1965;6:161–169.
34. Wretenberg P, Arborelius UP. Power and work produced in different leg muscle groups when rising from a chair. *Eur J Appl Physiol.* 1994;68:413–417.
35. Németh G, Ekholm J, Arborelius UP. Hip load moments and muscular activity during lifting. *Scand J Rehabil Med.* 1984;16:103–111.
36. Vakos JP, Nitz AJ, Threlkeld AJ, Shapiro R, Horn T. Electromyographic activity of selected trunk and hip muscles during a squat lift. *Spine.* 1994;19:687–695.
37. Joseph J, Williams PL. Electromyography of certain hip muscles. *J Anat.* 1957;91:286–294.
38. Paré EB, Stern JT, Schwartz JM. Functional differentiation within the tensor fasciae latae. *J Bone Joint Surg.* 1981;63A:1457–1471.
39. Jonsson B, Steen B. Function of the gracilis muscle. An electromyographic study. *Acta Morphol Neerl-Scand.* 1964;6:325–341.
40. Johnson CE, Basmajian JV, Dasher W. Electromyography of sartorius muscle. *Anat Rec.* 1972;173:127–130.
41. Basmajian JV, DeLuca CJ. *Muscles Alive: Their Functions Revealed by Electromyography.* 5th ed. Baltimore: Williams & Wilkins; 1985.
42. Inman VT. Functional aspects of the abductor muscles of the hip. *J Bone Joint Surg.* 1947;29:607–619.
43. Steindler A. *Kinesiology of the Human Body: Under Normal and Pathological Conditions.* Springfield, IL: Charles C Thomas; 1955.
44. Williams M, Wesley W. Hip rotator action of the adductor longus muscle. *Phys Ther Rev.* 1951;31:90–92.
45. Basmajian JV. *Muscles Alive: Their Functions Revealed by Electromyography.* 4th ed. Baltimore: Williams & Wilkins; 1978.
46. Soderberg GL. *Kinesiology: Application to Pathological Motion.* 2nd ed. Baltimore: Williams & Wilkins; 1997.
47. Basmajian JV. Electromyography of iliopsoas. *Anat Rec.* 1958;132:127–132.
48. Inman VT, Ralston HJ, Todd F. *Human Walking.* Baltimore: Williams & Wilkins; 1981.
49. Rab GT. Muscle. In: Rose J, Gamble JG, eds. *Human Walking.* 2nd ed. Baltimore: Williams & Wilkins; 1994.
50. Montgomery WH, Pink M, Perry J. Electromyographic analysis of hip and knee musculature during running. *Am J Sports Med.* 1994;22:272–278.

KNEE

▼ SURFACE ANATOMY (Fig. 7-1)

Structure	Location
1. Greater trochanter	With the tip of the thumb placed on the iliac crest at the midline and the tip of the third finger placed distally on the lateral aspect of the thigh, locates the superior border of the greater trochanter.
2. Patella	Large triangular sesamoid bone on the anterior aspect of the knee. The base is proximal and the apex distal.
3. Ligamentum patellae (patellar ligament or tendon)	Extends from the apex of the patella to the tibial tuberosity. As the patient attempts to extend the knee the edges of the tendon are palpable.
4. Tibial tuberosity	Bony prominence at the proximal end of the anterior border of the tibia and the insertion of the ligamentum patellae.
5. Tibial plateaus	The upper edges of the medial and lateral tibial plateaus are located in the soft tissue depressions on either side of the ligamentum patellae. Follow the plateau medially and laterally to ascertain the knee joint line.
6. Head of the fibula	A round bony prominence on the lateral aspect of the leg on a level with the tibial tuberosity.
7. Lateral malleolus	The prominent distal end of the fibula on the lateral aspect of the ankle.

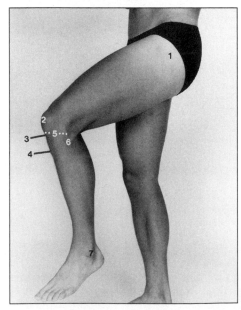

Figure 7-1. Anterolateral aspect of the lower limb.

ASSESSMENT PROCESS: THE KNEE

1. The therapist observes:
   a. Function
   b. Posture, body symmetry, atrophy, and skin condition
   c. Active range of motion (AROM) at the knee, the hip, and the ankle joints
2. The therapist assesses passive range of motion (PROM) by:
   a. Estimating joint PROM
   b. Determining the end feels at the joint
   c. Establishing the presence or absence of pain
   d. Determining the presence of a capsular or noncapsular pattern
3. The therapist measures PROM through goniometry.
4. The therapist assesses muscle strength through manual muscle testing.

TABLE
7-1

▼ JOINT STRUCTURE: KNEE MOVEMENTS

	Flexion	Extension	Internal Rotation	External Rotation
Articulation[1,2]	Femorotibial Femoropatellar	Femorotibial Femoropatellar	Femorotibial	Femorotibial
Plane	Sagittal	Sagittal	Horizontal	Horizontal
Axis	Frontal	Frontal	Longitudinal	Longitudinal
Normal limiting factors[1,3–6]	Tension in the rectus femoris (with the hip in extension); tension in the vasti muscles; soft tissue apposition of the posterior aspects of the calf and thigh or the heel and buttock	Tension in parts of both cruciate ligaments, the tibial and fibular collateral ligaments, the posterior aspect of the capsule, and the oblique posterior ligament	Tension in the cruciate ligaments[1]	Tension in the collateral ligaments[1]
Normal end feel[3,7,8]	Firm/soft	Firm	Firm	Firm
Normal AROM[9]	0–135°	135–0°	33°[10] total range (at 5° knee flexion)	
Capsular pattern[7,8]	Knee joint: flexion, extension			

▼ RANGE OF MOTION ASSESSMENT AND MEASUREMENT

The knee joint articulations and axes are illustrated in Figures 7-2 and 7-3. The joint structure is described in Table 7-1.

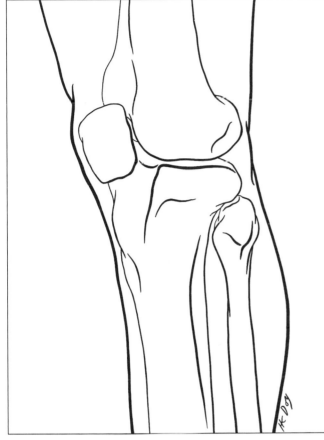

Figure 7-2.   Knee joint articulations.

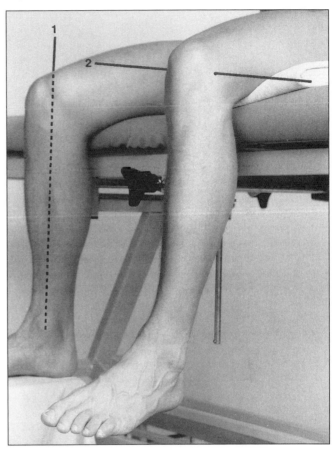

Figure 7-3.   Knee joint axes: (*1*) tibial internal external rotation; (*2*) flexion–extension.

KNEE FLEXION–EXTENSION

PROM Assessment

• **Start Position.** The patient is supine with the hip and knee in the anatomical position (Fig. 7-4). A towel is placed under the distal thigh.

• **Stabilization.** The pelvis is stabilized by the weight of the patient's body. The therapist stabilizes the femur.

• **Therapist's Distal Hand Placement.** The therapist grasps the distal tibia and fibula.

• **End Positions.** The therapist applies slight traction and moves the lower leg to flex the hip and knee (Fig. 7-5). Slight overpressure is applied at the limit of knee flexion.

The therapist applies slight traction and extends the knee, applying slight overpressure at the limit of knee extension/hyperextension (Fig. 7-6).

• **End Feels.** Flexion—firm/soft; extension/hyperextension—firm.

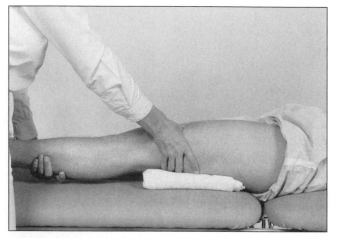

Figure 7-4.   Start position: knee flexion and extension or hyperextension.

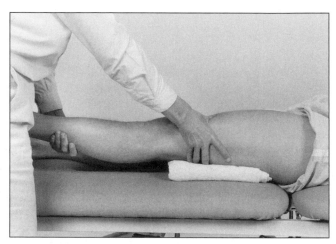

Figure 7-6.   Firm end feel at the limit of knee extension or hyperextension.

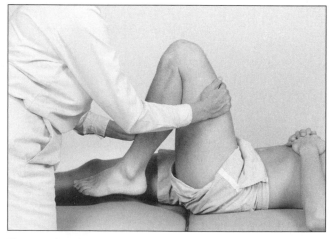

Figure 7-5.   Firm or soft end feel at the limit of knee flexion.

Measurement: Universal Goniometer

- **Start Position.** The patient is supine. The hip is in the anatomical position and the knee is in extension (0°) (Fig. 7-7). A towel is placed under the distal thigh.

- **Stabilization.** The pelvis is stabilized by the weight of the patient's body. The therapist stabilizes the femur.

- **Goniometer Axis.** The axis is placed over the lateral epicondyle of the femur.

- **Stationary Arm.** Parallel to the longitudinal axis of the femur, pointing toward the greater trochanter.

- **Movable Arm.** Parallel to the longitudinal axis of the fibula, pointing toward the lateral malleolus.

- **End Position.** From the start position of knee extension, the hip and knee are flexed (Fig. 7-8). The heel is moved toward the buttock to the limit of knee flexion (135°).

- **Hyperextension.** The femur is stabilized and the lower leg is moved in an anterior direction beyond 0° of extension (Fig. 7-9). Hyperextension from 0° to 10° may be present.

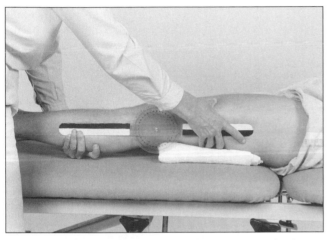

Figure 7-7. Start position: goniometer placement for knee flexion and extension/hyperextension.

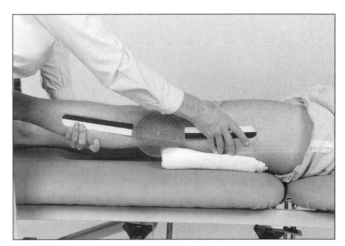

Figure 7-9. Knee hyperextension.

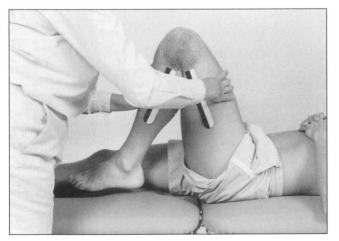

Figure 7-8. Knee flexion.

PATELLAR MOBILITY— DISTAL GLIDE

PROM Assessment

- Start Position. The patient is supine; a roll supports the knee joint in slight flexion (Fig. 7-10).

- Stabilization. The femur rests on the plinth.

- Procedure.[11] The heel of one hand is against the base of the patella with the forearm lying along the thigh. The other hand is placed on top and both hands move the patella in a distal direction to the end of the movement. Movement of the patella in a posterior direction compresses the patella against the femur and should be avoided. The therapist records whether the movement is full or restricted. The patella moves vertically a total of 8 cm from full flexion and to full extension of the knee.[12]

- End Feel. Firm.

PATELLAR MOBILITY— MEDIAL-LATERAL GLIDE

PROM Assessment

- Start Position. The patient is supine; a roll supports the knee joint in slight flexion (Fig. 7-11).

- Stabilization. The therapist stabilizes the femur and tibia.

- Procedure. The palmar aspects of the thumbs are placed on the lateral border of the patella. The pads of the index fingers are placed on the medial border of the patella. The thumbs move the patella medially and the index fingers move the patella laterally in a side-to-side motion. With the knee in extension, passive movement of the patella should average 9.6 mm medially and 5.4 mm laterally.[13] Excessive, normal, or restricted ROM is recorded.

- End Feel. Firm.

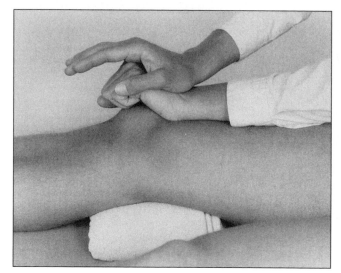

Figure 7-10.   Distal glide of the patella.

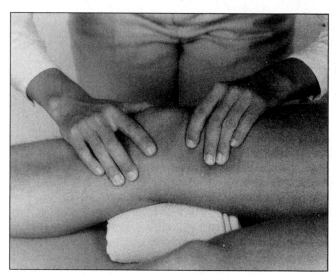

Figure 7-11.   Medial-lateral glide of the patella.

TIBIAL ROTATION

Tibial rotation is an essential component of normal ROM at the knee. Assessment of total rotation ROM is more reliable than assessment of internal and external tibial rotation because of the difficulty of defining the zero start position for the individual movements.[10] The greatest range of tibial rotation is available when the knee is flexed 90°.[14]

PROM Assessment

• **Start Position.** The patient is sitting, with the knee in 90° flexion and the tibia in full internal rotation (Fig. 7-12). A pad is placed under the distal thigh to maintain the thigh in a horizontal position.

• **Stabilization.** The therapist stabilizes the femur.

• **Procedure.** From full internal rotation, the therapist rotates the tibia externally through the full available ROM (Fig. 7-13). The total range of tibial rotation is observed (average total active range, about 58°[15]) and recorded as excessive, normal, or restricted.

• **End Feels.** Internal rotation—firm; external rotation—firm.

Measurement: OB Goniometer. The OB "Myrin" goniometer is used to measure tibial rotation ROM. Refer to Appendix A for a detailed description of the measurement technique using the OB "Myrin" goniometer.

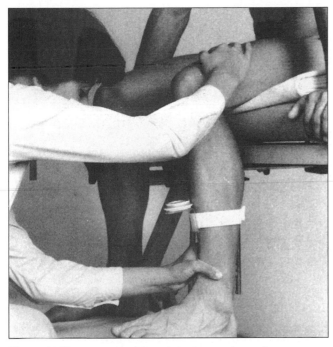

Figure 7-12.   Start position: tibial internal rotation.

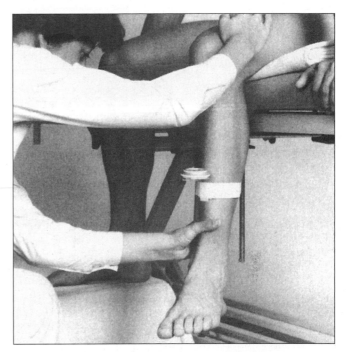

Figure 7-13.   End position: tibial external rotation.

Knee

MEASUREMENT OF MUSCLE LENGTH: HAMSTRINGS

• **Start Position.** The patient is sitting, grasps the edge of the plinth, and has the nontest foot supported on a stool (Fig. 7-14). A pad is placed under the distal thigh to maintain the thigh in a horizontal position. The ankle on the test side is relaxed in plantarflexion.

• **Stabilization.** The therapist stabilizes the femur.

• **Goniometer Placement.** The goniometer is placed the same as for knee flexion–extension.

• **End Position.** The knee is extended to the limit of motion so that hamstrings are put on full stretch (Fig. 7-15). The ankle is relaxed in plantarflexion throughout the test movement to prevent gastrocnemius muscle tightness from limiting knee ROM.

• **End Feel.** Hamstrings on stretch—firm.

• **Substitution/Trick Movement.** The patient leans back to posteriorly tilt the pelvis, extending the hip joint to place the hamstrings on slack and thus allow increased knee extension (Fig. 7-16).

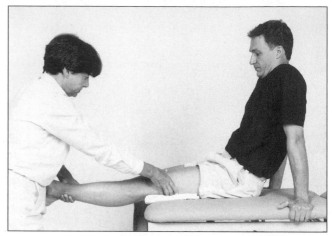

Figure 7-16.   Substitution/trick movement: backward lean during hamstrings length test.

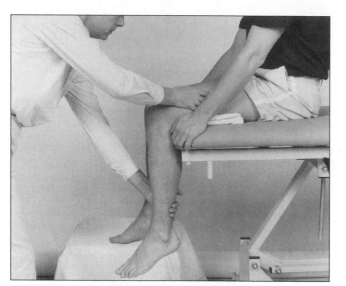

Figure 7-14.   Start position: length of hamstrings.

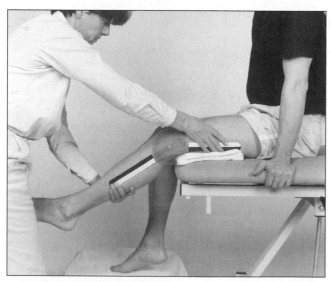

Figure 7-15.   Goniometer measurement: length of hamstrings.

MEASUREMENT OF MUSCLE LENGTH: RECTUS FEMORIS

- **Start Position.** The patient is prone. A towel is placed under the thigh to eliminate pressure on the patella. The leg is in the anatomical position with the knee in extension (0°) (Fig. 7-17).

- **Stabilization.** The therapist stabilizes the femur.

- **Goniometer Placement.** The goniometer is placed the same as for knee flexion-extension.

- **End Position.** The lower leg is moved in a posterior direction so that the heel approximates the buttock to the limit of knee flexion. Passive insufficiency of rectus femoris may restrict the range of knee flexion when the patient is prone (Fig. 7-18).

- **End Feel.** Rectus femoris on stretch—firm.

- **Substitution/Trick Movement.** The patient anteriorly tilts the pelvis and flexes the hip to place the rectus femoris on slack and thus allow increased knee flexion (Fig. 7-19).

- **Alternate Position**
- **Start Position.** The patient is supine near the end of the plinth and supports the hips and knees in flexion (Fig. 7-20).

- **Stabilization.** The patient maintains the nontest hip and knee in flexion to stabilize the pelvis in a posterior pelvic tilt. The therapist stabilizes the femur.

- **Goniometer Placement.** The goniometer is placed the same as for knee flexion-extension.

- **End Position.** The test leg is allowed to fall toward the plinth to the limit of movement. The knee is flexed to the limit of motion to put the rectus femoris on full stretch (Figs. 7-21 and 7-22).

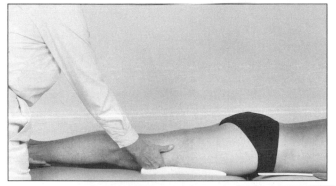

Figure 7-17.   Start position: length of rectus femoris.

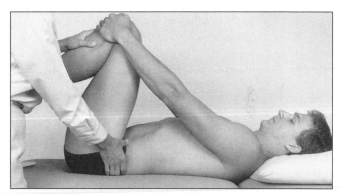

Figure 7-20.   Alternate start position: length of rectus femoris.

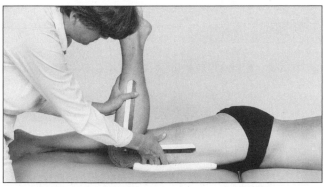

Figure 7-18.   Goniometer measurement: length of rectus femoris.

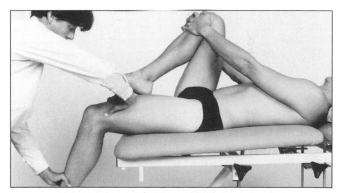

Figure 7-21.   End position: length of rectus femoris.

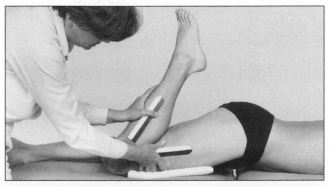

Figure 7-19.   Substitution/trick movement: anterior pelvic tilt and hip flexion placing rectus femoris on slack.

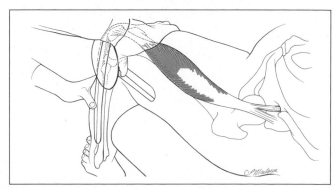

Figure 7-22.   Alternate goniometer measurement: length of rectus femoris.

KNEE

TABLE 7-2 ▼ MUSCLE ACTIONS, ATTACHMENTS, AND NERVE SUPPLY: THE KNEE[2]

Muscle	Primary Muscle Action	Muscle Origin	Muscle Insertion	Peripheral Nerve	Nerve Root
Hamstrings					
Semimembranosus	Knee flexion Internal rotation of the flexed knee	Superolateral aspect of the ischial tuberosity	Tubercle on the posterior aspect of the medial tibial condyle	Sciatic (tibial portion)	L5S12
Semitendinosus	Knee flexion Internal rotation of the flexed knee	Inferomedial impression on the superior aspect of the ischial tuberosity	Proximal part of the medial surface of the tibia	Sciatic (tibial portion)	L5S12
Biceps femoris	Knee flexion External rotation of the flexed knee	a. Long head: inferomedial impression of the superior aspect of the ischial tuberosity; lower portion of the sacrotuberous ligament b. Short head: lateral lip of the linea aspera and lateral supracondylar line	Head of the fibula; slip to the lateral condyle of the tibia; slip to the lateral collateral ligament	Sciatic (tibial and common peroneal portions)	L5S12
Quadriceps					
Vastus medialis	Knee extension	Lower part of the intertrochanteric line and the spiral line, medial lip of the linea aspera, proximal part of the supracondylar line, the adductor tendons of longus and magnus, and the intermuscular septum	Medial border of the patella, via the quadriceps tendon into the tibial tuberosity	Femoral	L234

Muscle	Primary Muscle Action	Muscle Origin	Muscle Insertion	Peripheral Nerve	Nerve Root
Vastus lateralis	Knee extension	Superior part of the intertrochanteric line, anterior and inferior borders of the greater trochanter, lateral lip of the gluteal tuberosity, and the upper half of the lateral lip of the linea aspera	Lateral border and base of the patella, via the quadriceps tendon into the tibial tuberosity	Femoral	L234
Vastus intermedius	Knee extension	Upper two thirds of the anterior and lateral surfaces of the femoral shaft	Base of the patella, via the quadriceps tendon into the tibial tuberosity	Femoral	L234
Rectus femoris	Hip flexion Knee extension	a. Straight head: anterior aspect of the anterior inferior iliac spinc b. Reflected head: groove above the acetabulum and the capsule of the hip joint	Base of the patella, via the quadriceps tendon into the tibial tuberosity	Femoral	L234

KNEE

KNEE FLEXION

Against Gravity: Biceps Femoris, Semitendinosus, and Semimembranosus

Accessory muscles: gastrocnemius, popliteus, gracilis, and sartorius.

Research[16, 17] appears to support the practice of testing the hamstrings as a group with the tibia positioned in neutral rotation and isolating the medial and lateral hamstrings by positioning the tibia in either internal or external rotation, respectively.

• **Start Position.** The patient is in the prone-lying position with a pillow under the abdomen (Fig. 7-23). The knee is in extension, the tibia is in neutral rotation, and the foot is over the end of the plinth. The rectus femoris may limit the range of knee flexion in the prone position.

• **Stabilization.** A pelvic strap stabilizes the pelvis. The therapist stabilizes the thigh.

• **Movement.** The patient flexes the knee through full ROM (Fig. 7-24).

• **Palpation.** Biceps femoris: proximal to the knee joint on the lateral margin of the popliteal fossa. Semitendinosus: proximal to the knee joint on the medial margin of the popliteal fossa. Semimembranosus: proximal to the knee joint on either side of the semitendinosus tendon.[18]

• **Substitution/Trick Movement.** Sartorius (producing hip flexion and external rotation) and gracilis (producing hip adduction).[4]

• **Resistance Location.** Applied proximal to the ankle joint on the posterior aspect of the leg (Fig. 7-25). Walmsley and Yang[19] found that with the hip at or near 0° a strong knee flexion contraction could not be performed beyond 90° because of discomfort. It is not uncommon to experience cramping of the hamstring muscles if too much resistance is applied as the knee moves into greater degrees of flexion.[20]

• **Resistance Direction.** Knee extension.

• **Isolation of the Medial Hamstrings.** The medial hamstrings (semitendinosus and semimembranosus) internally rotate the tibia during knee flexion. The patient holds the tibia in internal rotation and brings the heel toward the lateral aspect of the ipsilateral buttock (Figs. 7-26 and 7-27).

• **Resistance Direction.** Knee extension and tibial external rotation.

• **Isolation of the Lateral Hamstring.** The lateral hamstring (biceps femoris) externally rotates the tibia during knee flexion. The patient holds the tibia in external rotation and brings the heel toward the contralateral buttock (Figs. 7-28 and 7-29).

• **Resistance Direction.** Knee extension and tibial internal rotation.

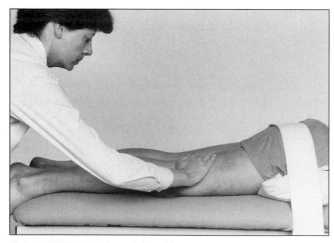

Figure 7-23.   Start position: biceps femoris, semitendinosus, and semimembranosus.

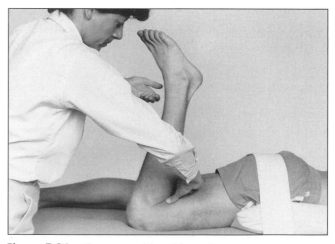

Figure 7-24.   Screen position: biceps femoris, semitendinosus, and semimembranosus.

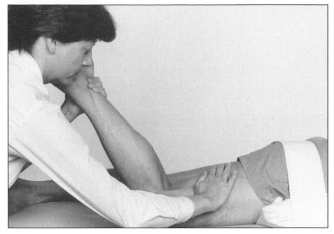

Figure 7-25. Resistance: biceps femoris, semitendinosus, and semimembranosus.

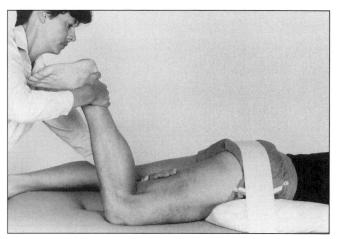

Figure 7-28. Resistance: biceps femoris.

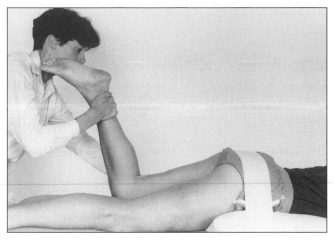

Figure 7-26. Resistance: semitendinosus and semimembranosus.

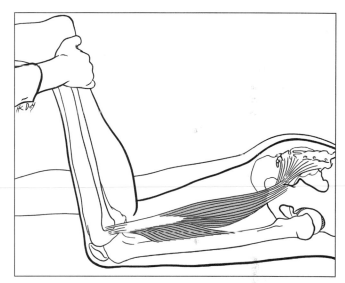

Figure 7-29. Biceps femoris.

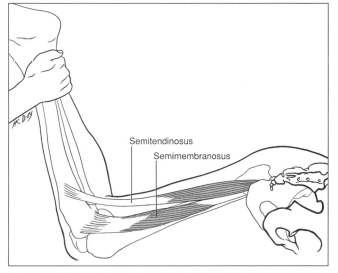

Semitendinosus
Semimembranosus

Figure 7-27. Semitendinosus and semimembranosus.

Gravity Eliminated: Biceps Femoris, Semitendinosus, and Semimembranosus

• **Start Position.** The patient is side lying on the nontest side (Fig. 7-30). The therapist supports the weight of the lower extremity. The hip is in anatomical position with the knee extended.

• **Stabilization.** The therapist stabilizes the thigh.

• **End Position.** The patient flexes the knee through full ROM (Fig. 7-31).

• **Substitution/Trick Movement.** Hip flexion resulting in passive knee flexion.

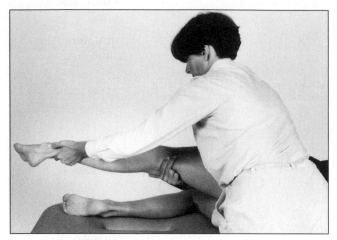

Figure 7-30. Start position: biceps femoris, semitendinosus, and semimembranosus.

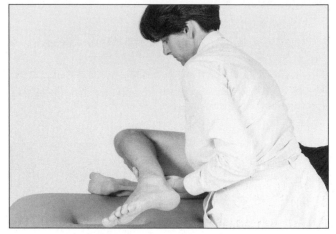

Figure 7-31. End position: biceps femoris, semitendinosus, and semimembranosus.

KNEE EXTENSION

Against Gravity: Rectus Femoris, Vastus Intermedius, Vastus Lateralis, and Vastus Medialis

• **Start Position.** The patient is sitting (Fig. 7-32). The knee is flexed and a pad is placed under the distal thigh to maintain the thigh in a horizontal position.

• **Stabilization.** The therapist stabilizes the thigh and the patient grasps the edge of the plinth.

• **Movement.** The patient extends the knee through full ROM (Fig. 7-33). If the hamstrings are tight, the patient may lean back to relieve the tension on the hamstrings during the movement. The patient may attempt to lean back during the test to place the rectus femoris muscle on stretch and increase the contribution from this muscle to produce knee extension.[18]

• **Palpation.** Rectus femoris: on the anterior midthigh. Vastus intermedius: too deep to palpate. Vastus lateralis: lateral aspect midthigh. Vastus medialis: distal medial aspect of the thigh. The quadriceps muscle group may be palpated proximal to the tibial tuberosity at the patellar tendon.

• **Substitution/Trick Movement.** Tensor fascia latae (observe internal rotation of the hip).[20]

• **Resistance Location.** Applied on the anterior surface of the distal end of the leg (Figs. 7-34 and 7-35). Ensure the patient does not lock the knee in full extension (close-packed position).

• **Resistance Direction.** Knee flexion.

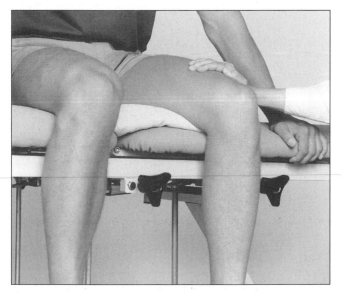

Figure 7-32.   Start position: rectus femoris, vastus intermedius, vastus lateralis, and vastus medialis.

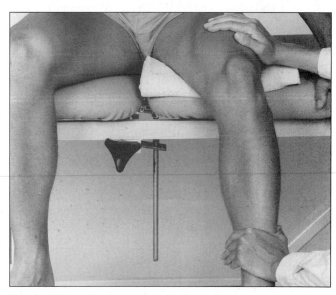

Figure 7-34.   Resistance: rectus femoris, vastus intermedius, vastus lateralis, and vastus medialis.

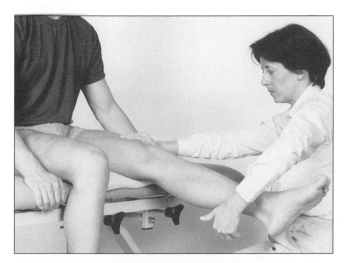

Figure 7-33.   Screen position: rectus femoris, vastus intermedius, vastus lateralis, and vastus medialis.

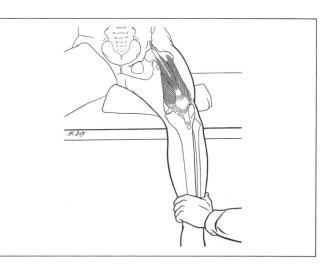

Figure 7-35.   Rectus femoris, vastus intermedius, vastus lateralis, and vastus medialis.

Knee

Gravity Eliminated: Rectus Femoris, Vastus Intermedius, Vastus Lateralis, and Vastus Medialis

• **Start Position.** The patient is side lying on the nontest side (Fig. 7-36). The therapist supports the weight of the lower extremity. The hip is in anatomical position with the knee flexed.

• **Stabilization.** The therapist stabilizes the thigh.

• **End Position.** The patient extends the knee through full ROM (Fig. 7-37).

• **Substitution/Trick Movement.** Hip extension from a flexed position can result in passive knee extension.[4]

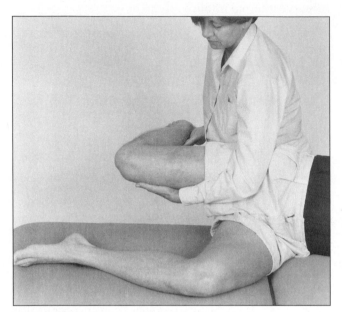

Figure 7-36.   Start position: rectus femoris, vastus intermedius, vastus lateralis, and vastus medialis.

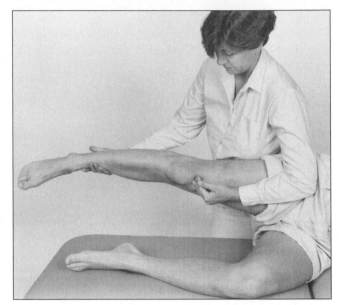

Figure 7-37.   End position: rectus femoris, vastus intermedius, vastus lateralis, and vastus medialis.

JOINT FUNCTION

The knee joint functions to support the body weight and to shorten or lengthen the lower limb.[14] Knee flexion with the foot planted lowers the body closer to the ground, whereas knee extension raises the body.[18] With the foot off the ground, foot orientation in space is provided[14] by flexing or extending the knee or rotating the tibia. The rotational mobility of the knee joint makes twisting movements of the body possible when the foot is planted on the ground.[18] In walking, the knee joint acts as a shock absorber, decreases the vertical displacement of the body, and through knee flexion shortens the lower limb to allow the toes to clear the ground during the swing phase of the gait cycle.[21,22]

FUNCTIONAL RANGE OF MOTION

The normal AROM at the knee is from 0° of extension to 135° of flexion. Although full extension is required for normal function, many daily activities require less than 135° of knee flexion. The fully extended (close-packed) position of the knee usually occurs in asymmetrical postures; for example, prolonged standing when one leg is used to support most of the body weight or when powerful thrusting motions[2] such as jumping are performed.

Daily activities involving ranges of knee motion up to an average of 117° of flexion include lifting an object off the floor (Fig. 7-38), sitting down in a chair (Fig. 7-39), climbing stairs (Fig. 7-40), and tying a shoelace[23] or pulling on a sock (Fig. 7-41). Many of the daily functions previously mentioned require on average less than 25° of tibial rotation.[23]

Livingston et al.[24] evaluated the knee flexion ROM required to ascend and descend three stairs of different dimensions. Depending on the stair dimensions, maximum knee flexion ROM requirements ranged between averages of 83° and 105° to ascend and 86° and 107° to descend the stairs. Minimum knee flexion ROM averages between 1° or 2° and 15° were required to ascend or descend stairs. It appears that changes of ROM at the knee joint, rather than the hip and ankle, are used to adjust to different stair dimensions.[24]

Gait

Walking requires an ROM from about 0° of knee extension as the leg advances forward to make initial contact with the ground to a maximum of about 60° of knee flexion at initial swing so that the foot clears the ground as the extremity is advanced forward (from the Rancho Los Amigos gait analysis forms as cited in Norkin and Levangie[14]). The tibia rotates internally on the femur at the end of the swing phase and maintains the position of internal rotation through the stance phase until preswing when the tibia externally rotates through to midswing.[25] An average of about 13° of tibial rotation is required for normal gait.[26] Refer to Appendix D for further description and illustrations of the positions and motions at the knee joint during gait.

Pink et al.[27] investigated and described the ROM requirement at the knee, for slow-paced (<8-minute mile) and fast-paced (>7.5-minute mile) running. Fast-paced running required a range of knee joint motion from an average of 11° flexion at terminal swing to an average 103° maximum knee flexion near the end of middle swing. Slower paced running required less flexion throughout most of the swing phase when compared to fast-paced running.

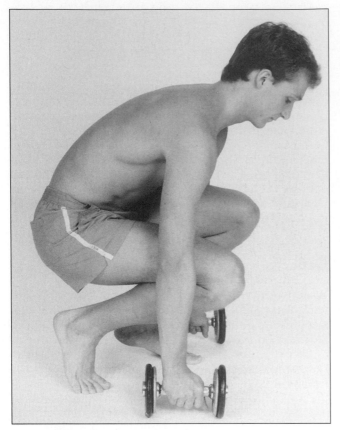

Figure 7-38. Lifting an object off the floor requires an average of 117° of knee flexion.[23]

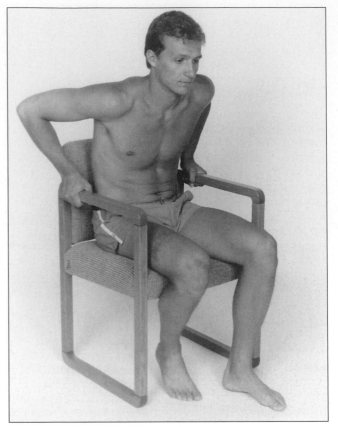

Figure 7-39. To sit down in a chair requires an average of 93° of knee flexion.[23]

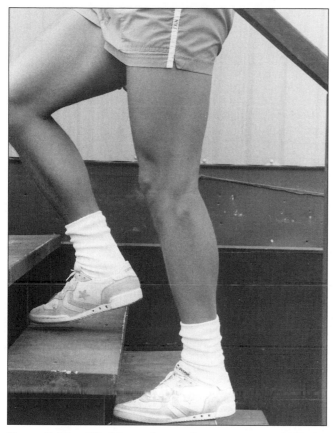

Figure 7-40. Climbing stairs requires an average of 83° of knee flexion.[23]

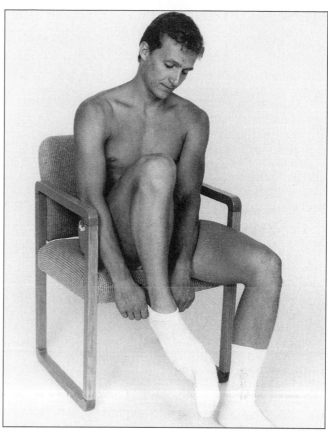

Figure 7-41. Knee range within the arc of 0° to 117° of flexion.

MUSCLE FUNCTION

Knee Flexors

The knee flexors include the biceps femoris, semitendinosus, semimembranosus, sartorius, gracilis, popliteus, and gastrocnemius. The popliteus and short head of biceps femoris are the only monoarticular knee flexors. The majority of the knee flexors are biarticular muscles and also produce movement at either the hip or ankle joints. With the exception of gastrocnemius, the knee flexors rotate the tibia. Biceps femoris contracts to externally rotate and flex the tibia on the femur. The other knee flexors internally rotate the tibia on the femur. The action of popliteus is negligible as a knee flexor, but the muscle functions to internally rotate the tibia on the femur,[28] contracting at the initiation of knee flexion to unlock the knee joint.[29] When loads are carried while walking downhill, popliteus activity is increased to stabilize the knee at midstance, from that of level or downhill walking.[30] When a crouch position is assumed, the popliteus contracts to prevent the forward displacement of the femur on the tibia[29] in activities such as squatting to pick up an object. The gastrocnemius flexes the knee joint and controls knee hyperextension.[12]

The action of the knee flexors is illustrated in sitting when the ankle is placed across the opposite thigh or when the legs are crossed at the ankles with the feet positioned under the chair. In standing, the knee flexors contract to allow one to inspect the sole of the foot. The flexors contract when knee flexion is forced at the end of the ROM, for example, when pulling on a sock. When walking or running, the knee flexors contract eccentrically to decelerate the leg as the knee extends to take a step forward. Activities such as ascending stairs do not require contraction of the knee flexors because the knee is flexed passively[12] due to active hip flexion. The knee flexors that function as rotators initiate and control knee rotation in activities such as running and turning.[18] These muscles are also active in squatting and kneeling when the trunk and upper extremities produce knee motions on the fixed tibia.[18]

Knee Extensors

The extensors of the knee are the rectus femoris, vastus medialis, vastus lateralis, and vastus intermedius. The rectus femoris acts at the hip and knee joints and is more effective as a knee extensor if the hip is extended and the muscle is placed on stretch.[5] Okamoto found that the hip must be stabilized for the rectus femoris to act fully as a knee extensor (cited in Basmajian and DeLuca[31]). The vastus medialis contracts with the other vasti muscles through the full ROM to perform knee extension.[32–35] The inferior oblique fibers of vastus medialis are thought to function at terminal extension to prevent the lateral displacement of the patella by drawing the patella medially.[31]

Two main patterns of movement occur in the lower limb during activities of daily living. One pattern includes hip flexion, knee flexion, and ankle dorsiflexion.[5]

In this pattern the knee extensors usually contract eccentrically to control knee flexion. This is illustrated in activities when the foot is fixed on the ground and the body is moved closer to the ground, such as squatting to lift an object off the floor, sitting down in a chair (see Fig. 7-39), and descending stairs (Fig. 7-42). The other common movement pattern of the lower limb consists of hip extension, knee extension, and ankle plantarflexion.[5] In this pattern the knee extensors normally contract concentrically to extend the knee joint. This synergy is illustrated when rising out of a chair, jumping, ascending stairs (see Fig. 7-40), and rising to get out of the bathtub.

When the foot is not fixed on the ground, the knee extensors contract when the knee is extended against resistance, including the weight of the leg. Kicking a ball, pulling on a pair of trousers, and swimming using the frog kick require contraction of the knee extensors.

Standing Posture

There is no contraction of the quadriceps in the standing position because the line of gravity tends to fall anterior to the knee joint. Using electromyography, Portnoy and Morin[36] found that the hamstrings and gastrocnemius muscles contract in standing. These muscles may function to prevent the knee from extending or hyperextending.[18]

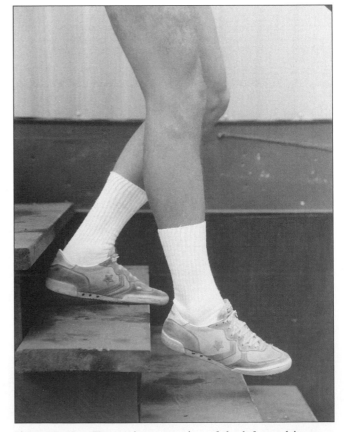

Figure 7-42. Eccentric contraction of the left quadriceps.

Gait

The knee extensors and flexors contract simultaneously to stabilize the knee in the extended position to prepare for initial contact.[37] During the first part of the stance phase, the quadriceps contract eccentrically to prevent knee flexion from occurring at initial contact and loading response as the weight is transferred to the limb. The quadriceps may or may not contract from loading response to midstance to extend the knee. At higher walking speeds, the quadriceps may contract to prevent excessive knee flexion and initiate knee extension at initial swing.[22] The hamstrings contract eccentrically at terminal swing to decelerate the forward-swinging limb.[37] The sartorius is active throughout the swing phase of the gait cycle, assisting with hip flexion required for toe clearance and external rotation of the hip as the pelvis rotates forward on the same side.[38] The gracilis contracts at the end of the stance phase and the beginning of the swing phase of the gait cycle.[39] The popliteus internally rotates the tibia on the femur and maintains this position from midswing through to preswing.[25]

Montgomery et al.[40] provide a description of the knee muscle activity during running.

REFERENCES

1. Kapandji IA. *The Physiology of the Joints.* Vol. 2. 2nd ed. New York: Churchill Livingstone; 1982.
2. Soames RW, ed. Skeletal system. Salmons S, ed. Muscle. *Gray's Anatomy.* 38th ed. New York: Churchill Livingstone; 1995.
3. Norkin CC, White DJ. *Measurement of Joint Motion: A Guide to Goniometry.* 2nd ed. Philadelphia: FA Davis; 1995.
4. Daniels L, Worthingham C. *Muscle Testing: Techniques of Manual Examination.* 5th ed. Philadelphia: WB Saunders; 1986.
5. Norkin CC, Levangie PK. *Joint Structure & Function: A Comprehensive Analysis.* Philadelphia: FA Davis; 1983.
6. Woodburne RT. *Essentials of Human Anatomy.* 5th ed. London: Oxford University Press; 1973.
7. Cyriax J. *Textbook of Orthopaedic Medicine, Vol. 1. Diagnosis of Soft Tissue Lesions.* 8th ed. London: Bailliere Tindall; 1982.
8. Magee DJ. *Orthopedic Physical Assessment.* 3rd ed. Philadelphia: WB Saunders; 1997.
9. American Academy of Orthopaedic Surgeons. *Joint Motion: Method of Measuring and Recording.* Chicago: Author; 1965.
10. Zarins B, Rowe CR, Harris BA, Watkins MP. Rotational motion of the knee. *Am J Sports Med.* 1983;11:152–156.
11. Kaltenborn FM. *Mobilization of the Extremity Joints: Examination and Basic Treatment Techniques.* 3rd ed. Oslo: Olaf Norlis Bokhandel; 1985.
12. Soderberg GL. *Kinesiology: Application to Pathological Motion.* 2nd ed. Baltimore: Williams & Wilkins; 1997.
13. Skalley TC, Terry GC, Teitge RA. The quantitative measurement of normal passive medial and lateral patellar motion limits. *Am J Sports Med.* 1993;21:728–732.
14. Norkin CC, Levangie PK. *Joint Structure & Function: A Comprehensive Analysis.* 2nd ed. Philadelphia: FA Davis; 1992.
15. Osternig LR, Bates BT, James SL. Patterns of tibial rotary torque in knees of healthy subjects. *Med Sci Sports Exerc.* 1980;12:195–199.
16. Fiebert IM, Haas JM, Dworkin KJ, LeBlanc WG. A comparison of medial versus lateral hamstring electromyographic activity and force output during isometric contractions. *Isokinetics and Exercise Science.* 1992;2:47–55.
17. Fiebert IM, Pahl CH, Applegate EB, Spielholz NI, Beernik K. Medial-lateral hamstring electromyographic activity during maximum isometric knee flexion at different angles. *Isokinetics and Exercise Science.* 1996;6:157–162.
18. Smith LK, Weiss EL, Lehmkuhl LD. *Brunnstrom's Clinical Kinesiology.* 5th ed. Philadelphia: FA Davis; 1996.
19. Walmsley RP, Yang JF. Measurement of maximum isometric knee flexor movement. *Physiother Can.* 1980;32:83–86.
20. Kendall FP, McCreary EK, Provance PG. *Muscles Testing and Function.* 4th ed. Baltimore: Williams & Wilkins; 1993.
21. Edelstein JE. Biomechanics of normal ambulation. *J Can Physiother Assoc.* 1965;17:174–185.
22. Inman VT, Ralston HJ, Todd F. *Human Walking.* Baltimore: Williams & Wilkins; 1981.
23. Laubenthal KN, Smidt GL, Kettelkamp DB. A quantitative analysis of knee motion during activities of daily living. *Phys Ther.* 1972;52:34–42.
24. Livingston LA, Stevenson JM, Olney SJ. Stairclimbing kinematics on stairs of differing dimensions. *Arch Phys Med Rehabil.* 1991;72:398–402.
25. Mann RA, Hagy JL. The popliteus muscle. *J Bone Joint Surg.* 1977;59A:924–927.
26. Kettelkamp DB, Johnson RJ, Smidt GL, Chao EYS, Walker M. An electrogoniometric study of knee motion in normal gait. *J Bone Joint Surg.* 1970;52A:775–790.
27. Pink M, Perry J, Houglum PA, Devine DJ. Lower extremity range of motion in the recreational sport runner. *Am J Sports Med.* 1994;22:541–549.
28. Basmajian JV, Lovejoy JF. Functions of the popliteus muscle in man. *J Bone Joint Surg.* 1971;53A:557–562.
29. Barnett CH, Richardson AT. The postural function of the popliteus muscle. *Ann Phys Med.* 1953;1:177–179.
30. Davis M, Newsam CJ, Perry J. Electromyograph analysis of the popliteus muscle in level and downhill walking. *Clin Orthop.* 1995;310:211–217.
31. Basmajian JV, DeLuca CJ. *Muscles Alive: Their Functions Revealed by Electromyography.* 5th ed. Baltimore: Williams & Wilkins; 1985.
32. Duarte Cintra AI, Furlani J. Electromyographic study of quadriceps femoris in man. *Electromyogr Clin Neurophysiol.* 1981;21:539–554.
33. Lieb FJ, Perry J. Quadriceps function. *J Bone Joint Surg.* 1971;53A:749–758.
34. Signorile JF, Kacsik D, Perry A, et al. The effect of knee and foot position on the electromyographical activity of the superficial quadriceps. *J Orthop Sports Phys Ther.* 1995;22:2–9.
35. Salzman A, Torburn L, Perry J. Contribution of rectus femoris and vasti to knee extension. *Clin Orthop.* 1993;290:236–243.
36. Portnoy H, Morin F. Electromyographic study of postural muscles in various positions and movements. *Am J Physiol.* 1956;186:122–126.
37. Rab GT. Muscle. In: Rose J, Gamble JG, eds. *Human Walking.* 2nd ed. Baltimore: Williams & Wilkins; 1994.
38. Johnson CE, Basmajian JV, Dasher W. Electromyography of sartorius muscle. *Anat Rec.* 1972;173:127–130.
39. Jonsson B, Steen B. Function of the gracilis muscle: an electromyographic study. *Acta Morphol Neerl-Scand.* 1964;6:325–341.
40. Montgomery WH, Pink M, Perry J. Electromyographic analysis of hip and knee musculature during running. *Am J Sports Med.* 1994;22:272–278.

KNEE

ANKLE AND FOOT

▼ **SURFACE ANATOMY** (Figs. 8-1 and 8-2)

Structure	Location
1. Head of the fibula	Round bony prominence on the lateral aspect of the leg level with the tibial tuberosity.
2. Anterior border of the tibia	Subcutaneous bony ridge along the anterior aspect of the leg.
3. Achilles tendon	Prominent ridge on the posterior aspect of the ankle; tendon edges are palpable proximal to the posterior aspect of the calcaneus.
4. Medial malleolus	Prominent distal end of the tibia on the medial aspect of the ankle.
5. Lateral malleolus	Prominent distal end of the fibula on the lateral aspect of the ankle.
6. Tuberosity of the navicular bone	About 2.5 cm inferior and anterior to the medial malleolus.
7. Base of the fifth metatarsal bone	Small bony prominence at the midpoint of the lateral border of the foot.
8. Head of the first metatarsal	Round bony prominence at the medial aspect of the ball of the foot, at the base of the great toe.
9. Calcaneus	Posterior aspect of the heel.

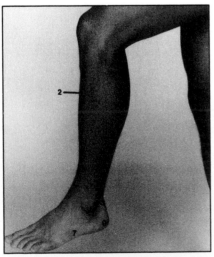

Figure 8-1. **Anterolateral aspect of the leg and foot.**

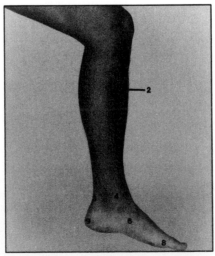

Figure 8-2. **Medial aspect of the leg and foot.**

▼ ASSESSMENT PROCESS: THE ANKLE AND FOOT

1. The therapist observes:
   a. Function
   b. Posture, body symmetry, atrophy, and skin condition
   c. Active range of motion (AROM) at the ankle, toes, and knee joints
2. The therapist assesses passive range of motion (PROM) by:
   a. Estimating joint PROM
   b. Determining the end feels at the joint
   c. Establishing the presence or absence of pain
   d. Determining the presence of a capsular or noncapsular pattern
3. The therapist measures PROM through goniometry.
4. The therapist assesses muscle strength through manual muscle testing.

TABLE
8-1 ▼ JOINT STRUCTURE: ANKLE AND FOOT MOVEMENTS

	Plantarflexion	Dorsiflexion	Inversion	Eversion
Articulation[1,2]	Talocrural	Talocrural	Subtalar	Subtalar
Plane	Oblique sagittal	Oblique sagittal	Oblique frontal	Oblique frontal
Axis	Oblique frontal	Oblique frontal	Oblique sagittal	Oblique sagittal
Normal limiting factors[1,3–6]	Tension in the anterior joint capsule, anterior portion of the deltoid, anterior talofibular ligaments, and the ankle dorsiflexors; contact between the talus and the tibia	Tension in the posterior joint capsule, the deltoid, calcaneofibular and posterior talofibular ligaments, and the ankle plantar flexors; contact between the talus and the tibia	Tension in the lateral collateral ligament, ankle evertors, talocalcaneal ligaments, and the lateral joint capsule	Contact between the talus and calcaneus; tension in the medial joint capsule, medial collateral ligaments, medial talocalcaneal ligament, tibialis posterior, flexor hallucis longus and flexor digitorum longus
Normal end feel[3,7,8]	Firm/hard	Firm/hard	Firm	Hard/firm
Normal AROM[9]	0–50°	0–20°	0–5° (forefoot 0–35°)	0–5° (forefoot 0–15°)
Capsular pattern[7,8]	Talocrural joint: plantarflexion, dorsiflexion Subtalar joint: varus (ie, inversion), valgus (ie, eversion)			

▼ RANGE OF MOTION ASSESSMENT AND MEASUREMENT

The joint articulations and axes of the ankle, foot, and toes are illustrated in Figures 8-3, 8-4, and 8-5. The structure of the joints is described in Tables 8-1 and 8-2.

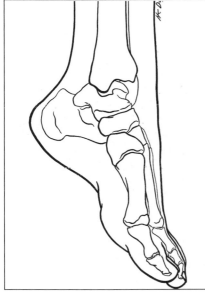

Figure 8-3. Ankle and foot articulations.

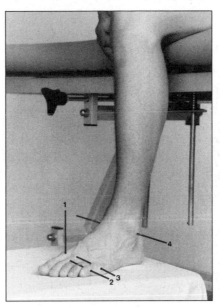

Figure 8-4. Ankle and foot axes: (*1*) metatarsophalangeal (MTP) joint abduction-adduction; (*2*) interphalangeal (IP) joint flexion-extension; (*3*) MTP joint flexion-extension; (*4*) talocrural joint dorsiflexion-plantarflexion.

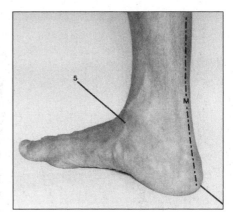

Figure 8-5. Subtalar joints axis: (*5*) inversion-eversion (*M*, midline of leg and heel).

TABLE
8-2 ▼ JOINT STRUCTURE: TOE MOVEMENTS

		Flexion	Extension	Abduction	Adduction
	Articulation[1,2]	Metatarsophalangeal (MTP), proximal interphalangeal (PIP), distal interphalangeal (DIP) (second to fifth toes)	MTP PIP DIP	MTP	MTP
	Plane	Sagittal	Sagittal	Horizontal	Horizontal
	Axis	Frontal	Frontal	Vertical	Vertical
	Normal limiting factors[1,3–6]	MTP: tension in the dorsal joint capsule, extensor muscles, collateral ligaments PIP: soft tissue apposition between the plantar aspects of the phalanges; tension in the dorsal joint capsule, collateral ligaments DIP: tension in the dorsal joint capsule, collateral ligaments and oblique retinacular ligaments	MTP: tension in the plantar joint capsule, plantar ligament, flexor muscles PIP: tension in the plantar joint capsule, plantar ligament DIP: tension in the plantar joint capsule, plantar ligament	Tension in the medial joint capsule, collateral ligaments, adductor muscles, fascia and skin between the web spaces, and the plantar interosseous muscles	Contact between the toes
	Normal end feel[3,7,8]	MTP firm PIP soft/firm DIP firm	MTP firm PIP firm DIP firm	Firm	
	Normal AROM[9]	Great toe MTP 0–45° IP 0–90° Toes 2–5 MTP 0–40° PIP 0–35° DIP 0–60°	MTP 0–70° IP 0° MTP 0–40° IP 0°		
	Capsular pattern[7,8]	First MTP joint: extension, flexion Second to fifth MTP joints: variable, tend to fix in extension with the interphalangeal (IP) joints in flexion			

ANKLE DORSIFLEXION AND PLANTARFLEXION

PROM Assessment

Ankle Dorsiflexion

• **Start Position.** The patient is supine. A roll is placed under the knee to position the knee in slight flexion and place the gastrocnemius on slack (Fig. 8-6A). The ankle is in the anatomical or neutral position with the foot perpendicular to the lower leg (Fig. 8-6B).

• **Stabilization.** The therapist stabilizes the tibia and fibula.

• **Therapist's Distal Hand Placement.** The therapist grasps the posterior aspect of the calcaneus and places the forearm against the plantar aspect of the forefoot.

• **End Position.** The therapist applies traction to the calcaneus and using the forearm moves the dorsal aspect of the foot toward the anterior aspect of the lower leg to the limit of ankle dorsiflexion (Fig. 8-7).

• **End Feel.** Dorsiflexion—firm/hard.

Ankle Plantarflexion

• **Start Position.** The patient is supine, a roll is placed under the knee and the ankle is in the neutral position (Fig. 8-8).

• **Stabilization.** The therapist stabilizes the tibia and fibula.

• **Therapist's Distal Hand Placement.** The therapist grasps the dorsum of the foot with the radial border of the index finger over the anterior aspects of the talus and calcaneus.

• **End Position.** The therapist applies slight traction to and moves the talus and calcaneus in a downward direction to the limit of ankle plantarflexion (Fig. 8-9).

• **End Feel.** Plantarflexion—firm/hard.

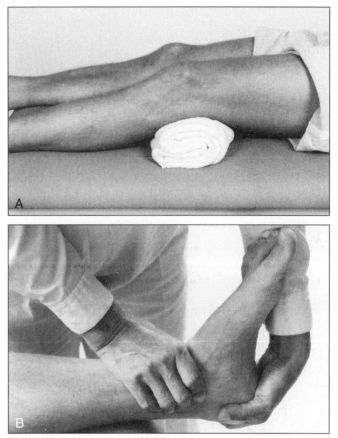

Figure 8-6. (*A*) Position of knee in slight flexion for assessment of ankle dorsiflexion. (*B*) Start position: ankle dorsiflexion.

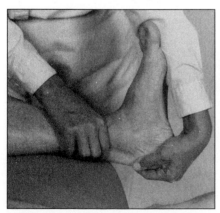

Figure 8-7. Firm or hard end feel at the limit of ankle dorsiflexion.

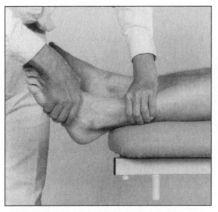

Figure 8-8. Start position: ankle plantarflexion.

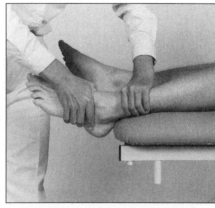

Figure 8-9. Firm or hard end feel at the limit of ankle plantarflexion.

Measurement: Universal Goniometer

Ankle Dorsiflexion and Plantarflexion

• **Start Position.** The patient is supine with a roll placed under the knee to maintain about 20° to 30° knee flexion and place the gastrocnemius on slack (Fig. 8-10). The ankle is in the anatomical position 0°. Alternatively, the patient may be sitting with the knee flexed to 90° and the ankle in anatomical position (Fig. 8-11).

• **Stabilization.** The therapist stabilizes the tibia and fibula.

• **Goniometer Axis.** The axis is placed inferior to the lateral malleolus. This measurement may also be obtained by placing the axis inferior to the medial malleolus (not shown).

• **Stationary Arm.** Parallel to the longitudinal axis of the fibula.

• **Movable Arm.** Parallel to the sole of the heel, to eliminate forefoot movement from the measurement. In the start position described, the goniometer will indicate 90°. This is recorded as 0°. For example, if the goniometer reads 90° at the start position for ankle dorsiflexion and 100° at the end position, ankle dorsiflexion PROM would be 10°.

• **End Positions.** Dorsiflexion (Fig. 8-12): The ankle is flexed with the dorsal aspect of the foot approximating the anterior aspect of the lower leg (20°). Plantarflexion (Fig. 8-13): The ankle is extended to the limit of motion (50°).

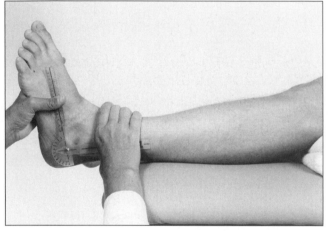

Figure 8-10.   Start position for ankle dorsiflexion and plantarflexion.

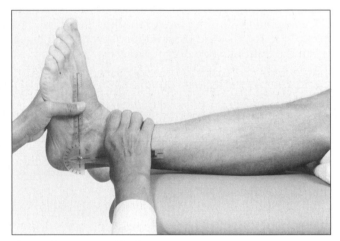

Figure 8-12.   Dorsiflexion.

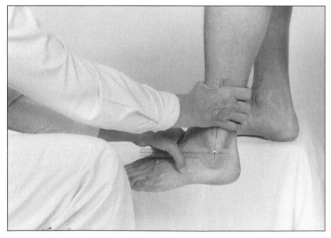

Figure 8-11.   Alternate start position for ankle dorsiflexion and plantarflexion.

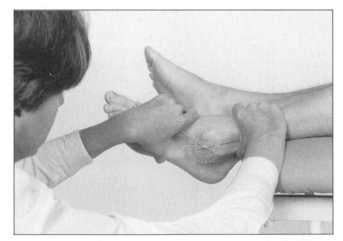

Figure 8-13.   Plantarflexion.

FOOT INVERSION AND EVERSION

PROM Assessment

• **Start Position.** The patient is supine. The ankle is in the neutral position (Fig. 8-14).

• **Stabilization.** The therapist stabilizes the talus immediately anterior and inferior to the medial and lateral malleoli.

• **Therapist's Distal Hand Placement.** The therapist grasps the posterior aspect and sides of the calcaneus.

• **End Positions.** The therapist applies slight traction to the calcaneus and moves the calcaneus inward to the limit of inversion (Fig. 8-15) and outward to the limit of eversion (Fig. 8-16).

• **End Feels.** Inversion—firm; eversion—firm/hard.

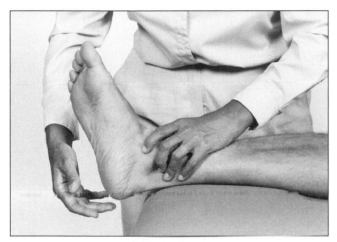

Figure 8-14.   Start position: inversion and eversion.

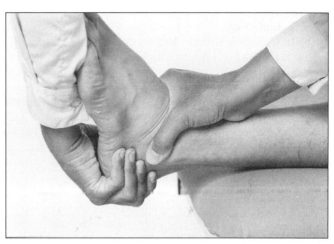

Figure 8-16.   Firm or hard end feel at the limit of eversion.

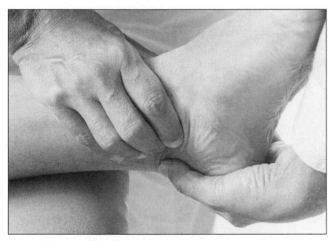

Figure 8-15.   Firm end feel at the limit of inversion.

Measurement: Universal Goniometer

• **Start Position.** The patient is supine (Fig. 8-17). A roll is placed under the knee to maintain slight flexion. The ankle is in the neutral position. A piece of paper, adhered to a flat surface, is placed under the heel. A flat-surfaced object (plexiglass or book) is placed against the full sole of the foot. A line is drawn along the plexiglass or book as shown in Figure 8-17.

• **Stabilization.** The therapist stabilizes the tibia and fibula.

• **End Positions.** The foot is placed in inversion to the limit of motion (Fig. 8-18). The plexiglass is again positioned against the full sole of the foot in this position and a line is again drawn along the plexiglass (Fig. 8-19). The process is repeated at the limit of eversion ROM (Figs. 8-20 and 8-21).

• **Goniometer Axis and Arms.** The goniometer is placed on the line graphics to obtain a measure of the arc of movement (Figs. 8-22 and 8-23).

Alternate Measurement

• **Start Position.** The patient is prone with the feet off the end of the plinth and the ankle in the neutral position. For alignment of the goniometer, the therapist marks the skin over the midlines of the superior aspect of the calcaneus posteriorly, and the inferior aspect of the heel pad posteriorly (Fig. 8-24A).

• **Stabilization.** The therapist stabilizes the tibia and fibula.

• **Goniometer Axis.** The axis is placed over the mark placed at the midline of the superior aspect of the calcaneus (Fig. 8-24B).

• **Stationary Arm.** Parallel to the longitudinal axis of the lower leg.

• **Movable Arm.** Lies along the midline of the posterior aspect of the calcaneus. Use the mark on the heel pad posteriorly to assist in maintaining alignment of the movable arm.

• **End Positions.** The calcaneus is inverted (Fig. 8-25) and then everted (Fig. 8-26) to the limits of motion.

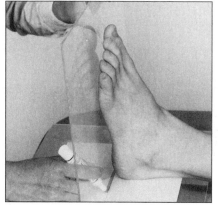

Figure 8-17. Start position for foot inversion and eversion.

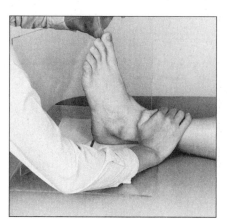

Figure 8-18. Placement of the foot in inversion.

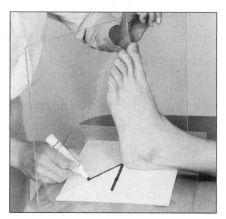

Figure 8-19. Inversion.

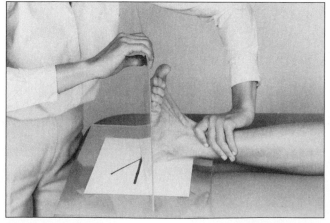

Figure 8-20. Placement of the foot in eversion.

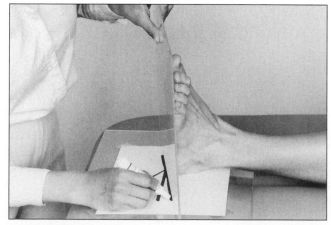

Figure 8-21. Eversion.

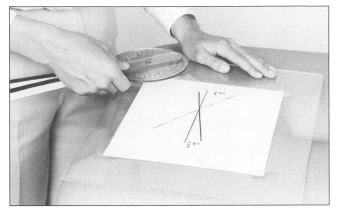

Figure 8-22. Completed measurement of inversion and eversion.

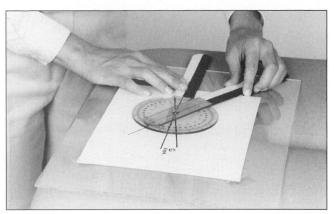

Figure 8-23. Goniometer placement for measurement of inversion.

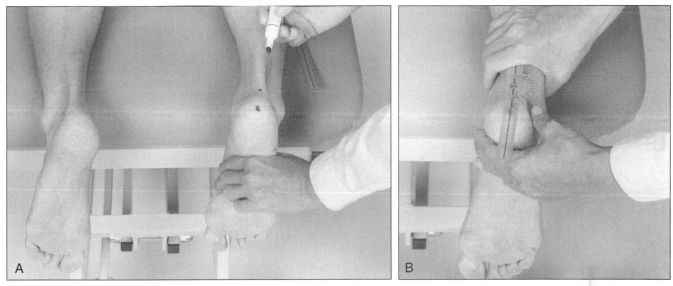

Figure 8-24. (*A*) Alternate measurement for inversion and eversion. Points marked for alignment of goniometer. (*B*) Goniometer alignment: inversion and eversion.

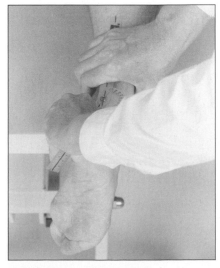

Figure 8-25. End position: measurement of inversion.

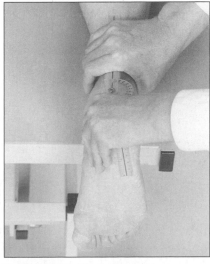

Figure 8-26. End position: measurement of eversion.

METATARSOPHALANGEAL JOINT FLEXION AND EXTENSION

PROM Assessment

• **Start Position.** The patient is supine. The ankle and toes are in the neutral position (Fig. 8-27).

• **Stabilization.** The therapist stabilizes the metatarsal of the MTP joint being assessed.

• **Therapist's Distal Hand Placement.** The therapist grasps the proximal phalanx.

• **End Positions.** The therapist applies slight traction to and moves the proximal phalanx to the limit of MTP joint flexion (Fig. 8-28) and MTP joint extension (Fig. 8-29).

• **End Feels.** MTP joint flexion—firm; MTP joint extension—firm.

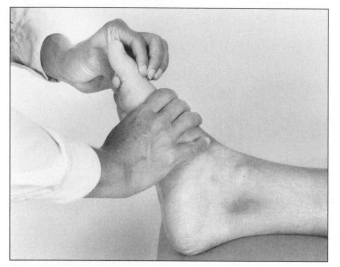

Figure 8-27. Start position: MTP joint flexion and extension.

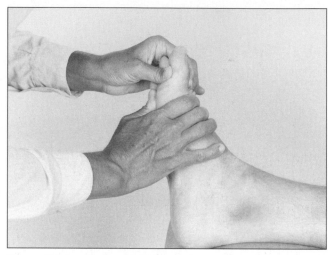

Figure 8-29. Firm end feel at limit of MTP joint extension of the great toe.

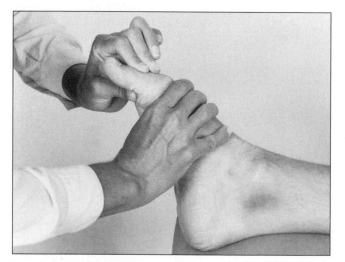

Figure 8-28. Firm end feel at limit of MTP joint flexion of the great toe.

Measurement: Universal Goniometer

- **Start Position.** The patient is supine or sitting. The ankle and toes are in the neutral position (Fig. 8-30).

- **Stabilization.** The therapist stabilizes the metatarsal of the MTP joint being measured.

- **Goniometer Axis.** The axis is placed over the dorsum of the MTP joint of the toe being measured. Alternatively, the axis can be placed over the medial or lateral aspect of the great and fifth toes, respectively.

    For MTP joint extension the goniometer is placed either along the sides of the joint as in measuring MTP joint flexion, or on the plantar aspect of the MTP joint being measured.

- **Stationary Arm.** Parallel to the longitudinal axis of the metatarsal of the toe being measured.

- **Movable Arm.** Parallel to the longitudinal axis of the proximal phalanx of the toe being measured.

- **End Positions.** The MTP joint is flexed to the limit of motion (45° for the great toe (Fig. 8-31) and 40° for the lateral four toes). The MTP joint of the toe being measured is extended to the limit of motion (70° for the great toe (Fig. 8-32); 40° for the lateral four toes).

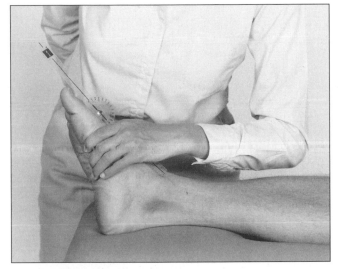

Figure 8-30.   Start position for MTP flexion.

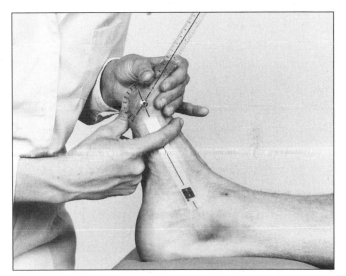

Figure 8-32.   MTP extension of the great toe.

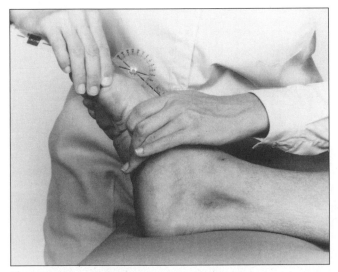

Figure 8-31.   MTP flexion of the great toe.

METATARSOPHALANGEAL JOINT ABDUCTION AND ADDUCTION OF THE GREAT TOE

PROM Assessment (MTP Joint Abduction)

• **Start Position.** The patient is supine. The ankle and great toe are in the neutral position.

• **Stabilization.** The therapist stabilizes the first metatarsal.

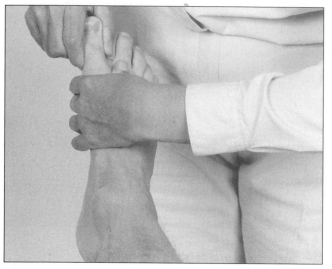

Figure 8-33.   Firm end feel at limit of MTP abduction.

• **Therapist's Distal Hand Placement.** The therapist grasps the proximal phalanx of the great toe.

• **End Position.** The therapist applies slight traction to and moves the proximal phalanx to the limit of MTP joint abduction (Fig. 8-33).

• **End Feel.** MTP joint abduction—firm.

Measurement: Universal Goniometer

• **Start Position.** The patient is supine or sitting. The ankle and toes are in the neutral position (Fig. 8-34).

• **Stabilization.** The therapist stabilizes the first metatarsal and the foot proximal to the MTP joint.

• **Goniometer Axis.** The axis is placed on the dorsum of the first MTP joint.

• **Stationary Arm.** Parallel to the longitudinal axis of the first metatarsal.

• **Movable Arm.** Parallel to the longitudinal axis of the proximal phalanx.

• **End Positions.** The MTP joint is abducted to the limit of motion (Fig. 8-35) and adducted to the limit of motion (Fig. 8-36).

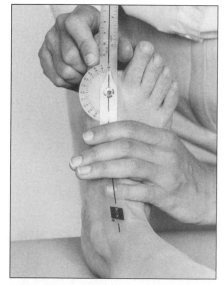

Figure 8-34.   Start position for MTP abduction and adduction.

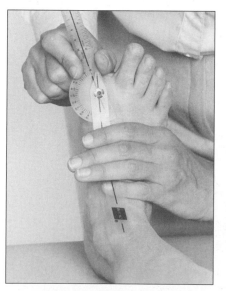

Figure 8-35.   MTP abduction.

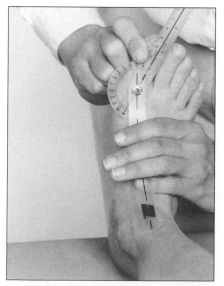

Figure 8-36.   MTP adduction.

INTERPHALANGEAL JOINT FLEXION/EXTENSION OF THE GREAT TOE

PROM Assessment

• **Start Position.** The patient is supine. The ankle and great toe are in the neutral position.

• **Stabilization.** The therapist stabilizes the proximal phalanx of the great toe.

• **Therapist's Distal Hand Placement.** The therapist grasps the distal phalanx of the great toe.

• **End Positions.** The therapist applies slight traction to and moves the distal phalanx to the limit of IP joint flexion (Fig. 8-37) and IP joint extension (Fig. 8-38).

• **End Feels.** IP joint flexion—soft or firm; IP joint extension—firm.

Measurement: Universal Goniometer

• **Start Position.** The patient is supine or sitting. The ankle and toes are in the neutral position (Fig. 8-39).

• **Stabilization.** The therapist stabilizes the proximal phalanx.

• **Goniometer Axis.** The axis is placed over the dorsal aspect of the IP joint for flexion and the plantar aspect of the IP joint for extension (not shown).

• **Stationary Arm.** Parallel to the longitudinal axis of the proximal phalanx.

• **Movable Arm.** Parallel to the longitudinal axis of the distal phalanx.

• **End Positions.** The IP joint is flexed to the limit of motion (90° for the great toe) (Fig. 8-40). The IP joint is extended to the limit of motion (0° for the great toe; not shown).

Flexion/extension of the lesser four toes is not measured using a universal goniometer. Flexion/extension of these toes is observed and ROM is recorded as either full or decreased (not shown).

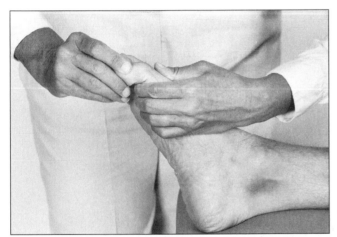

Figure 8-37. Soft or firm end feel at limit of IP joint flexion.

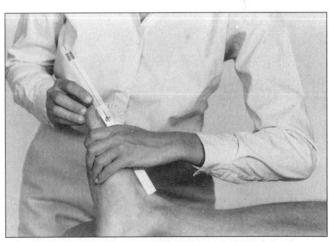

Figure 8-39. Start position for great toe IP flexion.

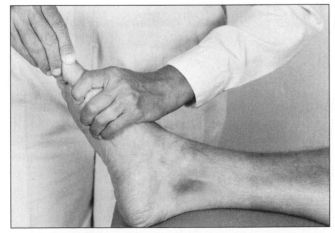

Figure 8-38. Firm end feel at limit of IP joint extension.

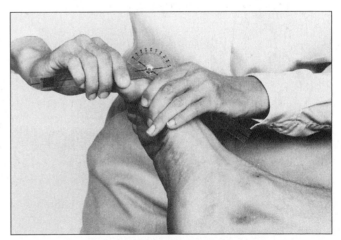

Figure 8-40. IP flexion of the great toe.

MEASUREMENT OF MUSCLE LENGTH: GASTROCNEMIUS

• **Start Position.** The patient is standing erect with the lower extremity in the anatomical position. The patient is positioned facing a plinth or wall.

• **End Position.** The patient leans forward to place the hands on the plinth or wall and places the nontest leg ahead of the test leg (Fig. 8-41). The patient is instructed to maintain the foot on the test side flat on the floor, with the toes pointing forward, and to keep the knee straight as the leg moves over the foot. The gastrocnemius is placed on full stretch as the patient leans closer toward the supporting surface.

• **Measurement.** If the gastrocnemius is shortened, ankle dorsiflexion ROM will be restricted proportional to the decrease in muscle length. The therapist measures and records the available ankle dorsiflexion PROM. The goniometer is placed as described for measuring ankle dorsiflexion ROM (Figs. 8-42 and 8-43). The patient may flex the knee during the test to place the gastrocnemius on slack. The knee must be maintained in extension.

Alternate Test

• **Start Position.** The patient is supine. The leg is in the anatomical position with the knee in extension (0°) (Fig. 8-44).

• **Stabilization.** The therapist stabilizes the lower leg.

• **End Position.** The foot is moved to the limit of ankle dorsiflexion (Fig. 8-45).

• **End Feel.** Gastrocnemius on stretch—firm.

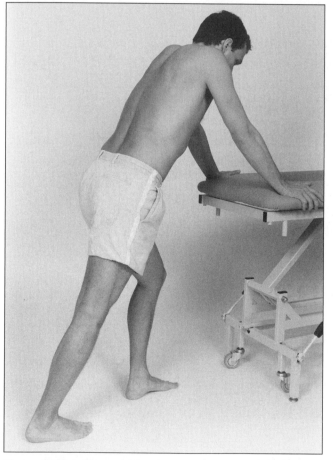

Figure 8-41.   Start position for measurement of the length of gastrocnemius.

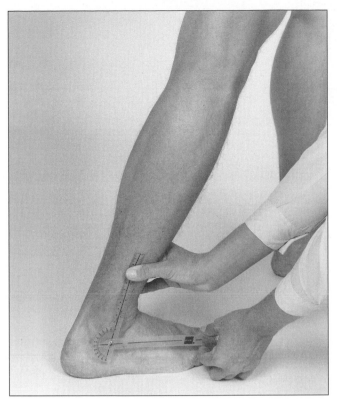

Figure 8-42. Goniometer measurement: length of gastrocnemius.

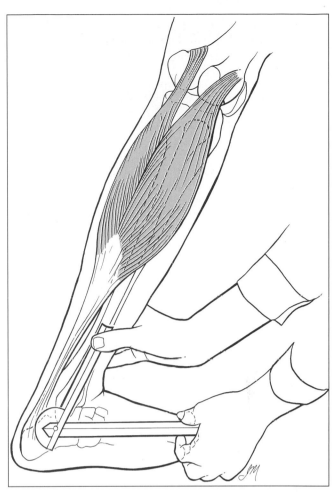

Figure 8-43. Gastrocnemius on stretch.

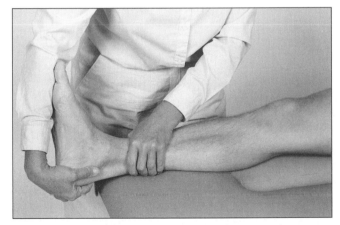

Figure 8-44. Alternate start position: gastrocnemius length.

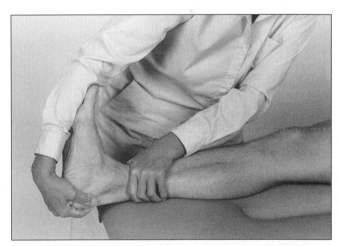

Figure 8-45. Gastrocnemius on stretch.

TABLE 8-3 ▼ **MUSCLE ACTIONS, ATTACHMENTS, AND NERVE SUPPLY: THE ANKLE AND FOOT[2]**

Muscle	Primary Muscle Action	Muscle Origin	Muscle Insertion	Peripheral Nerve	Nerve Root
Tibialis anterior	Ankle dorsiflexion Foot inversion	Lateral condyle of the tibia; proximal half of the lateral surface of the shaft of the tibia; anterior aspect of the interosseous membrane	Medial and inferior surfaces of the medial cunieform bone; medial aspect of the base of the first metatarsal bone	Deep peroneal	L45
Gastrocnemius	Ankle plantarflexion Knee flexion	a. Medial head: proximal and posterior aspect of the medial condyle of the femur posterior to the adductor tubercle b. Lateral head: lateral and posterior aspect of the lateral condyle of the femur; lower part of the supracondylar line	Via the Achilles tendon into the calcaneum	Tibial	S12
Soleus	Ankle plantarflexion	Posterior aspect of the head and proximal one fourth of the shaft of the fibula; soleal line and middle third of the medial border of the tibia	Via the Achilles tendon into the calcaneum	Tibial	S12

▼ MUSCLE ACTIONS, ATTACHMENTS, AND NERVE SUPPLY: THE ANKLE AND FOOT[2] *Continued*

Muscle	Primary Muscle Action	Muscle Origin	Muscle Insertion	Peripheral Nerve	Nerve Root
Tibialis posterior	Foot inversion	Upper two thirds of the posterolateral surface of the tibia below the soleal line; posterior surface of the interosseous membrane; medial aspect of the proximal two thirds of the fibula	Tuberosity of the navicular bone; expansions to the medial, intermediate, and lateral cuneiforms, the cuboid and the bases of the second, third and fourth metatarsals; tendinous band passes to the tip and distal margin of the sustentaculum tali	Tibial	L45
Peroneus longus	Foot eversion Ankle plantarflexion	Head and upper two thirds of the lateral surface of the fibula; a few fibers from the lateral condyle of the tibia	Lateral side of the base of the first metatarsal and medial cuneiform bones	Superficial peroneal	L5S1
Peroneus brevis	Foot eversion	Lower two thirds of the lateral surface of the fibula	Tubercle on the lateral aspect of the base of the fifth metatarsal bone	Superficial peroneal	L5S1
Flexor hallucis brevis	Flexion of the MTP joint of the great toe	Medial part of the plantar surface of the cuboid bone and adjacent part of the lateral cuneiform bone	Medial and lateral aspects of the base of the proximal phalanx of the great toe	Medial plantar	S12
Flexor hallucis longus	Flexion of the IP joint of the great toe	Distal two thirds of the posterior surface of the fibula; posterior surface of the interosseous membrane	Plantar aspect of the base of the distal phalanx of the great toe	Tibial	L5S12

Muscle	Primary Muscle Action	Muscle Origin	Muscle Insertion	Peripheral Nerve	Nerve Root
Flexor digitorum longus	Flexion of the DIP joints of the lateral four toes	Posterior surface of the middle three fifths of the tibia below the soleal line	Plantar aspects of the bases of the distal phalanges of the lateral four toes	Tibial	L5S1**2**
Flexor digitorum brevis	Flexion of the PIP joints of the lateral four toes	Medial process of the calcaneal tuberosity; plantar fascia	Medial and lateral aspects of the middle phalanges of the lateral four toes	Medial plantar	S1**2**
Flexor digiti minimi brevis	Flexion of the MTP joint of the fifth toe	Medial plantar aspect of the base of the fifth metatarsal; sheath of peroneus longus	Lateral side of the base of the proximal phalanx of the fifth toe	Lateral plantar	S**2**3
Lumbricales	Flexion of the MTP joints Extension of the IP joints of the toes	First lumbricalis: medial aspect of flexor digitorum longus tendon; Second to fourth lumbricales: adjacent sides of the flexor digitorum longus tendons	Medial aspects of the dorsal digital expansions on the proximal phalanges of the lateral four toes	First lumbricalis: medial plantar Second to fourth lumbricales: lateral plantar	S**2**3
Abductor hallucis	Abduction of the great toe	Medial process of the calcaneal tuberosity; flexor retinaculum and plantar aponeurosis	Medial aspect of the base of the proximal phalanx of the great toe	Medial plantar	S1**2**
Abductor digiti minimi	Abduction and flexion of the fifth toe	Medial and lateral processes of the calcaneal tuberosity; the bone between the tuberosities; plantar fascia	Lateral aspect of the base of the proximal phalanx of the fifth toe	Lateral plantar	S1**2**3

TABLE
8-3

▼ MUSCLE ACTIONS, ATTACHMENTS, AND NERVE SUPPLY: THE ANKLE AND FOOT[2] *Continued*

Muscle	Primary Muscle Action	Muscle Origin	Muscle Insertion	Peripheral Nerve	Nerve Root
Dorsal interossei	Abduction of the second, third, and fourth toes Flexion of the MTP joints	Adjacent sides of metatarsal bones	First interosseous: medial aspect of the base of the proximal phalanx of the second toe; second to fourth interossei: lateral aspects of the bases of the proximal phalanges of the second, third, and fourth toes; dorsal digital expansions	Lateral plantar	S23
Plantar interossei	Adduction of the third, fourth, and fifth toes Flexion of the MTP joints	Bases and medial aspects of the third, fourth, and fifth metatarsal bones	Medial aspects of the bases of the proximal phalanges of the third, fourth, and fifth toes; dorsal digital expansions	Lateral plantar	S23
Adductor hallucis	Adduction of the great toe	a. Oblique head: bases of the second, third, and fourth metatarsal bones; sheath of peroneus longus b. Transverse head: plantar MTP ligaments of the third, fourth, and fifth toes and the deep transverse metatarsal ligaments between them	Lateral sesamoid bone and the base of the first phalanx of the great toe	Lateral plantar	S23
Extensor hallucis longus	Extension of the IP joint of the great toe	Middle half of the medial surface of the fibula; anterior aspect of the interosseous membrane	Dorsal surface of the base of the distal phalanx of the great toe	Deep peroneal	L5

Muscle	Primary Muscle Action	Muscle Origin	Muscle Insertion	Peripheral Nerve	Nerve Root
Extensor digitorum longus	Extension of the MTP and IP joints of the lesser four toes	Lateral condyle of the tibia; proximal three fourths of the medial surface of the fibula; anterior surface of the interosseous membrane	Dorsal aspect of the base of the middle phalanx of the lesser four toes; dorsal aspect of the base of the distal phalanx of the lesser four toes	Deep peroneal	L5S1
Extensor digitorum brevis	Extension of the first MTP joint Extension of the phalanges of the middle three toes	Anterior superolateral surface of the calcaneum	Medial part of the muscle (extensor hallucis brevis): dorsal aspect of the base of the proximal phalanx of the great toe tendons to the second, third, and fourth toes: into the lateral aspect of the corresponding extensor digitorum longus tendons	Deep peroneal	L5S1

ANKLE DORSIFLEXION AND FOOT INVERSION

Against Gravity: Tibialis Anterior

• **Start Position.** The patient is sitting. The ankle is in plantarflexion and the foot is in slight eversion (Fig. 8-46).

• **Stabilization.** The lower leg is supported against the therapist's thigh and the therapist stabilizes the lower leg proximal to the ankle.

• **Movement.** The patient dorsiflexes the ankle and inverts the foot through full ROM (Fig. 8-47). The patient is instructed to keep the toes relaxed.

• **Palpation.** The tibialis anterior is the most medial tendon on the anteromedial aspect of the ankle joint or medial to the anterior border of the tibia.

• **Resistance Location.** Applied on the dorsomedial aspect of the forefoot (Figs. 8-48 and 8-49).

• **Resistance Direction.** Ankle plantarflexion and foot eversion.

• **Substitution/Trick Movement.** Extensor digitorum longus and extensor hallucis longus (toe extension); these muscles extend the toes before acting to dorsiflex the ankle.[10]

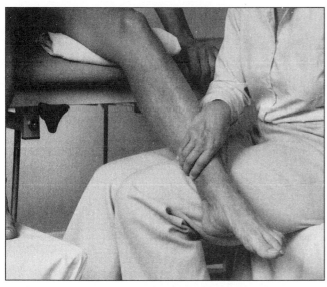

Figure 8-46.   Start position: tibialis anterior.

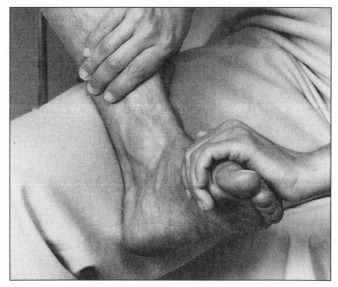

Figure 8-48.   Resistance: tibialis anterior.

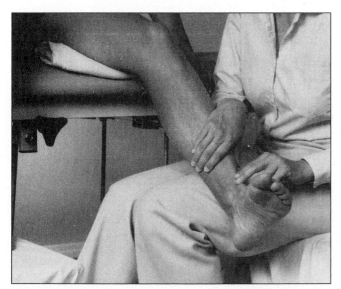

Figure 8-47.   Screen position: tibialis anterior.

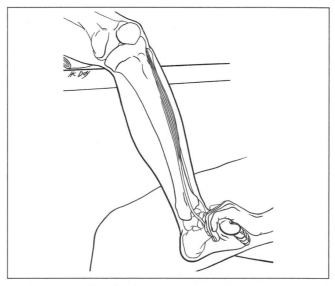

Figure 8-49.   Tibialis anterior.

Gravity Eliminated: Tibialis Anterior

- **Start Position.** The patient is in a side-lying position on the test side. The knee is flexed to place the gastrocnemius on slack, the ankle is in plantarflexion, and the foot is in slight eversion (Fig. 8-50).

- **Stabilization.** The therapist stabilizes the lower leg proximal to the ankle. By placing the hand underneath the leg the friction of the table is eliminated.

- **End Position.** The patient dorsiflexes the ankle and inverts the foot through full ROM (Fig. 8-51).

- **Substitution/Trick Movement.** Extensor hallucis longus and extensor digitorum longus (toe extension).

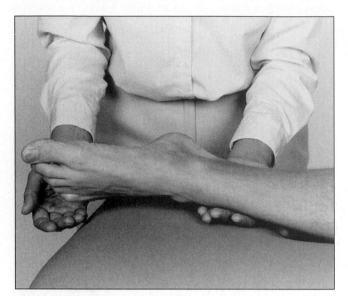

Figure 8-50.   Start position: tibialis anterior.

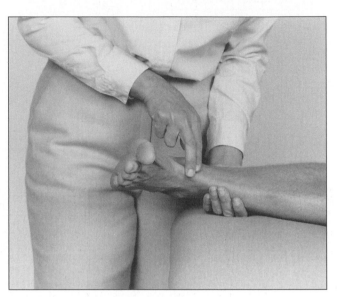

Figure 8-51.   End position: tibialis anterior.

ANKLE PLANTARFLEXION

The gastrocnemius and soleus muscles are tested when ankle plantarflexion is performed with the knee in extension. Gastrocnemius muscle activity and isometric ankle plantarflexion strength have been shown to decrease with increasing knee flexion, most significantly at knee flexion angles greater than 45°.[11] Therefore, the more specific testing of the soleus muscle strength is performed with the knee flexed to at least 45° when the gastrocnemius muscle is placed on slack.

Against Gravity: Gastrocnemius and Soleus

• **Start Positions.** Gastrocnemius (Fig. 8-52): The patient is prone with the knee extended and the feet are over the edge of the plinth. The ankle is dorsiflexed. Soleus (Fig. 8-53): The patient is prone with the knee on the test side flexed 90°. The ankle is dorsiflexed.

• **Stabilization.** The therapist stabilizes the lower leg proximal to the ankle.

• **Movement.** The patient plantarflexes the ankle through full ROM (Figs. 8-54 and 8-55). The patient is instructed to keep the toes relaxed.

• **Palpation.** Gastrocnemius: medial and lateral margin of the popliteal fossa distal to the knee joint. Soleus: on either side of gastrocnemius midway down the calf.

• **Resistance Location.** Applied on the posterior aspect of the calcaneum (Figs. 8-56–8-59).

• **Resistance Direction.** In a downward and anterior direction to dorsiflex the ankle.

• **Recording.** Record the grade indicating that this is a non–weight-bearing (NWB) test.

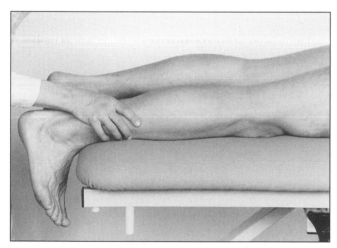

Figure 8-52.   Start position: gastrocnemius.

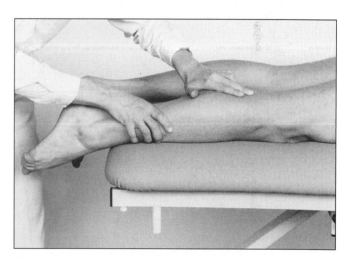

Figure 8-54.   Screen position: gastrocnemius.

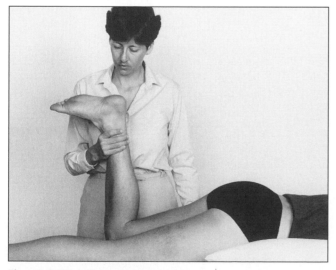

Figure 8-53.   Start position: soleus.

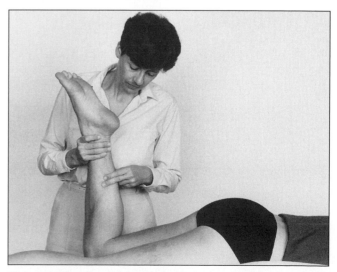

Figure 8-55.   Screen position: soleus.

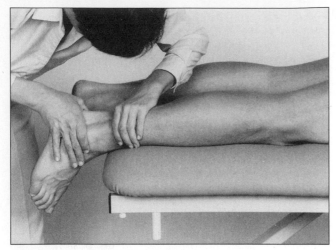

Figure 8-56.   Resistance: gastrocnemius.

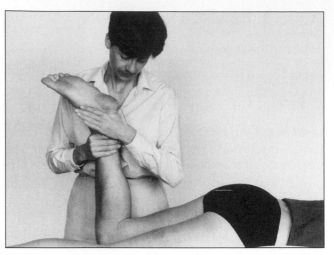

Figure 8-58.   Resistance: soleus.

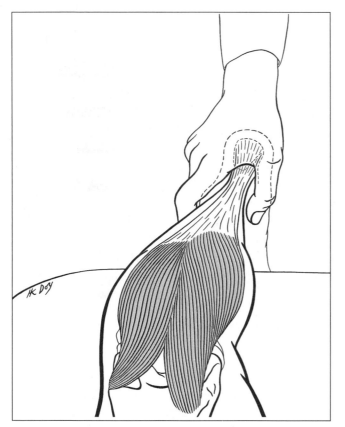

Figure 8-57.   Gastrocnemius.

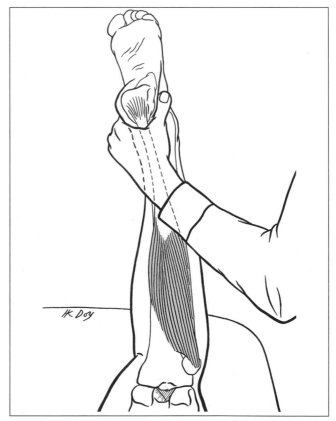

Figure 8-59.   Soleus.

Alternate Against Gravity: Gastrocnemius and Soleus. This test may be contraindicated for patients with poor standing balance or generalized or specific lower extremity weakness.

• **Start Positions.** Gastrocnemius (Fig. 8-60): The patient is standing. The patient raises the foot off the floor on the nontest side. The knee on the test side is in extension with the foot flat on the floor. Soleus (Fig. 8-61): The same position is assumed with the exception that the knee on the test side is flexed.

• **Stabilization.** The patient may use the parallel bars or other stable structure for balance but should be instructed not to bear weight through the hands. Alternatively, the therapist may provide this support.

• **Movement.** The patient plantarflexes the ankle (Figs. 8-62 and 8-63).

• **Resistance.** Body weight resists the movement.

• **Grading.** 5 = Maintaining the heel fully off the floor through more than six repetitions; 4 = maintaining the heel fully off the floor through three to five repetitions with subsequent attempts resulting in decreased range;

and 3 = maintaining the heel off the floor through one to two repetitions only with subsequent attempts resulting in decreased range.

(*Note:* Lunsford and Perry[12] studied 203 normal subjects between 20 and 59 years of age and recommended 25 standing heel-rise repetitions be required for a grade of 5. Parameters for other grades were not studied.)

The grading standard used to assess ankle plantarflexion strength should be recorded.

• **Substitution/Trick Movement.** (1) Soleus: flexion of the knee joint when testing gastrocnemius; (2) gastrocnemius: extension of the knee joint when testing soleus; (3) pushing down on parallel bars or other support (alternate test only); and (4) in non–weight-bearing testing, downward movement of the forefoot or toe flexion (through the action of tibialis posterior, peroneus longus, peroneus brevis, flexor hallucis longus, and flexor digitorum longus) giving the appearance of ankle plantarflexion. Ensure upward movement of the heel.

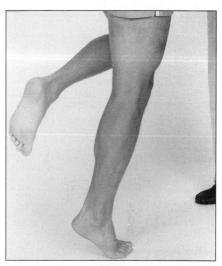

Figure 8-62.   End position: gastrocnemius.

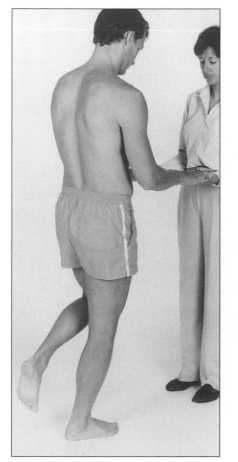

Figure 8-60.   Alternate start position: gastrocnemius.

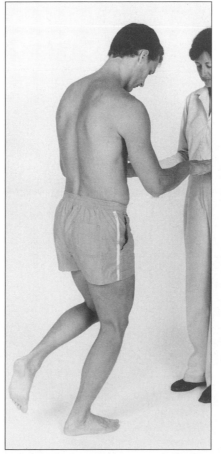

Figure 8-61.   Alternate start position: soleus.

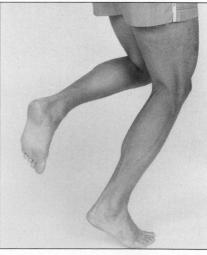

Figure 8-63.   End position: soleus.

Gravity Eliminated: Gastrocnemius and Soleus

• **Start Positions.** For both muscle tests the patient is in a side-lying position with the nontest side lower extremity flexed. Gastrocnemius (Fig. 8-64): the knee is extended and the ankle is dorsiflexed. Soleus (Fig. 8-65): the knee is flexed and the ankle is dorsiflexed.

• **Stabilization.** The lower leg is stabilized and supported proximal to the ankle joint.

• **End Position.** The patient plantarflexes the ankle through full ROM for gastrocnemius (Fig. 8-66) and for soleus (Fig. 8-67).

• **Substitution/Trick Movement.** Forefoot movement or toe flexion as described in the against gravity test.

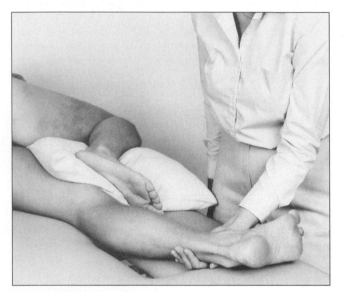

Figure 8-64.   Start position: gastrocnemius.

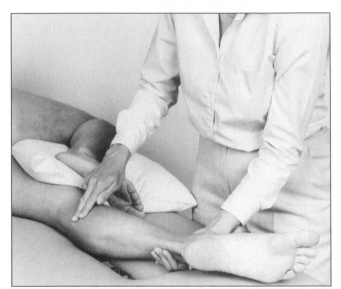

Figure 8-66.   End position: gastrocnemius.

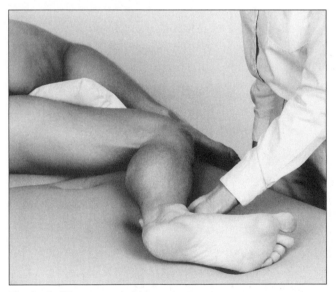

Figure 8-65.   Start position: soleus.

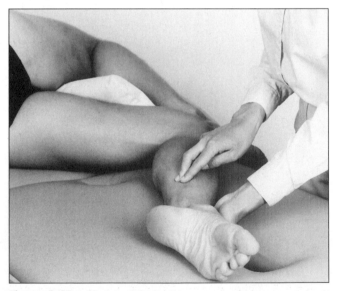

Figure 8-67.   End position: soleus.

FOOT INVERSION

Against Gravity: Tibialis Posterior

Accessory muscles: gastrocnemius, soleus, flexor digitorum longus, flexor hallucis longus, and tibialis anterior.

• **Start Position.** The patient is in a side-lying position on the test side with the knee slightly flexed (Fig. 8-68). The foot projects over the end of the plinth. Because the tibialis anterior can invert the foot only from an everted position to the neutral position,[10] the foot and ankle are positioned in neutral.

• **Stabilization.** The therapist stabilizes the lower leg proximal to the ankle.

• **Movement.** The patient inverts the foot through full ROM with slight plantarflexion (Fig. 8-69). The patient is instructed to keep the toes relaxed or slightly extended.

• **Palpation.** Between the tip of the medial malleolus and the navicular bone or proximal and posterior to the medial malleolus.

• **Substitution/Trick Movement.** Toe flexion.

• **Resistance Location.** Applied on the medial border of the forefoot (Figs. 8-70 and 8-71).

• **Resistance Direction.** Foot eversion.

Gravity Eliminated: Tibialis Posterior

• **Start Position.** The patient is supine. The heel is off the plinth and the foot and ankle are in neutral (Fig. 8-72).

• **Stabilization.** The therapist stabilizes the lower leg proximal to the ankle.

• **End Position.** The patient inverts the foot through full ROM with slight plantarflexion (Fig. 8-73).

• **Substitution/Trick Movement.** Toe flexion.

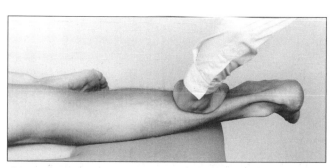

Figure 8-68. Start position: tibialis posterior.

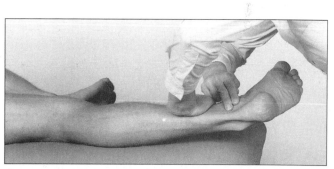

Figure 8-69. Screen position: tibialis posterior.

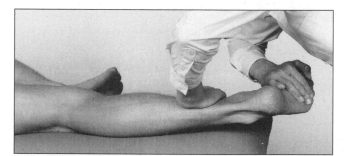

Figure 8-70. Resistance: tibialis posterior.

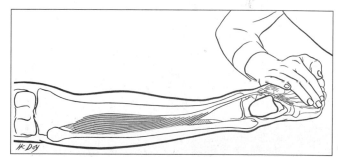

Figure 8-71. Tibialis posterior.

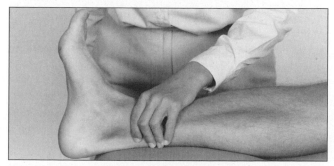

Figure 8-72. Start position: tibialis posterior.

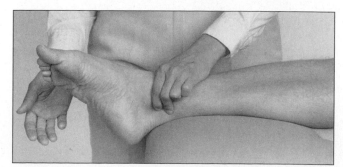

Figure 8-73. End position: tibialis posterior.

FOOT EVERSION

Against Gravity: Peroneus Longus and Peroneus Brevis

Accessory muscles: peroneus tertius and extensor digitorum longus.

• **Start Position.** The patient is in a side-lying position on the nontest side with the foot over the edge of the plinth (Fig. 8-74). The ankle is plantarflexed and the foot is inverted.

• **Stabilization.** The therapist stabilizes the lower leg proximal to the ankle.

• **Movement.** The patient everts the foot through full ROM while keeping the toes relaxed (Fig. 8-75).

• **Palpation.** Peroneus longus: posterior to the lateral malleolus or distal to the head of the fibula. Peroneus brevis: proximal to the base of the fifth metatarsal on the lateral border of the foot.

• **Substitution/Trick Movement.** Extensor digitorum longus and peroneus tertius.

• **Resistance Location.** Applied on the lateral border of the foot and on the plantar surface of the first metatarsal (Figs. 8-76, 8-77, and 8-78).

• **Resistance Direction.** Foot inversion and elevation of the first metatarsal.

Gravity Eliminated: Peroneus Longus and Peroneus Brevis

• **Start Position.** The patient is supine with the heel over the edge of the plinth. The foot and ankle are in the inverted position (Fig. 8-79).

• **Stabilization.** The therapist stabilizes the lower leg proximal to the ankle.

• **End Position.** The patient everts the foot through full ROM (Fig. 8-80).

• **Substitution/Trick Movement.** Peroneus tertius and extensor digitorum longus.

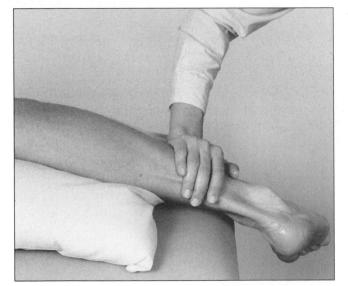

Figure 8-74. Start position: peroneus longus and brevis.

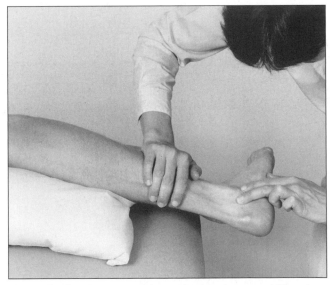

Figure 8-75. Screen position: peroneus longus and brevis.

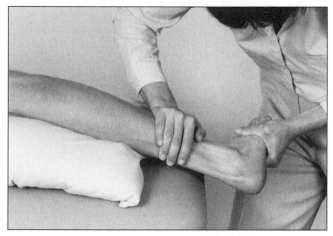

Figure 8-76. Resistance: peroneus longus and brevis.

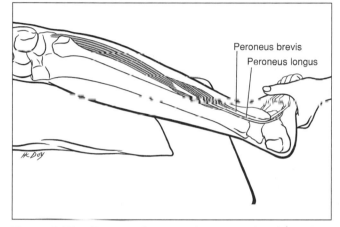

Peroneus brevis

Peroneus longus

Figure 8-77. Peroneus longus and peroneus brevis.

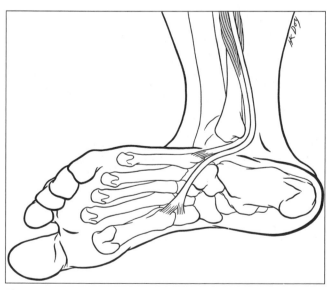

Figure 8-78. Insertions of peroneus longus and peroneus brevis.

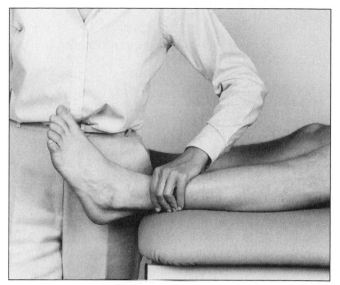

Figure 8-79. Start position: peroneus longus and brevis.

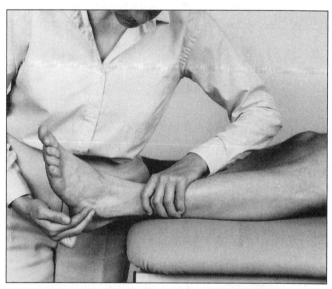

Figure 8-80. End position: peroneus longus and brevis.

TOE MOVEMENTS

Gravity is not considered to be a significant factor when testing the muscles of the toes. Isolated movement of the toes is rarely required for activities of daily living (ADL) and it may not be possible or practical to perform isolated movements for specific muscle testing of the foot, although these tests are described below.

METATARSOPHALANGEAL FLEXION

Flexor Hallucis Brevis: Great Toe and Lumbricales: Lesser Four Toes. Accessory muscles: flexor hallucis longus, flexor digitorum longus and brevis, abductor hallucis, abductor digiti minimi, and dorsal and plantar interossei.

• **Start Position.** The patient is supine. The foot, ankle, and toes are in the anatomical position (Fig. 8-81).

• **Stabilization.** The therapist stabilizes the metatarsals.

• **Movement.** The patient flexes the MTP joint(s) while maintaining extension at the IP joint(s). The great toe is tested independently (Fig. 8-82) of the lateral four toes.

• **Palpation.** The lumbricales are not palpable. Flexor hallucis brevis is palpated on the medial border of the sole of the foot.

• **Substitution/Trick Movement.** Great toe: flexor hallucis longus. Lesser four toes: flexor digitorum longus and brevis, flexor digiti minimi, and plantar and dorsal interossei.

• **Resistance Location.** Applied on the plantar surface of the proximal phalanges of the great toe (Figs. 8-83 and 8-84) and the lesser four toes (not shown).

• **Resistance Direction.** MTP joint extension.

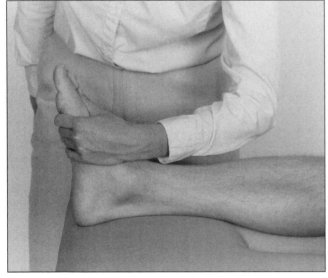

Figure 8-81.   Start position: flexor hallucis brevis.

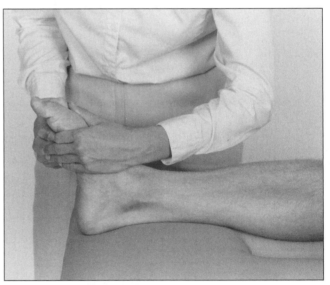

Figure 8-82.   Screen position: flexor hallucis brevis.

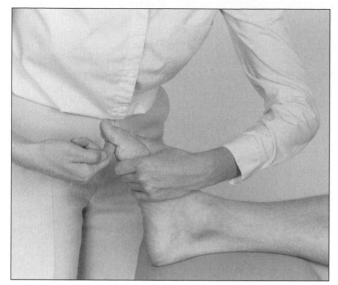

Figure 8-83.   Resistance: flexor hallucis brevis.

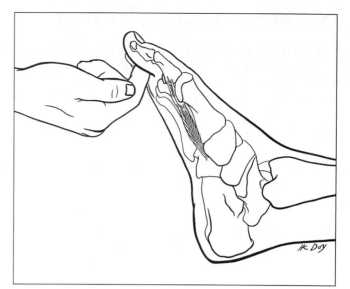

Figure 8-84.   Flexor hallucis brevis.

INTERPHALANGEAL FLEXION

Flexor Hallucis Longus: Flexion of the IP Joint of the Great Toe; Flexor Digitorum Longus: Flexion of the DIP Joints of the Lateral Four Toes; and Flexor Digitorum Brevis: Flexion of the PIP Joints of the Lateral Four Toes

• **Start Position.** The patient is supine. The foot, ankle, and toes are in the anatomical position (Figs. 8-85 and 8-86).

• **Stabilization.** The therapist stabilizes the MTP joints of each toe. If the gastrocnemius and soleus are paralyzed, the calcaneum should be stabilized to assist in fixing the origin of flexor digitorum brevis.

• **Movement.** The great toe is tested independently of the lateral four toes. The patient flexes the IP joint of the great toe through full ROM (Fig. 8-87). The patient flexes the PIP and DIP joints of the lateral four toes through full ROM (Fig. 8-88).

• **Palpation.** Flexor hallucis longus may be palpated on the plantar surface of the proximal phalanx of the great toe or inferior to the medial malleolus. The flexor digitorum brevis is not palpable. Flexor digitorum longus may be palpated on some individuals on the plantar aspect of the proximal phalanges.

• **Resistance Location.** Applied on the plantar surface of the distal phalanx of the great toe (Figs. 8-89 and 8-91). and the distal and middle phalanges of the lateral four toes (Figs. 8-90, 8-92, and 8-93).

• **Resistance Direction.** Toe extension.

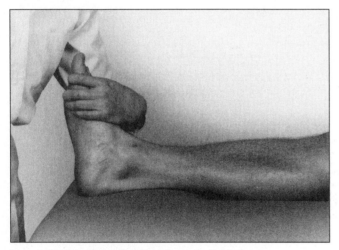

Figure 8-85.   Start position: flexor hallucis longus.

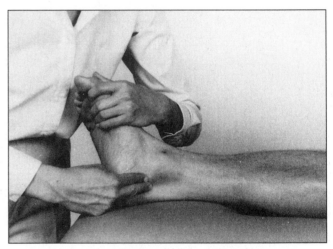

Figure 8-87.   Screen position: flexor hallucis longus.

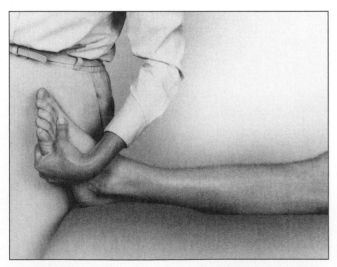

Figure 8-86.   Start position: flexor digitorum longus and brevis.

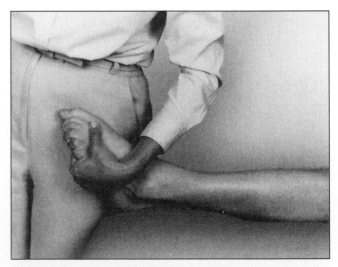

Figure 8-88.   Screen position: flexor digitorum longus and brevis.

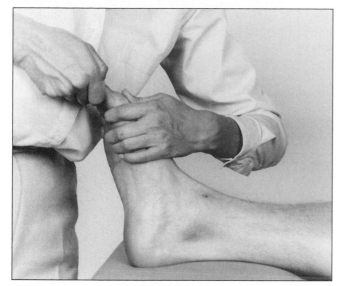

Figure 8-89.   Resistance: flexor hallucis longus.

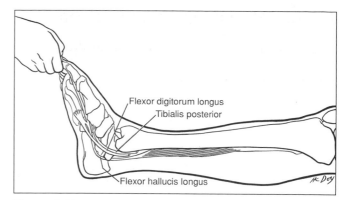

Flexor digitorum longus
Tibialis posterior
Flexor hallucis longus

Figure 8-91.   Flexor hallucis longus.

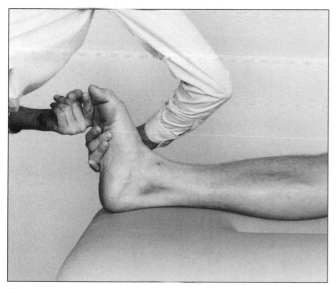

Figure 8-90.   Resistance: flexor digitorum longus and brevis.

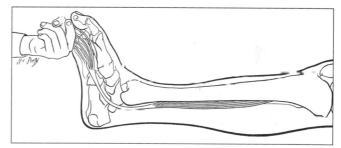

Figure 8-92.   Flexor digitorum longus.

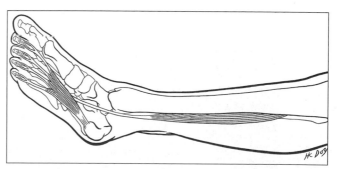

Figure 8-93.   Flexor digitorum longus and flexor digitorum brevis.

ANKLE AND FOOT

METATARSOPHALANGEAL ABDUCTION OF THE GREAT TOE (ABDUCTOR HALLUCIS)

• **Start Position.** The patient is supine. The ankle, foot, and toes are in the anatomical position (Fig. 8-94).

• **Stabilization.** The therapist stabilizes the first metatarsal bone.

• **Movement.** The patient abducts the great toe through full ROM (Fig. 8-95). The movement of abduction is accompanied by some flexion, as the abductor hallucis abducts and flexes the MTP joint of the great toe.

• **Palpation.** Medial border of the foot superficial to the first metatarsal bone.

• **Resistance Location.** Applied on the medial aspect of the proximal phalanx of the great toe (Figs. 8-96 and 8-97).

• **Resistance Direction.** Great toe adduction.

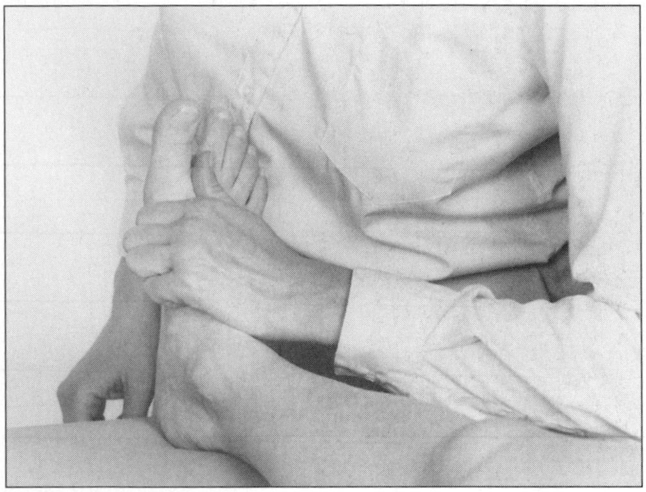

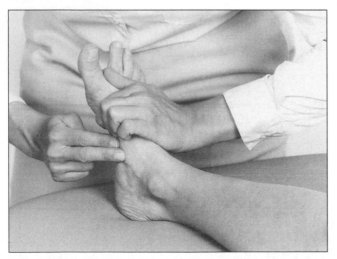

Figure 8-94.   Start position: abductor hallucis.

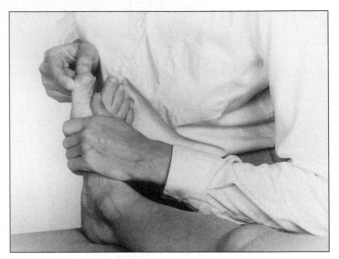

Figure 8-96.   Resistance: abductor hallucis.

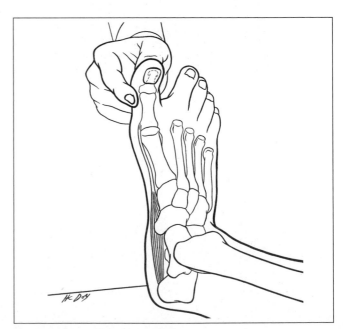

Figure 8-95.   Screen position: abductor hallucis.

Figure 8-97.   Abductor hallucis.

METATARSOPHALANGEAL ABDUCTION (ABDUCTOR DIGITI MINIMI AND DORSAL INTEROSSEI)

These two muscles are not isolated for grading. Function is determined through observation of abduction of the lateral three toes (Fig. 8-98). This movement is associated with flexion of the MTP joints. The therapist stabilizes the great toe.

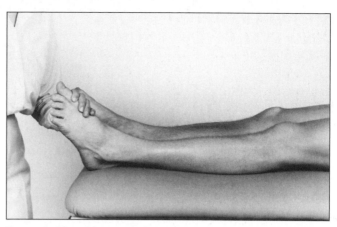

Figure 8-98.   Observation of abductor digiti minimi and dorsal interossei.

METATARSOPHALANGEAL AND INTERPHALANGEAL EXTENSION

Extensor Hallucis Longus: IP Extension of the Great Toe; Extensor Digitorum Brevis: MTP and IP Extension of the Middle Three Toes and MTP Extension of the Great Toe; and Extensor Digitorum Longus: MTP and IP Extension of the Lateral Four Toes

• **Start Position.** The patient is supine. The ankle is in the neutral position and the toes are flexed (Figs. 8-99 and 8-100).

• **Stabilization.** The therapist stabilizes the metatarsals.

• **Movement.** The patient extends the great toe through full ROM (Fig. 8-101). The patient extends the lateral four toes through full ROM (Fig. 8-102). It may be difficult for the patient to extend the great toe and the lateral four toes separately; therefore, the toes may have to be tested as a group.

• **Palpation.** The extensor hallucis longus is palpated on the dorsal aspect of the first MTP joint or on the anterior aspect of the ankle joint lateral to the tendon of tibialis anterior. Extensor digitorum brevis is palpated on the dorsolateral aspect of the foot anterior to the lateral malleolus. Extensor digitorum longus is palpated on the dorsal aspect of the metatarsal bones of the lateral four toes or on the anterior aspect of the ankle joint lateral to the tendon of extensor hallucis longus.

Note: The extensor digitorum brevis does not insert into the fifth toe; therefore, decreased extension strength of this toe indicates weakness of the extensor digitorum longus.[13] The portion of the extensor digitorum brevis that inserts into the base of the proximal phalanx of the great toe produces MTP joint extension of the great toe.

• **Resistance Location.** Extensor hallucis longus and extensor hallucis brevis (Figs. 8-103 and 8-104): applied over the dorsal aspect of the distal phalanx of the great toe. Extensor digitorum longus and brevis (Figs. 8-105 and 8-106): applied over the dorsal surface of the lateral four toes.

• **Resistance Direction.** Toe flexion.

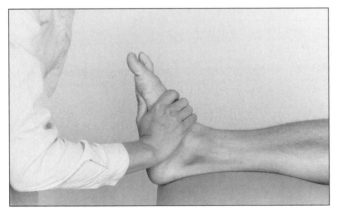

Figure 8-99.   Start position: extensor hallucis longus and extensor hallucis brevis.

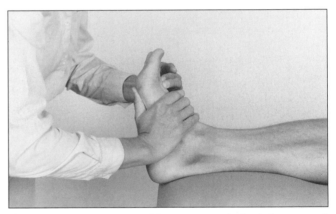

Figure 8-101.   Screen position: extensor hallucis longus and extensor hallucis brevis.

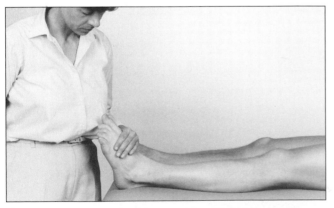

Figure 8-100.   Start position: extensor digitorum longus and brevis.

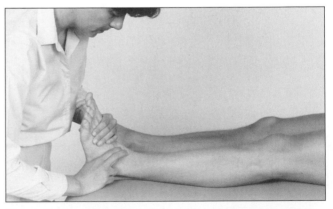

Figure 8-102.   Screen position: extensor digitorum longus and brevis.

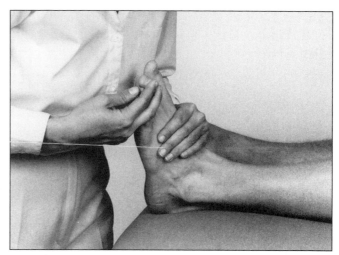

Figure 8-105. Resistance: extensor digitorum longus and brevis.

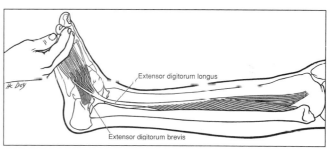

Figure 8-106. Extensor digitorum longus and extensor digitorum brevis.

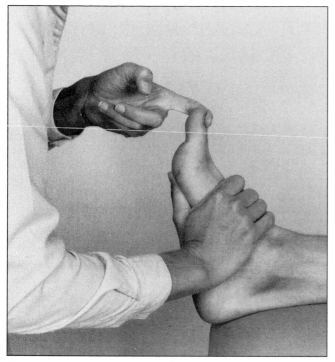

Figure 8-103. Resistance: extensor hallucis longus and brevis.

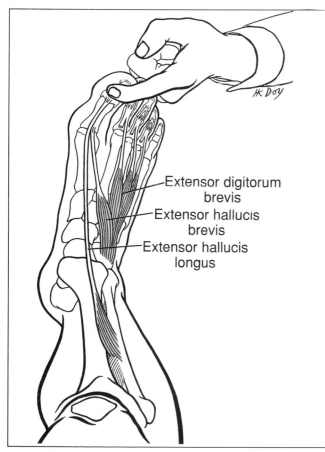

Extensor digitorum brevis
Extensor hallucis brevis
Extensor hallucis longus

Figure 8-104. Extensor hallucis longus and brevis and extensor digitorum brevis.

ANKLE AND FOOT

JOINT FUNCTION

The foot functions as a flexible base to accommodate rough terrain[10] and functions as a rigid lever during terminal stance of the walking pattern.[5] In transmitting forces between the ground and the leg the foot absorbs shock.[10] With the foot planted, the ankle and foot elevate the body and when off the ground, the foot is used to manipulate machinery.[10] When weight is taken through the foot, the MTP joints allow movement of the rigid foot over the toes.[5]

FUNCTIONAL RANGE OF MOTION

Ankle Dorsiflexion and Plantarflexion

The normal active ROM for the ankle (talocrural) joint is 20° dorsiflexion and 50° plantarflexion.

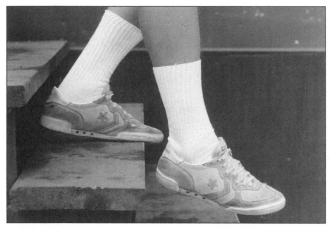

Figure 8-107.   Full range of ankle dorsiflexion is required to descend stairs.

The full range of ankle dorsiflexion is necessary to descend stairs (Fig. 8-107). Rising from sitting also requires significant ankle dorsiflexion ROM, that is, an average of 28°.[14]

Full ankle plantarflexion may be required when climbing, jumping, or reaching for an object on a high shelf. Less than the full range of ankle plantarflexion may be used to perform activities such as depressing the accelerator of a motor vehicle (Fig. 8-108) or the foot pedals of a piano and wearing high-heeled shoes.

To ascend and descend stairs, Livingston et al.[15] found maximum ankle dorsiflexion ROM requirements ranged between averages of 14° and 27° to ascend and 21° and 36° to descend stairs. The average maximum ankle plantarflexion ROM requirements ranged from 23° to 30° to ascend and 24° to 31° to descend stairs.[15]

Movements of the Foot

The active ROM of the subtalar joint is 5° each for inversion and eversion without forefoot movement. The ranges of inversion and eversion may be augmented by forefoot movement of 35° and 15°, respectively. The subtalar, transverse tarsal joints, and joints of the forefoot must be fully mobile to allow the foot to accommodate to varying degrees of rough terrain (Fig. 8-109). With the foot across the opposite thigh, inversion is required to inspect the foot for skin condition.

In standing, the MTP joints are in at least 25° extension due to the downward slope of the metatarsals.[2] Ranges approximating the full 90° of extension of the MTP joint of the great toe are required for many ADL.[16] Extension of the great toe and lesser four toes is essential for activities such as rising onto the toes to reach high objects (Fig. 8-110) and squatting. For most ADL only a few degrees of flexion are required at the great toe.[16] There appears to be no significant function that can be attributed to abduction and adduction at the MTP joints.[5]

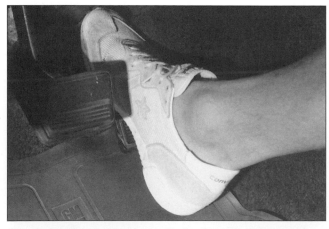

Figure 8-108.   Ankle plantarflexion is used to depress the accelerator of a motor vehicle.

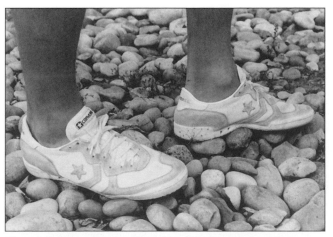

Figure 8-109.   The mobile joints of the ankle and foot accommodate rough terrain.

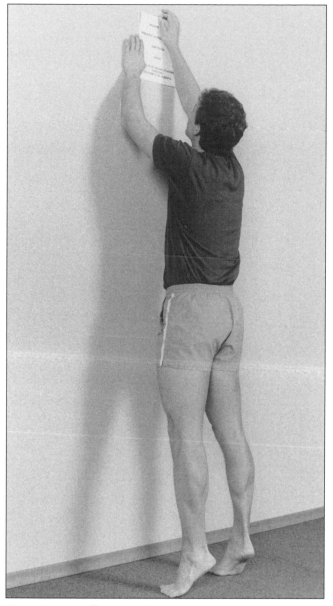

Figure 8-110. Toe extension and contraction of the ankle plantarflexor.

Gait

Normal walking (see Appendix D) requires a maximum of 10° of ankle dorsiflexion at midstance to terminal stance as the tibia advances over the fixed foot and a maximum of 20° of plantarflexion at the end of preswing (from the Rancho Los Amigos gait analysis forms as cited in Norkin and Levangie[5]). At the MTP joint of the great toe almost 90° of extension is required at preswing.[16] Extension is also required of the lesser four toes.[16] Extension of the toes stretches the plantar aponeurosis resulting in significant longitudinal arch support.[17]

Running requires a range of ankle joint motion from an average of 17° dorsiflexion at midstance to an average 32° maximum ankle plantarflexion at early swing.[18] Ankle ROM was the same when fast-paced running was compared to slow-paced running.[18]

MUSCLE FUNCTION

Ankle Plantarflexion

The triceps surae muscles, gastrocnemius and soleus, are the primary plantarflexors at the ankle joint. The gastrocnemius crosses the knee joint and is most effective as a plantarflexor when the knee is extended.[19] Gastrocnemius muscle activity and isometric ankle plantarflexion strength have been shown to decrease with increasing knee flexion, most significantly at knee flexion angles >45°. Herman and Bragin[20] found the gastrocnemius contributes to plantarflexion when the ankle is in the plantarflexed position, when tension is developed rapidly, and when strong contraction is required. The soleus is mainly active in plantarflexing the ankle when the ankle is in a dorsiflexed position and when the contraction is minimal.[20] Tibialis posterior, flexor hallucis longus, flexor digitorum longus, and peroneus longus and brevis act as accessory plantarflexors at the ankle joint. The actions of the plantarflexors are illustrated in activities where the ankle is plantarflexed against resistance, for example, rising onto the toes (see Fig. 8-110), jumping, and depressing the gas pedal of a motor vehicle (see Fig. 8-108). The ankle plantarflexors also contract when movement is forced at the extreme of plantarflexion, such as when pulling on a sock. With the foot fixed on the ground, the plantarflexors control ankle dorsiflexion when descending stairs[21] (see Fig. 8-107).

Ankle Dorsiflexion

The dorsiflexors of the ankle include the tibialis anterior, extensor hallucis longus, extensor digitorum longus, and peroneus tertius. The function of the tibialis anterior is to initiate ankle dorsiflexion.[22] The tibialis anterior and extensor hallucis longus are strong dorsiflexors compared to the extensor digitorum longus and peroneus tertius.[5] The dorsiflexors contract and maintain the ankle in a dorsiflexed position in activities such as cutting toenails or tying shoelaces. These muscles also contract to control ankle plantarflexion when lowering the foot onto the ground, as illustrated when slowly tapping the foot on the floor and at loading response in the gait cycle (see Appendix D). When rising from the sitting to the standing position with the foot planted on the ground, the dorsiflexors contract to stabilize the tibia on the tarsus.[23]

Inversion and Eversion

The tibialis posterior, flexor hallucis longus, flexor digitorum longus, soleus, gastrocnemius, and tibialis anterior are responsible for inversion. The tibialis posterior is the principle invertor of the foot. The gastrocnemius and soleus muscles produce inversion of the calcaneus with plantarflexion of the ankle.[10] Opinions vary concerning the contribution made by tibialis anterior in inverting the foot. The line of action of tibialis anterior is along the subtalar joint axis[19] for inversion and eversion. For this reason, Soderberg[19] indicates there is no motion produced by the tibialis anterior around the subtalar joint axis. Smith et al.[10] state that tibialis anterior and the long toes flexors may be weak invertors of the foot from a position of eversion to neutral position. O'Connell[22] concluded that the tibialis anterior only functions as an invertor when the medial border of the foot is elevated simultaneously. The action of the invertors is illustrated when the foot is positioned across the opposite thigh to inspect the foot for skin condition or when walking across rough terrain when the invertors assist in stabilizing the foot (see Fig. 8-109).

The peroneus longus and peroneus brevis, assisted by the extensor digitorum longus and peroneus tertius, perform eversion. The action of the evertors is illustrated when walking across rough ground (see Fig. 8-109).

Toe Flexion and Extension

The flexors of the great toe include the flexor hallucis longus, flexor hallucis brevis, and abductor hallucis brevis. The abductor hallucis brevis flexes the MTP joint and extends the IP joint of the great toe.[24] The flexor digitorum longus and flexor digitorum brevis flex the lesser four toes. The flexor digiti minimi and abductor digiti minimi also assist in flexion of the fifth toe. The toe flexors function so that the great toe presses firmly on the ground and the other four toes grip the ground to help maintain balance during unilateral stance[25] or when standing on the toes (see Fig. 8-110). The toe flexors contract eccentrically to control passive toe extension that occurs when crouching to pick up an object from the ground or walking.

The extensor apparatus of the foot is similar to the extensor apparatus of the hand. The extensors of the great toe include the extensor hallucis longus, extensor hallucis brevis, and abductor hallucis brevis. The extensor digitorum longus and extensor digitorum brevis extend the lesser four toes at the MTP joints. There is no extensor digitorum brevis to the fifth toe, but fibers from the abductor digiti minimi and flexor digiti minimi muscles make attachment to the dorsal digital expansion of the fifth toe[24] to assist with extension. The lumbricales and the interossei simultaneously flex the MTP joints and extend the IP joints of the lesser four toes. The toe extensors contract during walking and climbing stairs. The action of the toe extensors is illustrated when one extends the toes and maintains this position to cut the toenails.

Maintenance of the Arches

Unlike the hand, the intrinsic muscles of the foot do not perform specific functions but usually work as a group along with the extrinsic muscles to perform gross function. The intrinsic muscles function to stabilize the foot during propulsion.[26] Mann and Inman[26] explain that the main intrinsic muscles (abductor hallucis, flexor hallucis brevis, flexor digitorum brevis, and abductor digiti minimi) form the main muscle support

of the arch by exerting a strong flexion force on the forefoot, to help stabilize the transverse tarsal joint. The intrinsic muscles contract to stabilize the foot when weight is taken through the forefoot in activities such as standing on the toes (see Fig. 8-110) or ascending and descending stairs or a ramp. The triceps surae, peroneus longus and brevis, and tibialis anterior and posterior contract with the intrinsic muscles to make the foot more rigid for activities such as running and climbing.[16]

Standing Posture

In standing, the line of gravity falls anterior to the ankle joint axis creating a dorsiflexion torque.[5] The dorsiflexion torque is opposed by the soleus muscle as it contracts to pull the tibia in a posterior direction.[5] Muscle activity is not required to support the arches of the foot when standing.[26]

Gait

The following description of muscle function during the gait cycle is based on the work of Norkin and Levangie[5] and Inman et al.[27] The ankle dorsiflexors contract during the swing phase of the gait cycle to allow the foot to clear the ground. The tibialis anterior, extensor hallucis longus, and extensor digitorum longus contract concentrically to dorsiflex the ankle from preswing through midswing and then contract isometrically to hold the foot in this position. These same muscles contract eccentrically to control the lowering of the foot onto the floor from initial contact through loading response during the stance phase of the gait cycle.

The gastrocnemius and soleus muscles contract eccentrically from loading response to terminal stance to control ankle dorsiflexion produced by the forward movement of the tibia over the fixed foot as the body advances forward. In preswing the gastrocnemius, soleus, peroneus longus, peroneus brevis, and flexor hallucis longus contract concentrically and the heel is raised off the ground. Peroneus longus controls balance during normal gait, most notably at slower walking speeds.[28]

The intrinsic muscles of the foot contract during the stance phase of the gait cycle.[26] The contraction of the intrinsic muscles coincides with the period in the gait cycle when the foot requires maximal stability.

Reber et al.[29] describe the ankle muscle activity during running.

REFERENCES

1. Kapandji IA. *The Physiology of the Joints.* Vol 1. 5th ed. New York: Churchill Livingstone; 1982.
2. Soames RW, ed. Skeletal system. Salmons S, ed. Muscle. *Gray's Anatomy.* 38th ed. New York: Churchill Livingstone; 1995.
3. Norkin CC, White DJ. *Measurement of Joint Motion: A Guide to Goniometry.* 2nd ed. Philadelphia: FA Davis; 1995.
4. Daniels L, Worthingham C. *Muscle Testing: Techniques of*

Manual Examination. 5th ed. Philadelphia: WB Saunders; 1986.

5. Norkin CC, Levangie PK. *Joint Structure & Function: A Comprehensive Analysis*. 2nd ed. Philadelphia: FA Davis; 1992.

6. Woodburne RT. *Essentials of Human Anatomy*. 5th ed. London: Oxford University Press; 1973.

7. Cyriax J. *Textbook of Orthopaedic Medicine, Vol 1. Diagnosis of Soft Tissue Lesions*. 8th ed. London: Bailliere Tindall; 1982.

8. Magee DJ. *Orthopedic Physical Assessment*. 3rd ed. Philadelphia: WB Saunders; 1997.

9. American Academy of Orthopaedic Surgeons. *Joint Motion: Method of Measuring and Recording*. Chicago: Author; 1965.

10. Smith LK, Weiss EL, Lehmkuhl LD. *Brunnstrom's Clinical Kinesiology*. 5th ed. Philadelphia: FA Davis; 1996.

11. Fiebert IM, Correia EP, Roach KE, Carte MB, Cespedes J, Hemstreet K. A comparison of EMG activity between the medial and lateral heads of the gastrocnemius muscle during isometric plantarflexion contractions at various knee angles. *Isokinetics and Exercise Science*. 1996;6:71–77.

12. Lunsford BR, Perry J. The standing heel-rise test for ankle plantar flexion: criterion for normal. *Phys Ther*. 1995;75:694–698.

13. Janda V. *Muscle Function Testing*. London: Butterworth; 1983.

14. Ikeda ER, Schenkman ML, Riley PO, Hodge WA. Influence of age on dynamics of rising from a chair. *Phys Ther*. 1991;71:473–481.

15. Livingston LA, Stevenson JM, Olney SJ. Stairclimbing kinematics on stairs of differing dimensions. *Arch Phys Med Rehabil*. 1991;72:398–402.

16. Sammarco GJ. Biomechanics of the foot. In: Nordin M, Frankel VH. *Basic Biomechanics of the Musculoskeletal System*. 2nd ed. Philadelphia: Lea & Febiger; 1989.

17. Thordarson DB, Schmotzer H, Chon J, Peters J. Dynamic support of the human longitudinal arch. *Clin Orthop*. 1995;316:165–172.

18. Pink M, Perry J, Houglum PA, Devine DJ. Lower extremity range of motion in the recreational sport runner. *Am J Sports Med*. 1994;22:541–549.

19. Soderberg GL. *Kinesiology: Application to Pathological Motion*. 2nd ed. Baltimore: Williams & Wilkins; 1997.

20. Herman R, Bragin SJ. Function of the gastrocnemius and soleus muscles. *Phys Ther*. 1967;47:105–113.

21. Andriacchi TP, Andersson GBJ, Fermier RW, Stern D, Galante JO. A study of lower-limb mechanics during stairclimbing. *J Bone Joint Surg*. 1980;62A:749–757.

22. O'Connell AL. Electromyographic study of certain leg muscles during movements of the free foot and during standing. *Am J Phys Med*. 1958;37:289–301.

23. Houtz SJ, Walsh FP. Electromyographic analysis of the function of the muscles acting on the ankle during weight-bearing with special reference to the triceps surae. *J Bone Joint Surg*. 1959;41A:1469–1481.

24. Sarrafian SK, Topouzian LK. Anatomy and physiology of the extensor apparatus of the toes. *J Bone Joint Surg*. 1969;51A:669–679.

25. Caillet R. *Foot and Ankle Pain*. Philadelphia: FA Davis; 1968.

26. Mann R, Inman VT. Phasic activity of the intrinsic muscles of the foot. *J Bone Joint Surg*. 1964;46A:469–481.

27. Inman VT, Ralston HJ, Todd F. *Human Walking*. Baltimore: Williams & Wilkins; 1981.

28. Louwerens JWK, van Linge B, de Klerk LWL, Mulder PGH, Snijders CJ. Peroneus longus and tibialis anterior muscle activity in the stance phase. *Acta Orthop Scand*. 1995;66:517–523.

29. Reber L, Perry J, Pink M. Muscular control of the ankle in running. *Am J Sports Med*. 1993;21:805–810.

CHAPTER 9

RELATING TREATMENT TO ASSESSMENT

Although the guidelines for diagnosis and treatment protocols are beyond the scope of this text, this chapter links the methods used to assess deficiencies in active range of motion (AROM), passive range of motion (PROM), muscle length, and muscle strength with the methods, used when appropriate, to treat these deficiencies.

▼ SIMILAR ASSESSMENT AND TREATMENT METHODS

Similar assessment and treatment methods are categorized according to the type of movement used, that is, active, passive, and resisted movement as set out in Table 9-1.

Active movement when used as an assessment method is called active range of motion or AROM. When AROM is used specifically to assess muscle strength, it is called manual muscle testing (MMT). Active movement used as a treatment method is called active exercise and may be used to maintain or increase joint range of motion (ROM) and/or muscle strength.

Passive movement when used as an assessment method is called passive range of motion or PROM, and muscle length assessment. The therapist uses PROM to determine the ROM at a joint, end feel, and the length of muscles. This passive movement when used as a treatment method to maintain or increase joint ROM and muscle length is called relaxed passive movement and prolonged passive stretch.

Resisted movement is used to assess muscle strength. It is also used as a treatment method to maintain or increase muscle strength and when used for this purpose is called resisted exercise.

TABLE 9-1 ▼ A COMPARISON OF ASSESSMENT AND TREATMENT METHODS

Key Steps	Active Movement		Passive Movement				Resisted Movement	
	Active ROM (AROM) Assessment	Active Exercise Treatment	Passive ROM (PROM) Assessment	Relaxed Passive Movement Treatment	Muscle Length Assessment	Prolonged Passive Stretch Treatment	Muscle Strength Assessment	Resisted Exercise Treatment
PURPOSE	Assessment of: • AROM • muscle strength* • ability to perform ADL	Treatment to maintain/increase: • joint ROM • muscle strength • ability to perform ADL	Assessment of: • joint PROM • end feel	Treatment to maintain/increase: • joint ROM	Assessment of: • muscle length	Treatment to maintain/increase: • muscle length	Assessment of: • muscle strength*	Treatment to maintain/increase: • muscle strength
METHOD								
Explanation/Instruction	Verbal (clear, concise), demonstration and/or passive movement →→→							
Expose Area	Expose area and drape as required →→→							
Start Position	• safe, comfortable, adequate support • consider effect of gravity		• safe, comfortable, adequate support, relaxed				• safe, comfortable, adequate support • consider effect of gravity	
Stabilization**	• proximal joint segment(s) • muscle origins		• proximal joint segment(s)		• muscle origin(s)		• muscle origin(s)	
Movement**	• distal joint segment(s)		• distal joint segment(s)		• other joints crossed by muscle(s)		• muscle insertion(s) • none if isometric contraction	
Resistance	n/a		n/a		n/a		• distal end of segment muscle(s) inserts into	
End Position	• end of full or available AROM		• end of full or available PROM		• muscle(s) on full stretch		• end of full available PROM • start position if isometric contraction	
Substitute/Trick Movement	←——————————— Eliminate ———————————→							

METHOD PROCEDURE SPECIFIC TO PURPOSE							
• usually estimate and/or measure AROM	• active movement performed according to exercise prescription	• observe and/or measure joint PROM • note end feel	• passive movement performed according to treatment prescription	• visually observe and/or measure joint position at maximum stretch of muscle	• joint held at position of maximal muscle stretch for prescribed length of time	• determine the amount of resistance that can be applied and allow patient to move through movement	• resisted movement performed according to exercise prescription
CHARTING							
• joint AROM • MMT grade	• describe exercise prescribed • note any change in patient's condition	• joint PROM • end feel	• describe treatment prescribed • note any change in patient's condition	• joint position • end feel	• describe position of stretch and length of time stretch applied • note any change in patient's condition	• MMT grade	• describe exercise prescribed • note any change in patient's condition

* Manual muscle testing, depending on the method of testing used (ie, conventional, alternate), may fall under the assessment of AROM or the assessment of muscle strength if resistance is used to test the strength of the muscle.

** For ease of explanation and understanding, the proximal joint segment or site of attachment of the origin of the muscle is stabilized and the distal joint segment or site of attachment of the muscle described as the moving segment.

ADL, activities of daily living; MMT, manual muscle testing

Key steps when applying assessment and treatment methods are listed in order in the first column of Table 9-1. These steps are set out in detail for assessment in Chapter 1 and are summarized here and in Table 9-1 to compare with those for treatment.

PURPOSE

The therapist performs assessment methods to evaluate how an injury or disease affects the patient's status. Treatment methods, if appropriate, are used to eliminate or lessen the effects of injury or disease. The therapist repeats the assessment methods to evaluate the outcome of treatment.

METHOD

Explanation and Instruction. Before applying assessment or treatment methods, the therapist explains these to the patient and obtains the patient's informed consent before proceeding. When applying a method for the first time, the therapist explains and/or demonstrates the movement to be performed and/or asks the patient to relax and passively moves the patient's limb through the movement.

Expose Region. For assessment and treatment methods the therapist will expose the area to be assessed or treated and drape the patient accordingly.

Start Position. For assessment and treatment methods, ensure the patient is in a safe, comfortable position and is adequately supported. When positioning the patient, the effect of gravity on the movement or position held may be relevant.

Stabilization. For assessment and treatment methods, adequate stabilization is required to ensure only the desired movement or muscle contraction occurs. For all assessment and treatment methods, either (1) the proximal joint segment or site of attachment of the origin of the muscle(s) is stabilized or (2) the distal joint segment or site of insertion of the muscle(s) is stabilized.

Movement. For assessment and treatment methods, either (1) the distal joint segment or site of attachment of the insertion of the muscle(s) is moved, or (2) the proximal joint segment or site of origin of the muscle(s) is moved.

Resistance. For resisted movements used in assessment and treatment, the resistance is most often applied at the distal end of the segment into which the muscle or muscles are inserted.

End Position. For assessment and treatment methods the patient is instructed to move or the therapist passively moves the body segment(s) through either a selected part of or the full available ROM. When using active or resisted movement, the patient is instructed to maintain or hold a specified start position when using isometric contraction. For prolonged passive stretching, the point in the ROM that provides a maximal stretch to the soft tissue is maintained.

Trick or Substitute Movement. For assessment and treatment methods, the therapist must eliminate trick or substitute movements. Trick or substitute movement appears to exaggerate joint ROM and/or muscle strength and the patient's capacity to perform an exercise.

To eliminate unwanted movements, the therapist must provide adequate explanation and instruction to the patient regarding how the method is to be performed and the trick or substitute movements to be avoided. When applying the method, detailed attention should be paid to positioning and stabilizing the patient. Careful observation coupled with skill and experience enables the therapist to prevent trick movements and detect any that may occur.

METHOD PROCEDURE SPECIFIC TO PURPOSE

The active, passive, and resisted movement methods used for assessment and treatment are the same. However, to meet the purpose, modifications may be made in the way the method is applied, such as measuring, grading, or changing the number of times a movement is performed, the length of time a position is held, and/or the magnitude of the resistance used.

CHARTING

For each assessment method, any deviations from standardized testing procedure and the findings are noted in the chart. For each treatment method, details of the method used and any change in the patient's condition are noted in the chart.

EXAMPLES OF SIMILAR ASSESSMENT AND TREATMENT METHODS

The examples of similar assessment and treatment methods using active, passive, and resisted movement are demonstrated. *Note that for all similar assessment and treatment methods, the "Method" is the same but the "Purpose of the Method," "Method Procedure Specific to Purpose," and the "Charting" are different.* These examples apply to other joints and muscles in the body. In Table 9-1 and in these examples, the proximal joint segment or site of attachment of the origin of the muscle is stabilized and the distal joint segment or site of attachment of the insertion of the muscle is the moving segment.

KNEE EXTENSION:* AROM ASSESSMENT AND TREATMENT USING ACTIVE EXERCISE

Assessment AROM	Treatment Active Exercise

PURPOSE
To assess AROM, quadriceps muscle strength and determine the ability to perform ADL.

METHOD
Explanation/Instruction. The therapist explains, demonstrates, and/or passively moves the limb through knee extension. The therapist instructs the patient to straighten the knee as far as possible.
Expose Region. The patient wears shorts.
Start Position. The patient is sitting, grasps the edge of the plinth, and has the nontest foot supported on a stool (Fig. 9-1).
Stabilization. The patient is instructed to maintain the thigh in the start position or the therapist may stabilize the thigh.
Movement. The patient performs knee extension.
End Position. The knee is extended as far as possible through the ROM (Fig. 9-2). The hamstrings may restrict knee extension in this position.
Substitution/Trick Movement. The patient leans back to posteriorly tilt the pelvis and extend the hip joint.

METHOD PROCEDURE SPECIFIC TO PURPOSE
AROM is visually assessed or measured using the universal goniometer. Following the assessment of PROM, the therapist grades the strength of the knee extensors using AROM.

CHARTING
Knee extension AROM is recorded in degrees and/or the knee extensors are assigned a grade for strength.

PURPOSE
To maintain or increase AROM, quadriceps muscle strength, and the ability to perform ADL.

METHOD
Explanation/Instruction. The therapist explains, demonstrates, and/or passively moves the limb through knee extension. The therapist instructs the patient to straighten the knee as far as possible.
Expose Region. The patient wears shorts.
Start Position. The patient is sitting, grasps the edge of the plinth, and has the nontest foot supported on a stool (Fig. 9-1).
Stabilization. The patient is instructed to maintain the thigh in the start position or the therapist may stabilize the thigh.
Movement. The patient performs knee extension.
End Position. The knee is extended as far as possible through the ROM (Fig. 9-2). The hamstrings may restrict knee extension in this position.
Substitution/Trick Movement. The patient leans back to posteriorly tilt the pelvis and extend the hip joint.

METHOD PROCEDURE SPECIFIC TO PURPOSE
Knee extension is performed actively by the patient a predetermined number of times according to the exercise prescription.

CHARTING
The prescribed exercise is described and any change in the patient's condition is noted.

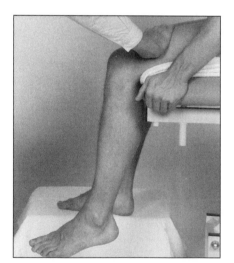

Figure 9-1.   Start position knee extension: AROM assessment and active exercise.

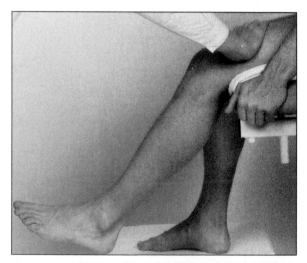

Figure 9-2.   End position: AROM assessment and active exercise. The therapist may stabilize the femur and/or palpate for contraction of the knee extensors.

---

* To show an example of movement performed against gravity.
  Note: Movement performed with gravity eliminated could also be used to illustrate the similarity between AROM assessment and active exercise.

▼ HIP FLEXION: PROM ASSESSMENT AND TREATMENT USING RELAXED PASSIVE MOVEMENT

Assessment	Treatment
PROM	Relaxed Passive Movement

PURPOSE
To assess hip flexion PROM and determine an end feel.

METHOD
Explanation/Instruction. The therapist explains, demonstrates, and/or passively moves the limb through hip flexion. The therapist instructs the patient to relax as the movement is performed.

Expose Region. The patient wears shorts and is draped as required.

Start Position. The patient is supine. The hip and knee on the test side are in the neutral position. The other hip is extended on the plinth (Fig. 9-3).

Stabilization. The therapist stabilizes the pelvis. The trunk is stabilized through body positioning.

Movement. The therapist raises the lower extremity off the plinth and applies slight traction to and moves the femur anteriorly to flex the hip.

End Position. The femur is moved to the limit of hip flexion (Fig. 9-4).

Substitution/Trick Movement. Posterior pelvic tilt and flexion of the lumbar spine.

METHOD PROCEDURE SPECIFIC TO PURPOSE
The therapist applies slight overpressure at the end of the PROM to identify the end feel. The therapist observes and measures the joint PROM.

CHARTING
The end feel and number of degrees of hip flexion PROM are recorded.

PURPOSE
To maintain or increase hip flexion ROM.

METHOD
Explanation/Instruction. The therapist explains, demonstrates, and/or passively moves the limb through hip flexion. The therapist instructs the patient to relax as the movement is performed.

Expose Region. The patient wears shorts and is draped as required.

Start Position. The patient is supine. The hip and knee on the test side are in the neutral position. The other hip is extended on the plinth (Fig. 9-3).

Stabilization. The therapist stabilizes the pelvis. The trunk is stabilized through body positioning.

Movement. The therapist raises the lower extremity off the plinth and applies slight traction to and moves the femur anteriorly to flex the hip.

End Position. The femur is moved to the limit of hip flexion (Fig. 9-4).

Substitution/Trick Movement. Posterior pelvic tilt and flexion of the lumbar spine.

METHOD PROCEDURE SPECIFIC TO PURPOSE
The hip is passively moved into flexion a predetermined number of times according to the treatment prescription.

CHARTING
The prescribed treatment is described and any change in the patient's condition is noted.

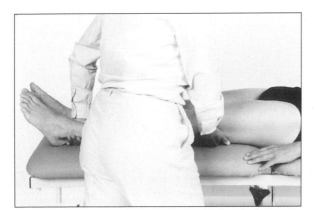

Figure 9-3. Start position hip flexion: PROM assessment and relaxed passive movement.

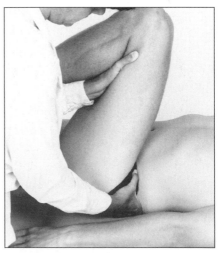

Figure 9-4. End position hip flexion: PROM assessment and relaxed passive movement.

LONG FINGER EXTENSORS: MUSCLE LENGTH ASSESSMENT AND TREATMENT USING PROLONGED PASSIVE STRETCH

Assessment Muscle Length	Treatment Prolonged Passive Stretch

PURPOSE

To assess the length of the long finger extensor muscles.

PURPOSE

To maintain or increase the length of the long finger extensor muscles.

METHOD

Explanation/Instruction. The therapist explains, demonstrates, and/or passively positions the patient in the stretch position. The therapist instructs the patient to relax as the movement is performed and held.

Expose Region. The patient wears a short-sleeved shirt.

Start Position. The patient is sitting. The elbow is extended, the forearm is pronated, and the fingers are flexed (Fig. 9-5).

Stabilization. The therapist stabilizes the radius and ulna.

Movement. The therapist applies slight traction to and flexes the wrist.

End Position. The wrist is flexed to the limit of motion so that the long finger extensors are fully stretched (Figs. 9-6 and 9-7).

Substitution/Trick Movement. Finger extension.

METHOD

Explanation/Instruction. The therapist explains, demonstrates, and/or passively positions the patient in the stretch position. The therapist instructs the patient to relax as the movement is performed and held.

Expose Region. The patient wears a short-sleeved shirt.

Start Position. The patient is sitting. The elbow is extended, the forearm is pronated, and the fingers are flexed (Fig. 9-5).

Stabilization. The therapist stabilizes the radius and ulna.

Movement. The therapist applies slight traction to and flexes the wrist.

End Position. The wrist is flexed to the limit of motion so that the long finger extensors are fully stretched (Figs. 9-6 and 9-7).

Substitution/Trick Movement. Finger extension.

METHOD PROCEDURE SPECIFIC TO PURPOSE

With the long finger extensors on full stretch, the angle of wrist flexion is observed and/or measured and the therapist identifies the end feel.

METHOD PROCEDURE SPECIFIC TO PURPOSE

The position of maximum wrist flexion is maintained so that the long finger flexors are placed on full stretch for a prescribed length of time and the therapist identifies the end feel.

CHARTING

The long finger extensors may be described as being shortened, and the angle of wrist flexion may be recorded. The end feel is noted.

CHARTING

The stretch position and the length of time the stretch is applied to the long finger extensors are recorded. Any change in the patient's condition is noted.

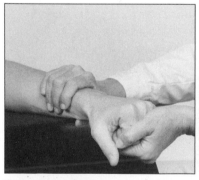

Figure 9-5. Start position long finger extensors: muscle length assessment and prolonged passive stretch.

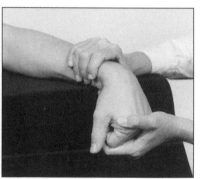

Figure 9-6. End position long finger extensors on stretch: muscle length assessment and prolonged passive stretch.

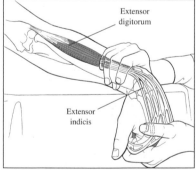

Figure 9-7. Long finger extensors on stretch.

ANTERIOR FIBERS DELTOID: MUSCLE STRENGTH ASSESSMENT AND TREATMENT USING RESISTED EXERCISE

Assessment Muscle Strength	Treatment Resisted Exercise

PURPOSE
To assess the strength of the anterior fibers deltoid.

METHOD
Explanation/Instruction. The therapist explains, demonstrates, and/or passively moves the patient through 90° shoulder flexion, with slight adduction and internal rotation. The therapist instructs the patient to work as hard as possible to raise the arm toward the ceiling as the therapist resists the movement.

Expose Region. The patient's shirt is removed. The patient is draped as required.

Start Position. The patient is sitting. The arm is at the side, with the shoulder in slight abduction and the palm facing medially (Fig. 9-8).

Stabilization. The therapist stabilizes the scapula and clavicle.

Movement. The patient flexes the shoulder, simultaneously slightly adducting and internally rotating the shoulder joint (Fig. 9-9 and 9-10).

Resistance Location. Applied on the anteromedial aspect of the arm just proximal to the elbow joint.

End Position. The patient flexes the shoulder to 90° shoulder flexion.

Substitution/Trick Movement. Scapular elevation, trunk extension.

METHOD PROCEDURE SPECIFIC TO PURPOSE
The therapist assesses the amount of manual resistance that can be applied and allow the patient to move smoothly through the movement (ie, shoulder flexion to 90°).

CHARTING
A grade of strength for the anterior fibers deltoid is recorded.

PURPOSE
To maintain or increase the strength of the anterior fibers deltoid.

METHOD
Explanation/Instruction. The therapist explains, demonstrates, and/or passively moves the patient through 90° shoulder flexion, with slight adduction and internal rotation. The therapist instructs the patient to work as hard as possible to raise the arm toward the ceiling as the therapist resists the movement.

Expose Region. The patient's shirt is removed. The patient is draped as required.

Start Position. The patient is sitting. The arm is at the side, with the shoulder in slight abduction and the palm facing medially (Fig. 9-8).

Stabilization. The therapist stabilizes the scapula and clavicle.

Movement. The patient flexes the shoulder, simultaneously slightly adducting and internally rotating the shoulder joint (Fig. 9-9 and 9-10).

Resistance Location. Applied on the anteromedial aspect of the arm just proximal to the elbow joint.

End Position. The patient flexes the shoulder to 90° shoulder flexion.

Substitution/Trick Movement. Scapular elevation, trunk extension.

METHOD PROCEDURE SPECIFIC TO PURPOSE
The anterior fibers of the deltoid are required to contract through the ROM against a predetermined resistance load a predetermined number of times according to the treatment prescription.

CHARTING
The prescribed exercise is described and any change in the patient's condition noted.

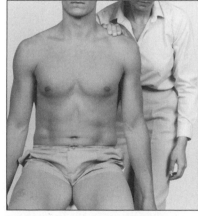
Figure 9-8. Start position for anterior fibers deltoid: MMT and resisted exercise.

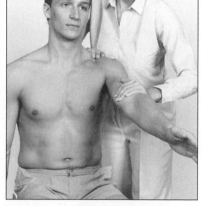
Figure 9-9. End position: for MMT anterior fibers deltoid and resisted exercise to strengthen anterior fibers deltoid.

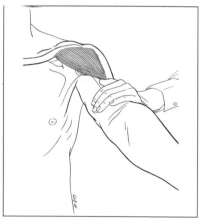
Figure 9-10. Anterior fibers deltoid.

OB "MYRIN" GONIOMETRY

The OB goniometer (Fig. A-1) can be used as an alternate instrument to the universal goniometer for assessing range of motion (ROM) at some joints. The OB goniometer consists of a fluid-filled rotatable container mounted on a plate.[1] The container has:

- A compass needle that reacts to the earth's magnetic field
- An inclination needle that is influenced by the force of gravity
- A scale on the container floor marked in 2° increments (eg, 1 minor unit = 2°; 1 major unit = 10°).[1]

The compass needle measures movements in the horizontal plane; the inclination needle measures movements in the frontal and sagittal planes.[1] Two straps with Velcro fastenings are supplied to attach the goniometer to the body segment, and two plastic extension plates are also supplied to position the goniometer for certain joint measurements.[1]

The advantages of the OB goniometer over the universal goniometer are:

- It is not necessary to align the goniometer with the joint axis.
- Rotational movements and assessment of trunk and neck ROM are measured with ease.
- There is little change in the alignment of the goniometer throughout the ROM.
- Passive ROM (PROM) is more easily assessed because the therapist does not have to hold onto the goniometer and can stabilize the proximal joint segment with one hand and passively move the distal segment with the other.

The disadvantages to the OB goniometer are:

- It is expensive and bulky compared to the universal goniometer.
- It cannot be used to measure the small joints of the hand and foot.
- Magnetic fields, other than those of the earth, will cause the compass needle to deviate and must be avoided.

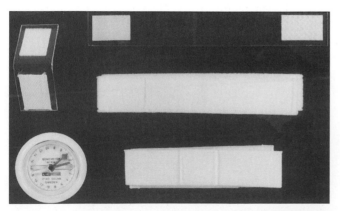

Figure A-1. The OB goniometer, Velcro straps, and plastic extension plates.

▼ MEASUREMENT PROCEDURE— OB GONIOMETER

Velcro strap and/or plastic extension plate: The Velcro strap is applied to the limb segment immediately distal to the joint being assessed. The appropriate plastic extension plate is attached to the Velcro strap for some ROM measurements.

OB goniometer: Attach the goniometer container to the Velcro strap or the plastic extension plate. The goniometer is positioned in relation to bony landmarks and placed in the same location on successive measurements.[2] With the patient in the start position, rotate the fluid-filled container until the 0° arrow lines up directly underneath either the inclination needle, if the moveent occurs in a vertical plane (ie, the sagittal or frontal planes) (Figs. A-2 and A-5), or the compass needle, if the movement occurs in the horizontal plane[1] (see Fig. A-11).

Ensure the inclination needle is free to swing during the measurement.[1] The therapist must not deviate the goniometer during the measurement by touching the strap or goniometer dial or by applying hand pressure to change the contour of the soft tissue mass near the OB goniometer.

At the end of the PROM or active ROM (AROM), the number of degrees the inclination needle (Figs. A-3 and A-6) or the compass needle (see Fig. A-12) moves away from the 0° arrow on the compass dial is recorded as the joint ROM.

The assessment of AROM for neck flexion, extension, lateral flexion, and rotation; and trunk rotation; and the assessment of PROM for tibial rotation, glenohumeral joint flexion and extension; forearm supination and pronation; hip internal and external rotation; and measurement of hamstring and gastrocnemius muscle length are described and illustrated as examples of how to apply the OB goniometer.

All normal AROM values in this appendix are referenced from the normal ROM values provided by the American Academy of Orthopaedic Surgeons[3] unless otherwise indicated.

NECK FLEXION AND EXTENSION (AROM)

• **Start Position.** The patient is sitting. The head and neck are in the anatomical position (see Fig. A-2).

• **Goniometer Placement.** The strap is placed around the head at the level of the forehead. The dial is placed on the lateral aspect of the head.

• **Stabilization.** The therapist stabilizes the trunk to prevent trunk flexion or extension.

• **End Positions.** The patient flexes (see Fig. A-3) and extends (Fig. A-4) the neck to the limit of motion (45° of flexion or extension).

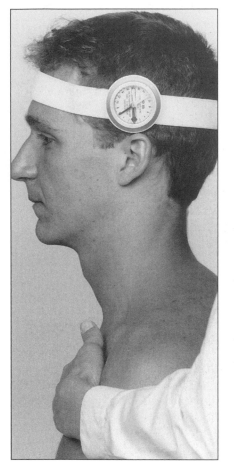

Figure A-2. Start position for neck flexion and extension.

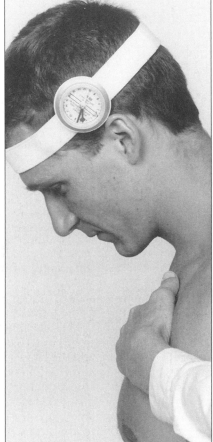

Figure A-3. Neck flexion.

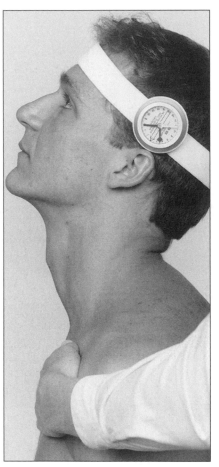

Figure A-4. Neck extension.

NECK LATERAL FLEXION (AROM)

• **Start Position.** The patient is sitting. The head and neck are in the anatomical position (Fig. A-5).

• **Goniometer Placement.** The strap is placed around the head at the level of the forehead. The dial is placed on the forehead.

• **Stabilization.** The therapist stabilizes the trunk to prevent trunk lateral flexion.

• **End Position.** The patient flexes the neck to the side to the limit of motion (45°) (Fig. A-6).

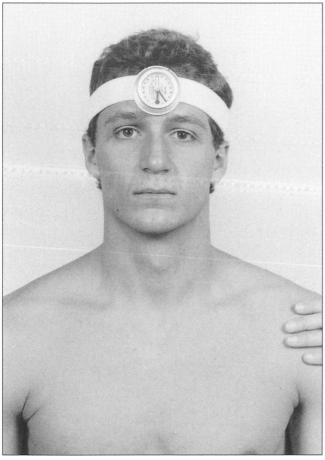

Figure A-5. Start position for neck lateral flexion.

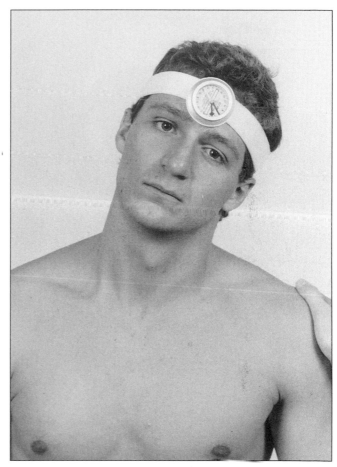

Figure A-6. Neck lateral flexion.

NECK ROTATION (AROM)

• **Start Position.** The patient is sitting. The head and neck are in the anatomical position (Fig. A-7).

• **Goniometer Placement.** One strap is placed around the head at the level of the forehead and the other strap is placed at the center of the top of the head. The dial is placed at the center of the top of the head.

• **Stabilization.** The therapist stabilizes the trunk to prevent trunk rotation.

• **End Position.** The patient rotates the neck to the limit of motion (60°) (Fig. A-8).

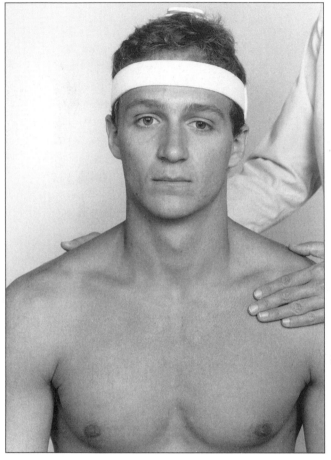

Figure A-7. Start position for neck rotation.

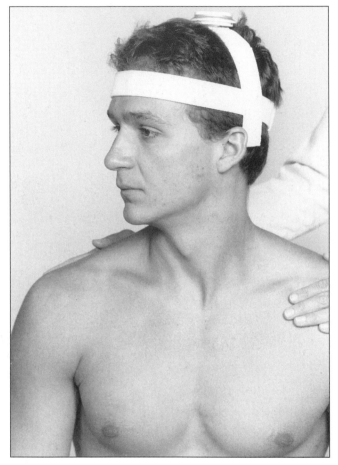

Figure A-8. Neck rotation.

TRUNK ROTATION (AROM)

• **Start Position.** The patient is sitting with the feet supported on a stool and the arms crossed in front of the chest (Fig. A-9).

• **Goniometer Placement.** The strap is placed around the forearm. The dial is placed on the posterior aspect of the forearm.

• **Stabilization.** The therapist stabilizes the pelvis.

• **End Position.** The patient rotates the trunk to the limit of motion (45°) (Fig. A-10).

• **Substitution/Trick Movement.** Trunk flexion, trunk extension, and shoulder extension on the side in the direction of trunk rotation.

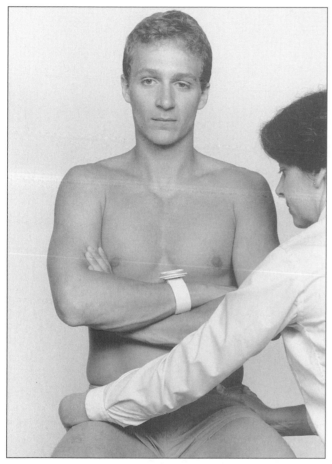

Figure A-9. Start position: trunk rotation.

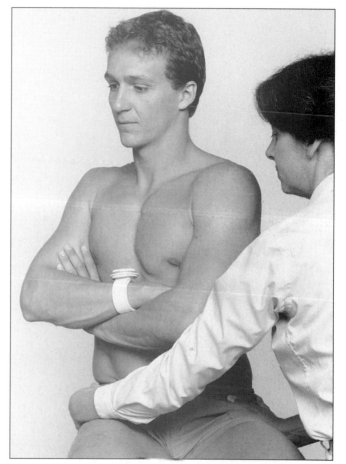

Figure A-10. End position: trunk rotation.

TIBIAL ROTATION

Total tibial rotation is assessed. Measurements of total rotation are more reliable than measurements of internal and external tibial rotation because of the difficulty of defining the zero start position for the individual measurements.[4] The greatest range of tibial rotation is available when the knee is flexed 90°.[5]

• **Goniometer Placement.** The strap is placed around the leg distal to the gastrocnemius muscle, and the dial is placed on the right angle extension plate on the anterior aspect of the leg.

• **Start Position.** The patient is sitting, with the knee in 90° flexion and the tibia in full internal rotation (Fig. A-11). A pad is placed under the distal thigh to maintain the thigh in a horizontal position.

• **Stabilization.** The therapist stabilizes the femur.

• **End Position.** From full internal rotation, the therapist rotates the tibia externally through the full available PROM (Fig. A-12). The total range of tibial rotation is observed (average total range, about 58°[6]).

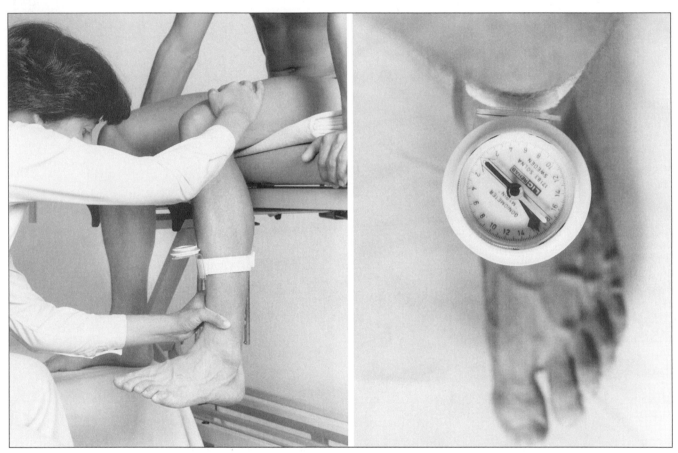

Figure A-11.   Start position for total tibial rotation: tibial internal rotation.

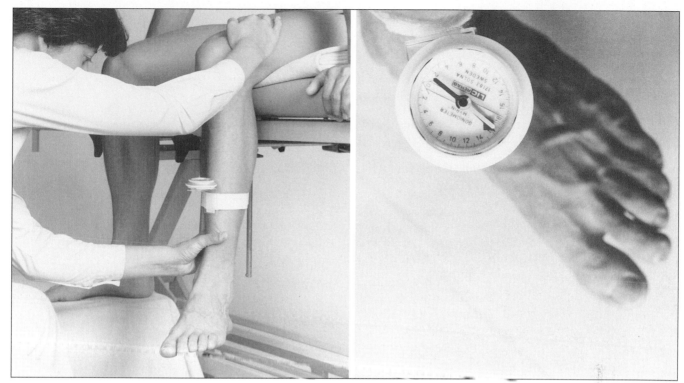

Figure A-12. End position for total tibial rotation: tibial external rotation.

GLENOHUMERAL JOINT FLEXION AND EXTENSION

- **Start Position.** The patient is sitting. The arm is by the side, with the palm facing medially (Fig. A-13).

- **Goniometer Placement.** The strap is placed around the distal portion of the upper arm, and the dial is placed on the lateral aspect of the arm.

- **Stabilization.** The therapist stabilizes the scapula to isolate glenohumeral joint motion.

- **End Positions.** The humerus is moved in an anterior direction to the limit of motion for glenohumeral joint flexion ($120°^5$) (Fig. A-14). The humerus is moved in a posterior direction to the limit of motion for shoulder extension (Fig. A-15).

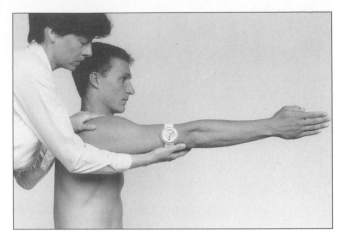

Figure A-14. Glenohumeral joint flexion.

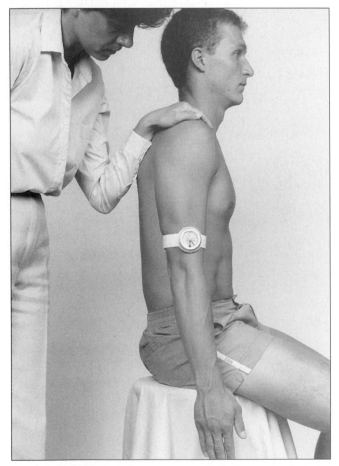

Figure A-13. Start position for glenohumeral joint flexion and extension.

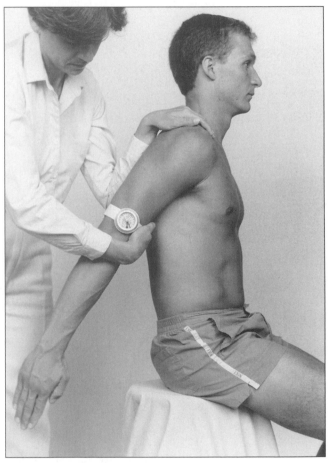

Figure A-15. Shoulder joint extension. *Note:* The elbow should be relaxed in flexion (not shown).

FOREARM SUPINATION AND PRONATION

• **Start Position.** The patient is sitting. The shoulder is adducted, and the elbow is flexed to 90° with the forearm in midposition. The wrist is in neutral, and the fingers are flexed (Fig. A-16).

• **Goniometer Placement.** The dial is placed on the right-angled plate. The plate is held between the patient's index and middle fingers.

• **Stabilization.** The therapist stabilizes the humerus.

• **Alternate Placement.** The strap is placed around the distal forearm. The dial is placed on the right-angled plate and attached on the radial side of the forearm (Fig. A-17).

• **End Position.** The forearm is rotated externally from midposition to the limit of motion for supination (Fig. A-18).

• **End Position.** The forearm is rotated internally from midposition to the limit of motion for pronation (Fig. A-19).

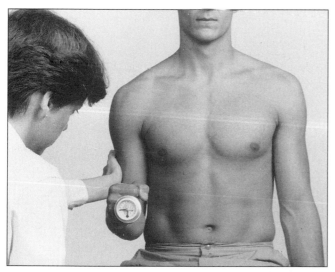

Figure A-16. Start position for supination and pronation.

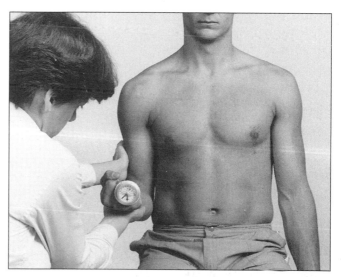

Figure A-18. Supination.

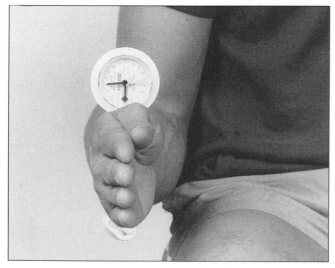

Figure A-17. Alternate goniometer placement for supination and pronation.

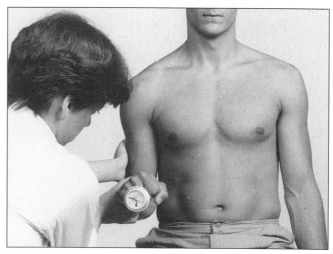

Figure A-19. Pronation.

HIP INTERNAL AND EXTERNAL ROTATION

• **Start Position.** The patient is sitting with the hip and knee flexed to 90°. The lower leg is hanging over the edge of the plinth (Fig. A-20). The contralateral hip is abducted and the foot is supported on a stool.

• **Alternate Start Position (not shown).** The patient is supine with the hip and knee flexed to 90°. The contralateral limb is extended.

• **Stabilization.** The therapist stabilizes the distal thigh taking care not to inhibit rotation of the thigh and thus hip rotation.

• **Goniometer Placement.** The strap is placed around the lower leg proximal to the ankle. The dial is placed on the anterior aspect of the lower leg.

• **End Positions.** The hip is internally rotated to the limit of motion (Fig. A-21). The hip is externally rotated to the limit of motion (Fig. A-22, alternate position).

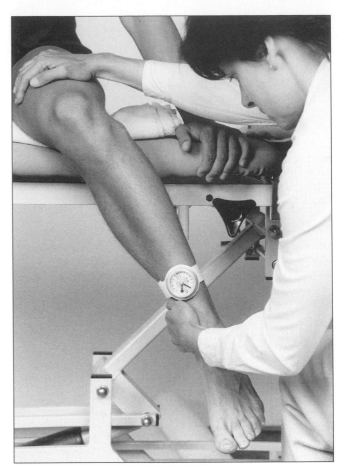

Figure A-21. Hip internal rotation.

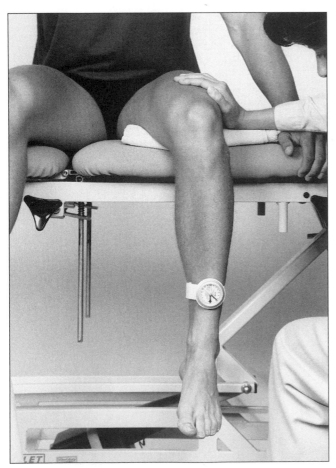

Figure A-20. Start position: hip internal and external rotation.

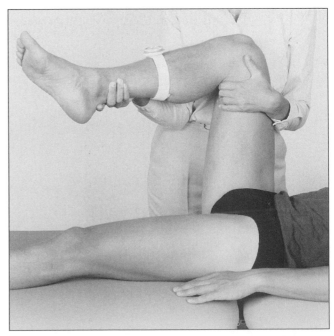

Figure A-22. Alternate position: hip external rotation.

MEASUREMENT OF HAMSTRINGS MUSCLE LENGTH

• **Start Position** (not shown). The patient is supine with the lower extremities in the anatomical position.

• **Stabilization.** The pelvis is stabilized by the patient's body weight and the contralateral thigh is held on the plinth with the use of a strap (not shown).

• **Goniometer Placement.** The strap is placed around the distal thigh. The dial is placed on the lateral aspect of the thigh.

• **End Position.** The hip is flexed to the limit of motion while maintaining knee extension so that the long head of biceps femoris, semitendinosus, and semimembranosus are put on full stretch (Fig. A-23).

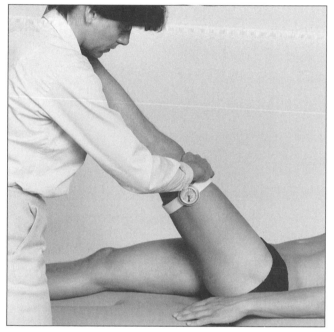

Figure A-23.   End position: for measurement of hamstrings length.

MEASUREMENT OF GASTROCNEMIUS MUSCLE LENGTH

• **Start Position** (not shown). The patient is standing erect, facing a wall or a plinth.

• **Stabilization.** The foot is stabilized by the patient's body weight.

• **Goniometer Placement.** The strap is placed around the lower leg proximal to the ankle. The dial is placed on the lateral aspect of the lower leg.

• **End Position.** The hands are placed on the plinth or on the wall, with the elbows in extension. The patient leans forward so that the gastrocnemius is put on full stretch (Fig. A-24). The knee must remain extended as the leg moves over the foot.

Note: If the contralateral leg is not placed ahead of the test leg, ensure the heel is raised slightly off the floor. This position ensures a true test for gastrocnemius tightness on the test side because the amount of forward lean the patient achieves will not be limited by contralateral gastrocnemius tightness, if present.

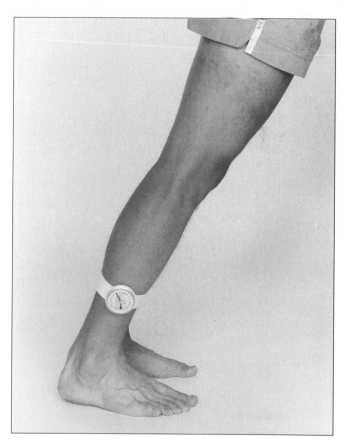

Figure A-24.   End position: for measurement of the length of gastrocnemius.

REFERENCES

1. *Instruction Manual: OB Goniometer "Myrin."* Available from OB REHAB AB ETT LIC-FORETAG S-171 38 Solna, Sweden.
2. Ekstrand J, Wiktorsson M, Oberg B, Gillquist J. Lower extremity goniometric measurements: a study to determine their reliability. *Arch Phys Med Rehabil.* 1982;63:171–175.
3. American Academy of Orthopaedic Surgeons. *Joint Motion: Method of Measuring and Recording.* Chicago: Author; 1965.
4. Zarins B, Rowe CR, Harris BA, Watkins MP. Rotational motion of the knee. *Am J Sports Med.* 1983;11:152–156.
5. Norkin CC, Levangie PK. *Joint Structure & Function: A Comprehensive Analysis.* 2nd ed. Philadelphia: FA Davis; 1992.
6. Osternig LR, Bates BT, James SL. Patterns of tibial rotary torque in knees of healthy subjects. *Med Sci Sports Exerc.* 1980;12:195–199.

SAMPLE NUMERICAL RECORDING FORM: RANGE OF MOTION MEASUREMENT

Patient's Name _____

Diagnosis _____

Therapist _____

Date of Birth _____

Date of Onset _____

Recording:

1. The Neutral Zero Method defined by the American Academy of Orthopaedic Surgeons[1] is used for measurement and recording.
2. Average ranges defined by the American Academy of Orthopaedic Surgeons[1] are provided in parentheses.

3. The columns designated with asterisks are used for indicating limitation of range of motion and referencing for summarization.
4. Space is left at the end of each section to record hypermobile ranges and comments regarding positioning of the patient or body part, edema, pain, and/or end feel.

Patient's Name _____   Therapist _____

Left Side			Date of Measurement	Right Side		
*		*	**Date of Measurement**	*		*
			Head, Neck and Trunk			
			Mandible: Depression			
			Protrusion			
			Lateral deviation			
			Neck: Flexion (0–45°)			
			Extension (0–45°)			
			Lateral flexion (0–45°)			
			Rotation (0–60°)			
			Trunk: Flexion (0–80°, 10 cm)			
			Extension (0–20–30°)			
			Lateral flexion (0–35°)			
			Rotation (0–45°)			
			Hypermobility:			
			Comments:			
			Scapula			
			Elevation			
			Depression			
			Abduction			
			Adduction			
			Shoulder Girdle			
			Flexion (0–180°)			
			Extension (0–60°)			
			Abduction (0–180°)			
			Horizontal abduction (0–45°)			
			Horizontal adduction (0–135°)			
			Internal rotation (0–70°)			
			External rotation (0–90°)			
			Hypermobility:			
			Comments:			
			Elbow and Forearm			
			Flexion (0–150°)			
			Supination (0–80°)			
			Pronation (0–80°)			
			Hypermobility:			
			Comments:			
			Wrist			
			Flexion (0–80°)			
			Extension (0–70°)			
			Ulnar deviation (0–30°)			
			Radial deviation (0–20°)			
			Hypermobility:			
			Comments:			

Patient's Name _____   Therapist _____

	*		*	Date of Measurement		*		*	
				Thumb					
				CM flexion (0–15°)					
				CM extension (0–20°)					
				abduction (0–70°)					
				MCP flexion (0–50°)					
				IP flexion (0–80°)					
				Opposition					
				Hypermobility:					
				Comments:					
				Fingers					
				MCP digit 2 flexion (0–90°)					
				extension (0–45°)					
				abduction					
				adduction					
				MCP digit 3 flexion (0–90°)					
				extension (0–45°)					
				abduction (radial)					
				abduction (ulnar)					
				MCP digit 4 flexion (0–90°)					
				extension (0–45°)					
				abduction					
				adduction					
				MCP digit 5 flexion (0–90°)					
				extension (0–45°)					
				abduction					
				adduction					
				PIP digit 2 flexion (0–100°)					
				3 flexion (0–100°)					
				4 flexion (0–100°)					
				5 flexion (0–100°)					
				DIP digit 2 flexion (0–90°)					
				3 flexion (0–90°)					
				4 flexion (0–90°)					
				5 flexion (0–90°)					
				Composite finger abduction/thumb extension—Distance between:					
				Thumb–digit 2					
				Digit 2–digit 3					
				Digit 3–digit 4					
				Digit 4–digit 5					
				Composite flexion—Distance between:					
				Finger pulp–distal palmar crease					
				Finger pulp–proximal plamar crease					
				Hypermobility:					
				Comments:					

Left Side · Right Side

APPENDIX B

Patient's Name _____   Therapist _____

Left Side			Date of Measurement	Right Side	
	*		*	*	*
			Hip			
			Flexion (0–120°)			
			Extension (0–30°)			
			Abduction (0–45°)			
			Adduction (0–30°)			
			Internal rotation (0–45°)			
			External rotation (0–45°)			
			Hypermobility:			
			Comments:			
			Knee			
			Flexion (0–135°)			
			Tibial rotation			
			Hypermobility:			
			Comments:			
			Ankle			
			Dorsiflexion (0–20°)			
			Plantarflexion (0–50°)			
			Inversion (0–35°)			
			Eversion (0–15°)			
			Hypermobility:			
			Comments:			
			Toes			
			MTP great toe flexion (0–45°)			
			extension (0–70°)			
			abduction			
			MTP digit 2 flexion (0–40°)			
			extension (0–40°)			
			MTP digit 3 flexion (0–40°)			
			extension (0–40°)			
			MTP digit 4 flexion (0–40°)			
			extension (0–40°)			
			MTP digit 5 flexion (0–40°)			
			extension (0–40°)			
			IP great toe flexion (0–90°)			
			PIP digit 2 flexion (0–35°)			
			PIP digit 3 flexion (0–35°)			
			PIP digit 4 flexion (0–35°)			
			PIP digit 5 flexion (0–35°)			
			Hypermobility:			
			Comments:			

Summary of Limitation:

Additional Comments:

[1]American Academy of Orthopaedic Surgeons: *Joint Motion: Method of Measuring and Recording.* Chicago: Author; 1965.

APPENDIX
C

SAMPLE RECORDING FORM: MANUAL MUSCLE STRENGTH ASSESSMENT

Patient's Name _____   Date of Birth _____

Diagnosis _____   Date of Onset _____

Therapist _____

Key: Conventional grading methodology used unless otherwise indicated in the "m" designated column.

- A.   Assisted against gravity grading
- P.   Palpation grading
- R.   Resisted gravity-eliminated grading

- H.   Isometric grading
- F.   Facial grading
- G.   Hand and toe grading

Patient's Name _____   Therapist _____

Left Side						Right Side		
	m		m	**Date of Measurement**		m		m
				Motion	**Muscle**	**Nerve supply**		
				Eye				
				Eyelid elevation	Levator palpebrae superioris	CN III		
				Eyelid closure	Obicularis oculi	CN VII		
				Eyeball elevation	Rectus superior Obliquus inferior	CN III CN III		
				Eyeball depression	Rectus inferior Obliquus superior	CN III CN IV		
				Eyeball abduction	Rectus lateralis	CN VI		
				Eyeball adduction	Rectus medialis	CN III		
				Eyebrows				
				Elevation	Epicranius	CN VII		
				Adduction	Corrugator supercilli	CN VII		
				Depression	Procerus	CN VII		
				Mandible				
				Elevation	Temporalis/masseter/ medial pterygoid	CN V		
				Depression	Lateral pterygoid/ suprahyoid	CN V		
				Protrusion	Pterygoids	CN V		
				Nasal Aperture				
				Dilation	Nasalis/depressor septi	CN VII		
				Constriction	Nasalis	CN VII		
				Lips/Mouth				
				Lip closure	Obicularis oris	CN VII		
				Cheek compression	Buccinator	CN VII		
				Elevation of angle	Levator anguli oris	CN VII		
				Retraction of angle	Zygomaticus major/ risorius	CN VII		
				Depression of angle	Platysma/depressor anguli oris/depressor labii inferioris	CN VII		
				Upper lip elevation	Levator labii superioris/zygomaticus minor	CN VII		
				Lower lip elevation	Mentalis	CN VII		
				Tongue				
				Protrusion	Genioglossus	CN XII		
				Neck				
				Hyoid bone depression	Infrahyoid group	Cervical		
				Flexion	Flexor group	Cervical		
					Sternomastoid	Cervical		
				Extension	Extensor group	Cervical		

Patient's Name _____   Therapist _____

	Left Side					Right Side			
	m		m		**Date of Measurement**		m		m	
				Motion	**Muscle**	**Nerve supply**				
				Scapula						
				Abduction Lateral rotation	Serratus anterior	Long Thoracic				
				Elevation	Upper trapezius Levator scapulae	Accessory, CN XI Dorsal Scapular				
				Adduction	Middle trapezius	Accessory, CN XI				
				Adduction Medial rotation	Rhomboids	Dorsal Scapular				
				Depression	Lower trapezius	Accessory, CN XI				
				Shoulder						
				Flexion	Anterior deltoid	Axillary				
				Flexion–Adduction	Coracobrachialis	Musculocutaneous				
				Extension	Latissimus dorsi Teres major	Thoracodorsal Subscapular				
				Abduction	Middle deltoid Supraspinatus	Axillary Suprascapular				
				Adduction	Pectoralis major Teres major Latissimus dorsi	Pectoral Subscapular Thoracodorsal				
				Horizontal adduction	Pectoralis major	Pectoral				
				Horizontal abduction	Posterior deltoid	Axillary				
				Internal rotation	Subscapularis	Subscapular				
				External rotation	Infraspinatus Teres minor	Suprascapular Axillary				
				Elbow/Forearm						
				Flexion	Biceps	Musculocutaneous				
					Brachioradialis Brachialis	Radial Musculocutaneous/ radial				
				Extension	Triceps	Radial				
				Supination	Supinator	Radial				
				Pronation	Pronator teres Pronator quadratus	Median				
				Wrist						
				Flexion	Flexor carpi radialis	Median				
					Flexor carpi ulnaris	Ulnar				
				Extension	Extensor carpi radialis longus	Radial				
					Extensor carpi radialis brevis	Radial				
					Extensor carpi ulnaris	Radial				

APPENDIX C

Left Side							Right Side			
	m		m	**Date of Measurement**			m		m	
				Motion	**Muscle**	**Nerve supply**				
				Fingers						
				MCP extension	Extensor digitorum	Radial				
					Extensor indicis proprius	Radial				
					Extensor digiti minimi	Radial				
				MCP abduction	Dorsal interossei	Ulnar				
					Abductor digiti minimi	Ulnar				
				MCP adduction	Palmar interossei	Ulnar				
				MCP flexion-IP extension	Lumbricales 1 and 2	Median				
					Lumbricales 3 and 4	Ulnar				
				5th MCP flexion	Flexor digiti minimi	Ulnar				
				PIP flexion digit 2	Flexor digitorum superficialis	Median				
				digit 3						
				digit 4						
				DIP flexion digit 2	Flexor digitorum profundus	Median				
				digit 3		Median				
				digit 4		Ulnar				
				digit 5		Ulnar				
				Thumb						
				IP flexion	Flexor pollicis longus	Median				
				MCP flexion	Flexor pollicis brevis	Ulnar				
				IP extension	Extensor pollicis longus	Radial				
				MCP extension	Extensor pollicis brevis	Radial				
				Radial abduction	Abductor pollicis longus	Radial				
				Palmar abduction	Abductor pollicis brevis	Median				
				Adduction	Adductor pollicis	Ulnar				
				Opposition	Opponens pollicis	Median				
					Opponens digiti minimi	Ulnar				
				Trunk						
				Flexion	Rectus abdominis	Thoracic				
				Rotation	External oblique	Thoracic				
					Internal oblique	Thoracic				
				Extension	Extensor group	Thoracic				
				Pelvic elevation	Quadratus lumborum	Lumbar				

Patient's Name _____   Therapist _____

	Left Side						Right Side		
m		m	**Date of Measurement**			m		m	
			Motion	**Muscle**	**Nerve supply**				
			Hip						
			Flexion	Psoas major	Lumbar				
				Iliacus	Femoral				
				Sartorius	Femoral				
			Extension	Gluteus maximus	Gluteal				
				Biceps femoris	Sciatic				
				Semitendinosus	Sciatic				
				Semimembranosus	Sciatic				
			Abduction	Gluteus medius	Gluteal				
				Gluteus minimus	Gluteal				
				Tensor fascia latae	Gluteal				
			Adduction	Adductor group	Obturator				
			Internal rotation	Gluteus medius	Gluteal				
				Gluteus minimus	Gluteal				
				Tensor fascia latae	Gluteal				
			External rotation	External rotator group	Sacral/lumbar				
			Knee						
			Flexion	Biceps femoris	Sciatic				
				Semitendinosus	Sciatic				
				Semimembranosus	Sciatic				
			Extension	Quadriceps	Femoral				
			Ankle						
			Dorsiflexion	Tibialis anterior	Peroneal				
			Plantarflexion	Gastrocnemius	Tibial				
				Soleus	Tibial				
			Inversion	Tibialis posterior	Tibial				
			Eversion	Peroneus longus	Peroneal				
				Peroneus brevis	Peroneal				
			Toes						
			MTP flexion	Flexor hallucis brevis	Tibial				
				Lumbricales	Tibial				
			IP flexion	Flexor hallucis longus	Tibial				
				Flexor digitorum longus	Tibial				
				Flexor digitorum brevis					
			MTP abduction	Abductor hallucis	Tibial				
				Abductor digiti minimi	Tibial				
				Dorsal interossei	Tibial				
			Extension	Extensor hallucis longus	Peroneal				
				Extensor digitorum brevis					
				Extensor digitorum longus					

APPENDIX C

APPENDIX D

GAIT

The gait cycle consists of a series of motions that occur between consecutive initial contacts of one leg.[1] The gait cycle is divided into two phases: the stance phase, when the foot is in contact with the ground and the body advances over the weight-bearing limb, and the swing phase, when the limb is unweighted and advanced forward in preparation for the next stance phase. Each phase is further subdivided into a total of eight instants[1] or freeze frames. Five instants occur in the stance phase and three occur in the swing phase of the gait cycle. The description of the normal gait pattern is provided so that the implications of the findings on assessment of joint range of motion and manual muscle strength can be understood in relation to gait. The average positions and the motions of the joints during the gait cycle that are reported in this appendix were adapted from the Rancho Los Amigos gait analysis forms as cited in Norkin and Levangie.[2] The right leg is used to illustrate the joint positions and motions of the lower limb throughout the gait cycle.

The lower limb is advanced in front of the body during the swing phase and the stance phase begins at initial contact (Fig. D-1) when the heel makes the first contact between the foot and the ground. At initial contact the pelvis is rotated forward on the stance side and the trunk is rotated backward on the same side. The rotation of the pelvis counteracts the trunk rotation to prevent excessive trunk motion. The upper extremity on the opposite side is flexed at the shoulder. As the body advances over the supporting limb through the stance phase, the pelvis rotates backward and the trunk rotates forward on the same side. As the weight-bearing leg extends at the hip, the upper limb on the opposite side extends. The positions and motions in the sagittal plane of the right lower limb are described and illustrated.

Motion from *A* to *B* (Figs. D-1 and D-2): *hip:* extension (from 30 to 25° flexion); *knee:* flexion (from 0 to 15° flexion); *ankle:* plantarflexion (from 0 to 15° plantarflexion); *MTP joints of toes:* 0°.

Motion from *B* to *C* (Figs. D-2 and D-3): *hip:* extension (from 25 to 0° flexion); *knee:* extension (from 15 to 5° flexion); *ankle:* dorsiflexion (from 15° plantarflexion to 5 to 10° dorsiflexion); *MTP joints of toes:* remain at 0°.

Motion from *C* to *D* (Figs. D-3 and D-4): *hip:* extension (from 0° flexion to 10 to 20° extension); *knee:* extension (from 5° flexion to 0°); *ankle:* dorsiflexion (from 5 to 10° dorsiflexion to 0° dorsiflexion); *MTP joints of toes:* extension (from 0 to 20° extension).

Motion from *D* to *E* (Figs. D-4 and D-5): *hip:* flexion (from 10 to 20° extension to 0°); *knee:* flexion (from 0 to 30° flexion); *ankle:* plantarflexion (from 0 to 20° plantarflexion); *MTP joints of toes:* extension (from 30° extension to 50 to 60° extension).

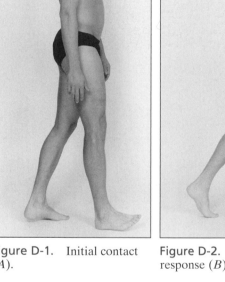

Figure D-1. Initial contact (*A*).

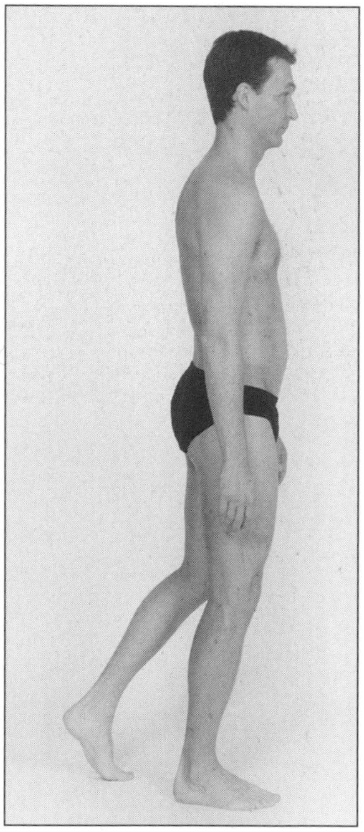

Figure D-2. Loading response (*B*).

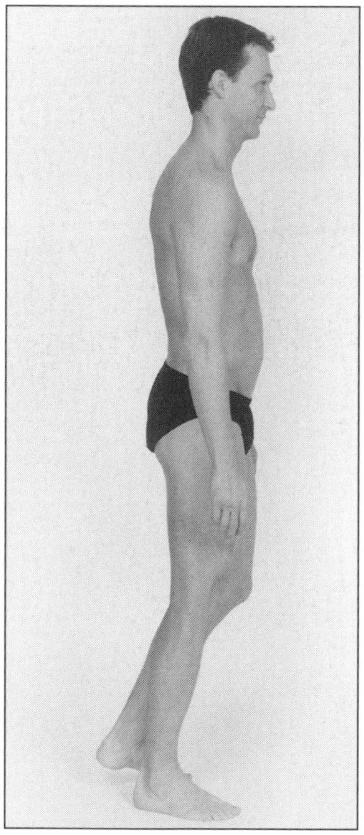

Figure D-3. Midstance (*C*).

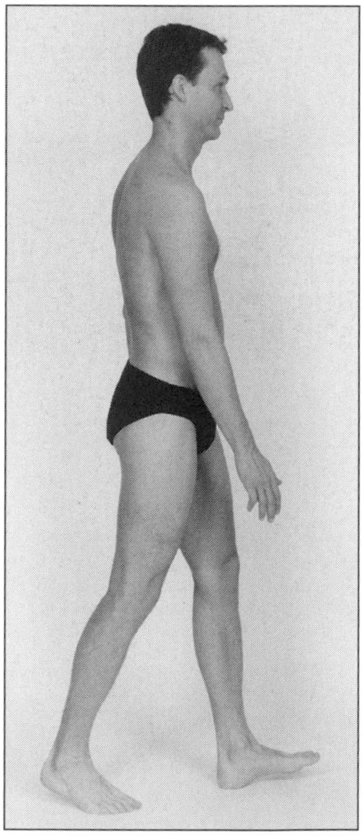

Figure D-4. Terminal stance (*D*).

▼ SWING PHASE

The swing phase begins after preswing when the foot leaves the ground and is advanced forward in the line of progression in preparation for initial contact. The positions and motions of the right lower limb are described and illustrated.

Motion from *E* to *F* (Figs. D-5 and D-6): *hip:* flexion (from 0 to 20° flexion); *knee:* flexion (from 30° flexion to 60° flexion); *ankle:* dorsiflexion (from 20° plantarflexion to 10° plantarflexion).

Motion from *F* to *G* (Figs. D-6 and D-7): *hip:* flexion (from 20° flexion to 30° flexion); *knee:* extension (from 60° flexion to 30° flexion); *ankle:* dorsiflexion (from 10° plantarflexion to 0°).

Motion from *G* to *H* (Figs. D-7 and D-8): *hip:* remains flexed at 30°; *knee:* extension (from 30° flexion to 0°); *ankle:* remains at 0°.

Motion from *H* to *A* (Figs. D-8 and D-1): *hip:* remains flexed at 30°; *knee:* remains extended at 0°; *ankle:* remains at 0°.

REFERENCES

1. Koerner I. *Observation of Human Gait.* Edmonton, Alberta: Health Sciences Media Services and Development, University of Alberta; 1986.
2. Norkin CC, Levangie PK. *Joint Structure & Function: A Comprehensive Analysis.* 2nd ed. Philadelphia: FA Davis; 1992.

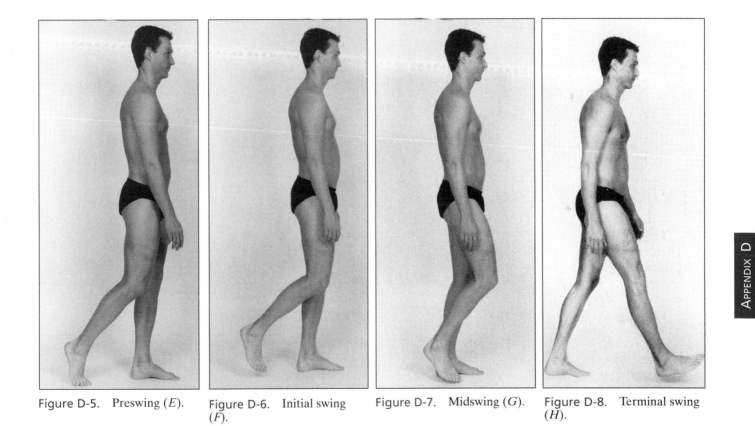

Figure D-5. Preswing (*E*).

Figure D-6. Initial swing (*F*).

Figure D-7. Midswing (*G*).

Figure D-8. Terminal swing (*H*).

APPENDIX D

INDEX

Note: Page numbers in *italics* denote figures; those followed by *t* denote tables.